Refugee Health

An approach to emergency situations

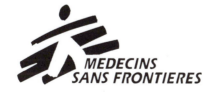

MEDECINS
SANS FRONTIERES

MACMILLAN

First published 1997 by
MACMILLAN EDUCATION LTD
London and Basingstoke
Companies and representatives throughout the world

ISBN 0-333-72210-8

10   9   8   7   6   5   4   3   2
06   05   04   03   02   01   00   99

This book is printed on paper suitable for recycling and
made from fully managed and sustained forest sources.

Printed in Hong Kong

A catalogue record for this book is available from the
British Library.

Cover photograph by Roger Job

Coventry University

CONTENTS

APPENDICES

ACKNOWLEDGEMENTS

General Editor:
Germaine HANQUET

Editorial committee:
Jean RIGAL, Egbert SONDORP, Fabienne VAUTIER

Authors:
Antoine BIGOT, Lucie BLOK, Marleen BOELAERT, Yves CHARTIER, Piet CORIJN, Austen DAVIS, Murielle DEGUERRY, Tine DUSAUCHOIT, Florence FERMON, André GRIEKSPOOR, Myriam HENKENS, Jean-Pierre HUART, François JEAN, Alain MOREN, Jean-Pierre MUSTIN, Bart OSTYN, Christophe PAQUET, Françoise SAIVE, Pim SCHOLTE, Nathalie SOHIER, Willem VAN DE PUT, Saskia VAN DER KAM, Stefaan VAN DER BORGHT, Stefaan VAN PRAET, Françoise WUILLAUME

With additional contribution from:
Richard BEDELL, Marc BIOT, Dirk BOGAERT, Laurence BONTE, Kate BURNS, Mathilde CORONAT, Maud COUDRAY, Martine DEDEURWAERDER, Benoît DENEYS, Dominique DUBOURG, François ENTEN, Marie-Christine FERIR, Marc GASTELLU-ETCHEGORY, Eric GOESSENS, David GOETGEBUER, Mario GOETHALS, Pim de GRAAF, Peter HAKEWILL, Benson HAUSMAN, Dennis HEIDEBROEK, Bernard HODY, Guy JACQUIER, William KLAUS, Karim LAOUABDIA-SELLAMI, Bruce LAURENCE, Barend LEEUWENBERG, Serge MALÉ, Ginette MARCHANT, Francine MATTHYS, Stephany MAXWELL, Marie-Pierre POUX, André SASSE, Gill SIMONS, Marie-Paule SPIELMAN, Carl SUETENS, Mike TOOLE, Francis VARAINE, Dineke VENEKAMP, Bechara ZIADE

The English text has been thoroughly revised and corrected by
Alison MARSCHNER and Trevor LINES

MSF would like to thank the Italian donors who provided the funding for this book.

Layout by:
Annie ARBELOT-LACHIEZE

Preface

Since World War II, up to one hundred million civilians have been forced to flee persecution or the violence of war to seek refuge either in neighbouring countries or in different areas of their own country. During the past two decades, the number of persons meeting the international definition of a refugee has steadily increased from approximately 5 million in 1980 to a peak of more than 20 million in 1994; at least an equal number were displaced within their own country. The optimism that accompanied the end of the Cold War was short-lived as an 'epidemic' of civil conflicts erupted in several continents. In 1993 alone, 47 conflicts were active of which 43 were internal wars. Armed conflicts have increasingly affected civilian populations, resulting in high casualty rates, widespread human rights abuses, forced migration, famine, and in some countries the total collapse of governance.

The public health consequences of armed conflict and population displacement have been well documented during the past 20 years. The major determinants of high death rates among affected populations and the major priorities for action have also been identified. The provision of adequate food, clean water, sanitation, and shelter have been demonstrated to be more effective interventions than most medical programmes. The focus of emergency health programmes has shifted to community-based disease prevention, health promotion, nutritional rehabilitation, and epidemic preparedness, surveillance and control. Refugee health has developed into a specialized field of public health with its own particular technical policies, methods, and procedures.

The front-line field workers in emergency situations are usually volunteers working for a range of different international non-governmental organizations and local health professionals. They require knowledge and practical experience in a broad range of subjects, including food and nutrition, water and sanitation, public health surveillance, immunization, communicable disease control, epidemic management, and maternal and child health care. They should be able to conduct rapid needs assessments, establish public health programme priorities, work closely with affected communities, organize and manage health facilities and essential medical supplies, train local workers, coordinate with a complex array of relief organizations, monitor and evaluate the impact of their programmes, and efficiently manage scarce resources. In addition, they need to function effectively in a different cultural context and an often hostile and dangerous environment. Such skills are specific to emergencies and are not necessarily acquired in the average medical or nursing school.

When Médecins Sans Frontières published a manual 'Emergency care in catastrophic situations' in 1979, more than 75% of the contents were devoted to surgical and resuscitative procedures; the remainder covered epidemiology, nutrition, water & sanitation, and immunization. In subsequent years, technical manuals were published on a range of subjects covering diagnostic and treatment guidelines, nutrition, and environmental health. The comprehensive range of issues covered by 'Refugee Health' reflects the lessons learned in the past two decades and illustrates the major shift in thinking that has occurred not just within the international MSF movement but within the general relief community. This is not a text-book but a guide for the relief worker which firmly places operational priorities in the context of today's complex humanitarian emergencies. It is a timely contribution to improving the quality, effectiveness, and sustainability of international emergency response efforts.

Michael J Toole
Vice-President of MSF Australia

Introduction

This book is a collective accomplishment of the different sections of Médecins Sans Frontières (MSF), and has been written to consolidate the broad experience of MSF in refugee programmes. It deals with refugees and internally displaced persons, and what a health agency can do to relieve their plight. It focuses on policies rather than on practical aspects, and is meant to act as a guide to decision-makers.

The terms 'refugee' and 'internally displaced person' have wide implications for the people concerned, particularly regarding their rights to protection and assistance, which are embedded in international law. Refugees have crossed an international border; internally displaced persons have not. The United Nation's High Commissioner for Refugees (UNHCR) is mandated by the international community to protect and assist refugees only; due to considerations of state sovereignty, the internally displaced have not been included within UNHCR's mandate. Only on an ad hoc basis has UNHCR been involved in the protection and assistance of the internally displaced, i.e. at the request of the state concerned or of the Secretary General of the United Nations. However, both groups have been forced to leave their homes and undergo physical or mental trauma before their departure or during their flight. They are then often forced to settle in an unhealthy environment, where they are unlikely to be in a position to take responsibility for their own welfare. A humanitarian health agency will try to obtain access to both groups, wherever they are, and the references to 'refugees' in the book should therefore usually be taken to indicate both categories.

The book is written from the perspective of a non-governmental health agency with a primary role in assistance, and protection as a secondary objective. It is intended to provide a public health perspective; the social, political and financial aspects are not dealt with here. Nevertheless, health care does not take place in a vacuum, and this is recognized in the two introductory chapters. The first covers the political implications of refugee situations and the role of the various agencies involved; the second focuses on the socio-cultural aspects of a refugee community.

More specifically, the book deals with health care during the emergency phase, when priority is given to actions that aim to prevent or reduce excess mortality. These intervention priorities have been labelled 'The ten top priorities'. This label proves to be a useful tool, providing a structure for the main part of the book and eventually serving as a kind of checklist during field operations. The basic assumption is that if all 10 priorities are properly addressed, excess mortality will be reduced.

In the post-emergency phase, a degree of stability has been reached, although the overall equilibrium is still fragile. Excess mortality is under control, but there remains a risk of the situation deteriorating. However, now is the time to draw up new plans, set new priorities and envisage some new programmes. This is all dealt with in Part III.

The final part of the book deals with issues related to repatriation and resettlement. An extended appendix then describes specific diseases that may be encountered during the emergency or post-emergency phases and aims to give guidance in what to do should an outbreak threaten, or actually occur.

Readers are encouraged to read the introductions to Parts II and III in order to have an overview of the book, and then decide which chapters might be the most useful to read at that particular moment. Many of the chapters are reference texts and are intended to stand on their own. Fuller technical details in regard to programme implementation can be found in the references which are appended to every chapter.

The book focuses attention on refugee health in camp situations but this does not mean that Médecins Sans Frontières favours the establishment of camps in refugee situations. Unfortunately, health agencies are often confronted with refugees who are already settled in a camp, for reasons beyond their control. Where refugees and internally displaced persons are somehow dispersed among the local population rather than living in camps, the basic principles described in this book do still apply, but will almost certainly have to be adapted to the particular situation.

Although this book deals with refugee and displaced persons, relief workers should be aware that the local population living in the area is also affected, and at several levels. On the one hand, the arrival of refugees in an environment where resources are limited brings up an additional burden on the local residents: competition for water, wood and farming land, drainage of health staff and negative environmental impacts have been regularly observed. However on the other hand, the resident population may also benefit from the relief programmes: they may receive direct aid (food ration, access to services) or they will benefit indirectly, from the larger availability of goods on the market, employment etc. The UNHCR has defined a policy for the 'refugee affected areas', and it is essential that relief agencies take this aspect into account when they provide aid to refugee populations. Specific issues related to the local population are tackled in several chapters of this book.

PART I

Refugee and displaced populations

Political aspects

Socio-cultural aspects

Political aspects

Refugees are a tragic reminder of the wars, oppression and famine that continue to taint our rapidly changing world, forcing millions of uprooted people into exile and focusing international attention onto forgotten conflicts and isolated, little-known countries. Over the past few years, hundreds of thousands of Somalis, Sudanese, Tajiks, Burmese Rohingyas, Serbs, Croats, Bosnian Moslems, Burundians and Rwandans have swollen the number of refugees worldwide to about 23 millions (1994 UNHCR figures) while a further 26 million people are forced to live as displaced persons within the borders of their own countries (1994 US Committee for Refugees figures)[1].

Background history

Refugee crises are not a new problem, but rather one that dates back to the earliest days of humanity, for history books are full of episodes of the forced movements of populations. However, the term 'refugee' seems to have first been coined in 1573, when it was used to describe Calvinists fleeing political repression in the Spanish-controlled Netherlands to seek refuge with their co-religionists in France. But refugees were not only defined as victims of persecution; they were also seen as individuals with political, religious, economic or other affiliations that aroused solidarity among those supporting similar interests in other countries and a corresponding sense of responsibility towards them.

This tendency continued into the beginning of the 20th century, but by the end of the First World War and the foundation of the League of Nations, a transition was taking place and the previously selective responses to refugees by interested sections of the community began to be institutionalized. Now, it is seen as the collective duty of the 'international community' to provide aid and protection to refugees, defined by the League as groups of people whose lives would be at risk if they returned to their home countries. In 1921, the League appointed Fridtjof Nansen to the newly-created post of High Commissioner for Russian Refugees in response to the waves of refugees fleeing the Russian Revolution and the subsequent civil war. However, the League soon had to extend his mandate to cover other categories, such as Assyrians, Turks, Greeks, Armenians, Spaniards, Austrian and German Jews, etc., and the initial preoccupation with travel problems and identity documents (the famous Nansen passport) was extended to protective measures in regard to employment rights and safeguards against expulsion.

The League of Nations was superseded by the United Nations (UN) at the end of the Second World War, and in 1946 the UN created the International Refugee Organization (IRO). In addition to the refugees which the international community had already taken responsibility for between the two World Wars, the IRO was mandated to take care of a further 20 million people scattered throughout Europe as a result of World War II. At first, the IRO's main focus was on repatriation, but Soviet repression of certain groups of repatriated refugees and the increased tensions at the beginning of the Cold War brought about a different approach and its efforts were re-directed towards resettlement in a third country. This covered all those who had a 'valid reason' not to return to their countries of origin because of 'persecution, or fear of persecution, for reasons of race, nationality or political opinion'.

The protection system for refugees

In 1951, the IRO was replaced by the United Nations' High Commissioner for Refugees (UNHCR), mandated by a UN General Assembly resolution in December 1950 to encourage countries to receive refugees, prevent them from being forcibly returned, provide assistance and protection, and seek lasting solutions to the problem. The Convention Relating to the Status of Refugees was also drawn up in 1951 and this was a decisive step towards institutionalizing the refugee question. The Convention, which has the force of law and has been ratified by almost 120 countries, defines a refugee as follows[2]:

'any person who, owing to a well-founded fear of being persecuted for reasons of race, religion, nationality, membership in a particular social group or political opinion, is outside the country of his nationality and is unable or, owing to such fear, is unwilling to avail himself of the protection of that country; or who, not having a nationality and being outside the country of his former habitual residence as a result of such events, is unable or, owing to such fear, is unwilling to return to it'.

Moreover, the Convention stresses the basic principle of non-refoulement, according to which refugees may not be forcibly returned to a country where they have reason to fear persecution.

More than forty years after its adoption, the 1951 Convention is still the cornerstone of the international system for protecting refugees. However, it bears the marks of the historical background against which it was worked out and has had to be supplemented by instruments better adapted to the evolution of the whole refugee question. The Convention's definition of a refugee, basically focusing on individual cases of persecution, reflects the concerns of post-war Europe. During the Cold War that began in the early 50s, Europe was firmly divided into two opposing blocs and refugees were seen as dissidents escaping from totalitarian regimes into democratic countries. The preferred solution was permanent resettlement in a European country, or in the United States, with a legal status and civil rights very similar to those of native citizens. The liberal asylum policies of countries in the West reflected both the very positive light in which refugees were seen as «choosing freedom» and the relative ease with which they integrated into host countries which generally shared the same cultural background as the countries from which they originated. In fact, until the end of the 50s, the refugee problem, covered by the 1951 Refugee Convention, was essentially an internal European problem, consisting mainly of movements from the East to the West. The refugee situations which existed at the time in other continents were not covered either by the scope or the formal range of the

Convention. Only in 1967, the 'Protocol Relating to the Status of Refugees' abolished the geographic and temporal restrictions on the scope of the Convention.

In the early 60s, national wars of liberation and then other, post-independence conflicts in Africa and Asia gave rise to large-scale refugee movements. After the period of decolonization, UNHCR, as well as other UN organizations, turned its attention to the developing world and the new reality of refugee movements from one country to another in the southern hemisphere as well as the large-scale internal population displacements caused by war and insecurity. In contrast to the dissidents from behind the Iron Curtain who came to the West on an individual basis, these refugees represented collective movements of people fleeing from conflict and generalized unrest who, more often than not, were only looking for temporary asylum in a neighbouring country. In response to this new situation, UNHCR's responsibilities were enlarged by the UN General Assembly in order to enable it to deal with large-scale exodus. Its mandate came to include de facto refugees, i.e. those people who flee generalized danger instead of individual persecution and who come in large groups. The refugee definition in the 1951 Convention was never adapted to this new reality.

This wider UNHCR definition was formalized to a certain extent in 1969 by the Organization of African Unity (OAU) which convened to discuss the problems of refugees in Africa. The 'Convention Governing the Specific Aspects of Refugee Problems in Africa', which was adopted at its meeting, included in its refugee definition those refugees who are forced to leave their native countries, not only because of persecution, but also due to 'aggression, occupation by an outside force, foreign domination or events seriously disturbing the peace in a part or all of the country of origin'. In 1984, Latin American countries adopted the Cartagena Declaration which extended the OAU definition to include victims of 'massive human rights violations'. This enlarged definition acknowledges that any person fleeing war and insecurity qualifies for refugee status and thus enables many people who would not have been covered by the 1951 Convention to benefit from international protection. This has proved invaluable in situations of large-scale exodus where it is impossible to examine every individual request for refugee status. In such situations, this so-called *prima facie* procedure enables groups of refugees to be recognized collectively and to receive aid and protection from the host state, UNHCR and the international community at large[2].

The specific problem of the internally displaced

This international protection does not cover groups who have fled from their homes for the same reasons as refugees and seek safety in the outskirts of towns or other areas where there is less violence and insecurity, but within the borders of their own countries. Displaced by fighting or repression, their situation is generally even more precarious than that of refugees; yet they do not qualify for any form of international protection. Humanitarian organizations are sometimes able to provide assistance, but this is often random and inadequate as the displaced may well be trapped by fighting and inaccessible to international help; when war is the reason for population displacements, it is also the obstacle preventing relief operations from reaching them. It is not only insecurity and related transport problems that have to be overcome: there may also be a determined refusal by some of the belligerents to allow any aid to reach populations sheltering in 'hostile' zones. Faced with such a situation, relief agencies have to prove their impartiality towards any of the parties involved in the conflict and convince armed groups that they will maintain a neutral and independent stance.

Refugee camps

Since the end of the 60s, the majority of refugees originate from countries in the southern hemisphere and seek refuge in neighbouring countries. Often, they settle in camps set up by the host country with support from the international community. Between the late 70s and the end of the 80s, the largest concentrations of refugees were to be found in those areas of tension and open conflict where the two sides of the Cold War played out their surrogate East-West power struggle (Southeast Asia, Afghanistan, the Horn of Africa, Southern Africa and Central America). More recently, refugees have been fleeing from countries torn apart by their own internal conflicts (Burma, Afghanistan, Tajikistan, Azerbaijan, Georgia, former Yugoslavia, Liberia, Somalia, Sudan, Burundi, Rwanda, etc.). The main response of the international community to the increased scale of refugee movements has been humanitarian assistance. This is usually provided within the setting of refugee camps while their exiled populations wait out the months, if not years, in the hope that they will eventually be able to return home 'in dignity and security'.

As already indicated, refugees escaping war, famine or insecurity usually form mass influxes to countries that neighbour their own. The exodus of the Kurds from Iraq, the Rohingyas from Burma, as well as Somalis, Burundians or Rwandans are striking examples of the scale and violence of refugee movements over the past few years. Only rapid action by the international community makes it possible to deal with such floods of refugees into regions which are sometimes difficult to reach and where food, water, shelters, sanitary equipment, etc. must be urgently transported under very difficult conditions. International aid is all the more necessary when it is the only hope of survival of refugees arriving destitute and weakened by lengthy periods of travel in areas where nothing has been foreseen for receiving them and where conditions are already extremely precarious.

The assistance which is supplied on such occasions by non-governmental organizations (NGOs) may in itself constitute an element of protection. In many situations, the rapid release of international aid and the early arrival of relief teams are far from negligible factors in ensuring that a host country does not forcibly return refugees, but allows them to remain. In this regard, assistance and protection are indissociably linked and mutually reinforcing.

Once the emergency phase has been brought under control, which implies a rapid reaction by aid agencies, these organizations must be prepared to commit themselves in the long term, for refugee camps that are set up as temporary structures have a tendency to stay. Refugees have remained in camps in Thailand, Pakistan and Sudan for periods as long as 10 to 15 years before being able to contemplate returning home. Refugee populations deprived of their traditional means of subsistence, and assembled into camps located on the borders of countries in conflict are dependent on the ability of the international humanitarian organizations to bring them appropriate and sufficient aid.

While those living in closed camps depend entirely on outside assistance, refugees settled in open camps, where they have a greater degree of contact with the local population, may be able to supplement aid through some kind of income-generating activity or by what they are able to trade.

In some cases, refugees may live in fully open situations, and may even be integrated into village communities with which they have traditional links: for example, Liberian refugees in Guinea or Ivory Coast and Chechens in Ingushkaya or Daghestan. However, humanitarian organizations have to be more vigilant in dealing with these situations, where needs are less easily identified than in closed camps. In addition, both refugees and native villagers are at risk as a result of the imbalance caused by the exodus the refugees have endured, and their artificial integration into the local population.

The role of relief agencies

The well-being of refugees, sometimes their very survival, depends on 4 key factors: water and sanitation, food, shelter and health care. UNHCR, whose mandate it is to coordinate assistance to refugees, operates in all these fields in close cooperation with other UN agencies, with the host government, and with the different specialized NGOs. The World Food Programme (WFP) is responsible for bringing in food aid, which is then distributed under the supervision of UNHCR. As far as health and sanitation is concerned, the work is shared between the NGOs that are in the field and the line ministries of the host government, in partnership with and under the general co-ordination of UNHCR.

The humanitarian organizations must always be on their guard to prevent the situation in the refugee settlement from deteriorating. The experience of the last few years has shown that refugees are very sensitive to anything lacking in their food ration that might provoke malnutrition or vitamin deficiencies. Likewise, they are very vulnerable to epidemics that can decimate a refugee population living in the conditions of overcrowding and poor sanitation that encourage the spread of disease. Surveillance is essential, and the humanitarian agencies must closely observe changes in the situation and be prepared to react swiftly to any problems. This may involve putting pressure on UNHCR and the WFP to persuade them to fully assume their responsibilities; for whatever the failings of UNHCR - and it is certainly one of the most operationally effective of the UN agencies - it is essential to keep in mind that it has a dual mandate of aid and protection. UNHCR should therefore be strongly encouraged to fulfil its mandate in regard to aid coordination; if it does not take on this central responsibility, it will not be able to successfully perform the task of refugee protection that only UNHCR is qualified to assume.

Refugee camps: humanitarian sanctuaries

The role that the international community has given UNHCR in regard to protecting refugees - a role which goes further than defending asylum rights and the principle of non-refoulement (preventing forced return or repatriation) - is absolutely essential. Even if refugee camps represent a refuge, they are themselves the product of violence, and the fact of crossing a border is not enough to isolate them from the tensions and fighting that are tearing apart their home country. Refugee populations are not composed of thousands of victims with no past history: they reconstitute their complex societies in the new setting, often reproducing the divisions and power struggles of the home country, possibly further exacerbated by those of the host country.

In many instances, armed groups control the refugee camps and their populations. Guerrilla movements may benefit from the aid and may use the camps to legitimize their power base by exploiting the refugee population, diverting aid distributions to build up their economic base, and using the camps as a source of fresh fighters and porters. This well-known phenomenon of 'humanitarian sanctuary' remains a key factor in perpetuating conflicts. In Pakistan and Honduras, in Sudan and in Thailand, the aid economy of refugee camps has indirectly funded a number of armed movements. Western countries have not been innocent dupes in this manipulation; indeed, it was noticeable that some of them increased their aid to specific camps in the early 80s, when swings in popular ideology transformed the image of the guerrilla fighter into that of the 'freedom fighter'.

The humanitarian organizations, confronted with the negative side effects of some of their operations, have sometimes been forced to face some painful dilemmas. For example, in 1979, aid that was essential for the survival of Cambodians forced into exile by the Khmer Rouge actually enabled this totalitarian movement to get back on its feet. The Khmer Rouge has since continued to carry out a war of attrition against the government of Phnom Penh, using the refugee camp sanctuaries in Thailand as bases. Likewise, the international aid which, in the summer of 1994, was supplied to the Rwandan refugees who fled to Burundi, Tanzania and Zaire following the genocide which took place in Rwanda in April 1994, was not always used for the right purposes. It enabled the former authorities of Rwanda, some of whom are the perpetrators of the genocide and who are still remaining in the camps today, to reinforce their control over the refugee population, and prepare to re-conquer Rwanda.

Such use of aid by armed movements, or by local power groups, is neither new nor exclusive to refugee situations. Humanitarian aid is not deployed in the philanthropic clouds in which it may originally have been conceived, but on political battlefields. As a result, it may itself become one of the stakes to be fought over in crisis situations. This is the root of the dilemma for those involved in humanitarian assistance, who have an obligation to assist the victims even where this might mean that they inevitably strengthen the hand of the aggressors. It is a dilemma with no simple solution. The background context, the nature of those in power and the scale of abuses all are determining factors that have to be taken into account in working out a response. But the major implication of this ambiguity is that those involved in humanitarian work have a special responsibility to try and ensure that aid is not diverted from its intended objectives and used against those it is intended to help. It is therefore essential that relief agencies should be given complete independence to assess needs and monitor distributions in order to ensure that these are used for the benefit of the victims.

Permanent solutions

Refugee camps have become a chronic problem and, combined with the prospect of an indefinite extension of the humanitarian status quo, this raises crucial questions in regard to solutions that might go beyond immediate aid. As the problem has evolved over the last few years, of the 3 possibilities for 'permanent solutions' that are usually proposed - integration into the host country, resettlement in a third country and repatriation to the country of origin - the principal donor countries consider repatriation to be the only option.

Although many countries, especially in Africa, keep their borders relatively open to refugee movements, integration into the host country is less and less often considered a realistic solution. More often than not, the host countries are poor and unstable, without the means or the necessary internal cohesion to integrate thousands of refugees. They also see how the wealthier countries of the northern hemisphere, which are supposed to set the example in respecting asylum rights, are becoming more and more reluctant to do so, and resist allowing refugees to integrate into their societies. Over the past 10 years, the refugee image has evolved. During the Cold War, refugees had a political significance - they had 'voted with their feet'; and with a positive connotation - they had 'chosen freedom'. Now they are perceived as 'undesirable'. The time has passed when Vietnamese boat people were welcomed with open arms in the West, and, since the summer of 1994 even Cubans have lost the right of refuge in the United States. Cold War certainty has given way to deep concern in the face of upheavals all over the globe and fear of mass migrations. Since the mid-80s, the West has become even more reluctant to open its doors when faced with ever-increasing numbers of asylum-seekers. This changing situation has brought about very significant changes in policy. Against a background of growing confusion over the difference between a refugee and a migrant, the West is now dissuading asylum seekers and putting an increasingly narrow interpretation on the 1951 Convention. Whereas the refugee question was previously seen as a human rights issue, it is now perceived as a problem of migration.

The scale of refugee movements and the increasing numbers of refugees seeking asylum in the West have reopened the debate on the refugee question. The chronic situation of refugee camps shows the inadequacies of aid policies in regard to countries in the southern hemisphere, while the reluctance of countries in the northern hemisphere to take in refugees demonstrates the limits of their resettlement policies. The aid/resettlement package that has been at the heart of refugee policy for 3 decades is now replaced by the new key words of prevention and repatriation.

The question of repatriation

Ultimately, repatriation is probably the best solution to the refugee problem; certainly, an indefinitely prolonged stay in a camp is neither humanely acceptable nor politically desirable. However, when in addition to spontaneous repatriation, the international community wants to facilitate the return home of other refugees, some criteria for the repatriation to be legitimate should be carefully guarded. Preferably on the basis of an agreement between UNHCR, the host country and the country of origin, a repatriation programme should only be set up when the circumstances in the home country have changed fundamentally. The repatriation programme should ensure that the refugees make their choice to return on a purely voluntary basis, and that they are aware of the right to refuse to go home. In order to be able to make the choice, sufficient information should be available to them about the situation back home (see Part IV, *Repatriation and Re-settlement*). On many occasions, these guarantees, which have been formulated by UNHCR, have not been observed. In recent years, many repatriation programmes have been set up to countries where the existence of fundamental changes was highly questionable: refugees returned to situations of conflict, repression or generalized violence that did not differ much from the situation that provoked their flight in the first place (for example, refugees repatriated to Sri Lanka, Burma and Rwanda). Moreover, the principle of voluntary return is increasingly replaced by the notion of a 'safe return', but it is UNHCR and the governments concerned, rather than the refugees themselves who decide whether the conditions for this are in place. Given this context, the humanitarian organizations present in the camps must keep a critical eye on repatriation operations. Without locking themselves into a pattern of systematic opposition, they must preserve their freedom to assess and witness to the situation. At a time when repatriation is increasingly regarded as a priority by fund-raisers, humanitarian organizations have an essential role to play in reminding UNHCR that it should safeguard its own guarantees.

The ambiguities of prevention

The growing UNHCR presence as an accompaniment to repatriation operations in the countries to which refugees return, further reinforces the other facet of the new refugee policy: prevention. This poses a 'political' problem for the international community in the face of the repressive regimes and internal conflicts that provoke major movements of refugees and displaced persons in the first place. At the beginning of the 90s, in the euphoria of post-Wall Berlin, the idea spread that the international community should act to re-establish peace and prevent large-scale human rights violations from taking place. But the evolving events of these past few years have shown that any debate on intervention is limited by the reluctance of governments to become involved in the internal conflicts of other countries in order to break the cycle of violence and protect their populations. What is requested in the way of protection exceeds by far what is offered in the way of intervention and the international community reacts selectively, influenced by political interests, media visibility and the pressure of public opinion. Prevention policies, although a popular subject for discussion in international forums, are usually delayed and essentially defensive: failing to deal with a situation at source, the donor countries of the West are finally left struggling to contain the disastrous consequences that result.

Humanitarian organizations and military interventions

The international community's preoccupation with avoiding any new refugee problem was well illustrated by the situation in Iraq in the spring of 1991, when it was even prepared to provide a safe haven - though only, of course, as a 'temporary solution' - to encourage repatriated refugees to remain in their own country. In a defeated country that had supposedly been placed under international surveillance, coalition forces stood with lowered arms in the face of the bloody repression of Shia and Kurdish uprisings. But once a whole population passed before us on our television screens as it spilled over the frontiers into neighbouring countries, western governments were pushed to intervene *in extremis*. Presented as a purely humanitarian intervention, the objective was to persuade the Kurds to pull back from the Turkish border and return home in exchange for the offer of temporary protection and humanitarian assistance in the north of Iraq.

The international reaction to the Kurdish exodus is certainly the most complete example of a new policy of containment based on a three-pronged approach of repatriation, the provision of safety areas and humanitarian aid. This policy aimed at supporting refugees in camps inside a country in crisis - if necessary, by exerting pressure to get them there - into areas that are de facto neutralized through an international presence and supplied by aid convoys. The result of this policy is a de facto extension to the UNHCR's mandate in order to be able to intervene in a country at war, i.e. bring aid to a displaced population to prevent them from fleeing further or even encouraging them to return. With the examples of Iraq, former Yugoslavia and Rwanda, it appears that this is becoming a generally accepted policy. However, it is raising new questions for the humanitarian world at large, how best to assist and protect refugees and displaced persons.

Humanitarian organizations are increasingly faced with the presence of international forces in crisis areas. In classic peacekeeping operations, based on agreements with the warring parties and the non-use of force, this coexistence does not present enormous problems, although the humanitarian organizations must keep a certain distance from UN forces in order to preserve their independence and freedom of action. But conducting aid operations in active crisis situations where intervention is taking place without the agreement of the combatants is quite another question, and it is therefore essential that humanitarian workers can be clearly distinguished from the military. The examples of Somalia and former Yugoslavia show how interventions that combine military logic and humanitarian objectives under the same flag limit the possibilities for action by the humanitarian relief agencies. There is a confusion between the military and the humanitarian imperatives which casts a shadow over the principles of neutrality and impartiality held by humanitarian organizations that are essential for establishing a climate of confidence with the combatants and ensuring access to those in need.

The problem is all the more serious in that these 'military-humanitarian' interventions provide no real protection to the civilian populations in danger. The resolutions adopted by the UN Security Council during the course of the last few years concentrate on protection for humanitarian operations but are silent in regard to the protection of victims. Throughout the war in Bosnia, UN forces had been prepared to protect aid convoys but had never taken any initiative likely to put an end to shelling, massacres and 'ethnic cleansing'. They had not even proved powerful enough to protect the 'safety areas' set up by the United Nations itself, which were either turned into prison-towns dependent on the goodwill of those besieging them or lost to determined large-scale offensives.

The mediocre results of intervention over the last few years reveal the difficulty of ensuring a real protection for displaced populations in countries at war. They also highlight the ambiguity of the current policies favoured by the international community in attempting to limit refugee movements. Under cover of prevention, there is a very considerable risk that the countries of the West will make it harder and harder for people to find refuge in a safe country and will prefer to send them back to their home countries and to the precarious status of displaced people. Creating 'safety areas' and organizing aid convoys cannot serve as an alibi for the refusal to grant asylum to populations in danger.

➤ References

1. International Federation of Red Cross and Red Crescent Societies. *World disasters report.* Oxford: Oxford University Press, 1996.

2. UNHCR. *Handbook on procedures and criteria for determining refugee status.* Geneva: UNHCR, 1992.

3. UNHCR. *The state of the world's refugees - in search of solutions.* Oxford: Oxford University Press, 1995.

4. Cohen, R. *Refugees and human rights.* Washington DC: Refugee Policy Group: Center for policy analysis and research on refugees issues, 1995.

Socio-cultural aspects

Introduction

Emergency assistance to refugee and displaced persons often implies huge logistical operations, particularly when large-scale population movements occur. Food, shelter, safe water, sanitation and medical facilities have to be provided in the shortest possible time in order to save lives and little attention is paid to discovering the specific needs of the refugee community. The priority is to meet the most basic human needs, without consideration for the individual social and cultural backgrounds of different refugee populations. Although the current philosophy of development programmes is to foster self-sufficiency among the populations and encourage their active participation, emergency assistance tends to leave such concepts on the shelf. Refugees are usually seen as 'victims' and it is therefore assumed that treating them as such will result in a quicker and more efficient response to the situation.

However, if refugees do not participate during the planning and implementation stages, assistance programmes may well fail in several ways. Without refugee involvement and the information this brings in regard to culture, religion and traditional differences between groups, some services may prove inaccessible to part of the population; for example, refugees have been known to boycott distribution systems that were not organized in a culturally acceptable way.[1]

Refugees are usually seen as temporary visitors to a host country, an attitude which results in a short-term planning approach that may be maintained for years after their arrival. Consequently, encouraging self-reliance is not seen as a first-order priority and is certainly not taken into account at the beginning. Yet experience has shown that small refugee or displaced populations receiving very little international support often prove capable of developing a sustainable life for themselves within a reasonably short time.

It is important that aid workers do not make the mistake of considering refugees and displaced people as helpless individuals totally dependent on outside assistance. Despite the outward appearance of exhaustion, sickness, malnutrition and poverty - and apathy as a result of these factors in combination - it should not automatically be assumed that they are incapable of any independent action and unable to organize themselves in any way. They may have lost their jobs and belongings, but they did not lose their education and skills. Although they have been forced to leave their homes and their habitual roles, they will redefine similar roles for themselves within the context of the new community: some as leaders and some as dependents, relying on the leadership of others. It is therefore important to encourage them to build a new life for themselves as quickly as possible, even if it is hoped that this will only be a temporary one.

Refugees are often traumatized by their recent experiences; they may have lost relatives and friends, and they have certainly been forced to abandon homes and possessions, and a way of life. Their best hope for dealing with all this trauma is to start to create a new and worthwhile life. And to do this, they should be allowed to participate actively in the planning and implementation of assistance programmes. This will help them to regain their shattered self-esteem and will encourage the emotional healing process, thereby avoiding the worst extremes of apathy, aggression or even psychiatric disorders (see *Psycho-social and Mental Health* in Part III). Refugees should be given the opportunity to express their needs and priorities and say how they want to live. Helping them to help themselves should be the principle behind relief assistance; given responsibility for their own future, they are more likely to have hope in that future.

The refugee community

It should always be remembered that every refugee population consists of individuals, each with his or her own background and history. If assistance programmes are only planned within the context of a whole social entity seen in terms of total number of families, males, females and children, there is no guarantee that each of these individuals will be reached. Programmes planned from this approach are also likely to neglect culture, religion and tradition with consequent negative effects on the acceptability of the assistance provided.

ETHNIC BACKGROUND, CULTURE AND RELIGION

Although it is essential to have general demographic information (numbers, age distribution, etc.), more specific information is also necessary in order to obtain a clear picture of the refugee community: for example, information about family structures, the number of single people, elderly, disabled and other vulnerable groups. It is important to know what support mechanisms exist for vulnerable individuals within the community and whether these are still functioning, whether the population is composed of one or several different ethnic groups and, if so, which ones, their size and their home area. Knowledge of such details can be very important in preventing potentially dangerous situations from escalating into violence. For example, information about different sections of the population in the El Wak refugee camp in Kenya made it possible to organize the camp in such a way that hostile groups were not settled close to each other and to take advantage of a 'neutral' group of Bantu origin. It is also indispensable to be well-informed about the recent political and social situation in the refugees' home country in order to understand why they are now living in exile.

Information about ethnic background is important because this has implications in terms of cultural and religious beliefs, and ignorance of these may have major consequences on whether or not the different services provided are accessible to all. In some populations, women will not be allowed to visit a clinic unless there are separate departments for men and women, or women will not be allowed to consult male doctors. In Afghanistan, low attendance in a feeding programme for malnourished children was found to be due to the fact that women were not allowed to leave their own neighbourhood block without being escorted and therefore could not bring their children to the centre every day. During a measles epidemic in Southern Sudan, it was discovered that mothers were hiding children with diarrhoea and measles as they believed the food and drink the health workers were giving them was poisonous.

As it is clearly important to acquire information early on so that assistance can be genuinely effective and relief workers less often frustrated by an inability to reach objectives, a good level of communication must be maintained with the refugee community from the start. They will be able to recognize potential cultural and religious constraints on planned programmes better than any outsider. However, as a refugee community is rarely homogenous, it is important to have a broad forum when discussing strategies for implementing programmes. This should include representatives from all ethnic groups and from all categories: the elderly and the young, men and women; for example, it may happen that the men are willing to compromise on certain traditional beliefs in the light of current circumstances, but women are afraid to abandon their practices and customs; or vice versa.

Additional problems can arise when different ethnic groups are forced to live together. Not only do cultural practices and religious beliefs differ, but old hostilities will still be present in the new situation. They may even be reinforced, as one group is pitted against another in a fight for scarce resources and the daily struggle for survival takes priority over feelings of solidarity in a shared disaster. There may also be a certain level of hostility between the refugee and host communities because of profound differences between their respective cultures and traditions; this may seriously affect the security of the refugee population and may also influence whether or not the local health services are accessible to all the refugees.

THE COMMUNITY AND ITS LEADERS

The role of each individual within the structure of a community is usually well defined; but when the community is displaced, the well-established system is disrupted and a new structure has to be created. A refugee settlement will often bring together members of different communities - and certainly there will be members missing from all of them. Some refugees will find it relatively easy to fulfil their customary role; others will take on new roles. The community elders, who may have been regarded as leaders in the home country, may well have difficulty in adapting to a new situation and become dependent on the leadership of stronger and younger men. Indeed, young, dynamic and educated refugees often come to play more important roles as they are more likely to be employed by the relief agencies or given a position within the camp administration, and are therefore in a position to control the information to and from the community[11]. However, it must also be noted that some refugee communities are able to resist the force of circumstances and do manage to retain their original social structures intact.

VULNERABLE GROUPS

Special account must be taken of all groups of vulnerable people in order to ensure that they have full access to health and other services. These groups include:

> ### *Potential vulnerable groups*
> – women and female-headed households,
> – children,
> – the elderly,
> – the disabled,
> – ethnic, religious or political minority groups,
> – urban refugees in a rural environment.

This list is not valid for every situation, nor is it necessarily complete. An anthropological assessment of the population will be required in order to identify vulnerable groups that may not immediately be obvious to outsiders.

Women

In most communities, women play a particular role both within the family and outside: they are responsible for preparing food, collecting water and cooking fuel, caring for children, the sick and the elderly. This means that women are one of the best sources of information on the various needs within the population. They may also play a role in decision-making, though often only discreetly, expressing their concerns and needs either through their husbands or through established community networks. But such family and community structures are usually disrupted and, as a result, their input is often missing.

The traditional caring role of women and the need to obtain food, water and other essential commodities for the family in an environment where these are not readily available makes them more vulnerable to abuse and sexual assaults. This is particularly true where reponsibility for registration and distributions is in the hands of male community leaders. Sexual abuse has been documented in several refugee situations and probably occurs more often than it is reported (as victims and their families are usually reluctant to report such sensitive issues, especially if there is fear of reprisals). As a result, rapes and assaults may well remain unnoticed unless relief workers are actively aware of the likely risks.

Women and children are extremely vulnerable in times of limited resources. Studies shows particularly high rates of mortality, morbidity and malnutrition compared with men. This cannot be explained by physical vulnerability alone; discrimination is clearly a major factor[2]. It has been clearly documented that female-headed households have a lower level of access to food and other distributed commodities and higher malnutrition rates than those headed by a male. This was seen most recently in the Rwandan refugee camps near Goma[9].

Involving women in planning all refugee programmes and taking account of their concerns when implementing them, may well help to protect them in regard to the risks of abuse and of any bias in distributions. Enrolling women as health workers and home-visitors should also help to ensure that all services are accessible to them; some recommend that more than half of those employed should be women[3]. UNHCR's mandate is to ensure protection for all refugees and their guidelines provide valuable information on the protection of women, and relief workers should take these into account[4]. It is up to the NGOs to reinforce the protection effort by reporting assaults, planning proper programmes of assistance and enforcing priorities that support women's safety and well-being.

Children

As stated above, children are not only physically vulnerable but are often discriminated against in times of scarcity, when the principle of 'survival of the fittest' applies. Children have special needs and may face additional risks that should be identified as early as possible. Unaccompanied minors are particularly vulnerable. The 1994 Rwandan refugee crisis produced great numbers of unaccompanied children with an excessively high mortality rate among them.

An effort must be made to identify children who may have been orphaned, become separated from their family, or deliberately abandoned by parents who feel they can no longer care for them. Support should be given to communities and families to foster these children as this is better for them in the long-run than placing them in orphanages or children's homes.

Elderly and disabled

Elderly and disabled people are also at particular risk during crisis situations and may be just as dependent on family care as children are. Reduced mobility means that they are not very visible among the refugee population and their voice may not be heard. They may have difficulty in attending distributions and be unable to make use of health services if they have become separated from their families during a displacement and have nobody else to assist them.

The same rule applies for this group as for unaccompanied minors: they should remain in the community and support should be given to families that are willing to care for them.

Ethnic and religious minorities

Minority groups with a different ethnic or religious background from that of the majority are often found among refugee poulations. If these groups are not integrated, they may well have reduced access to services. For example, if they are not well-represented among the community leaders responsible for food distributions, they could well be left out. This happened in a Sudanese refugee camp in Northern Uganda in 1993, where a minority

Dinka group protested that they had no real access to health services because all the staff were from another ethnic group; a combination of cultural differences and old hostilities made them distrustful of the care they would receive.

Vulnerable groups and their specific needs and difficulties should be identified as early as possible and all assistance programmes should be designed in such a way that these needs are covered and all refugee services are accessible to them.

Encouraging and supporting a strong refugee community will help to ensure that mechanisms operate within it to care for those who are dependent on others (see *Psycho-social and Mental Health* in Part III).

REFUGEES AND THE HOST POPULATION

A refugee or displaced population should never be regarded as separate from the host community. Refugees may arrive in large or small numbers, be settled in camps or dispersed amongst the host community, but there will always be some interaction between the two.

The host community may provide initial assistance by sharing their food, water and accommodation. However, these resources can gradually become scarce and the prices of essential commodities rise; therefore, some local people may see refugees as an opportunity to make extra money, and others may suffer as a result of their presence.

Another problem may arise once aid arrives and distributions have got under way: the local economy may be disrupted if basic commodities suddenly start flooding onto the local market as refugees barter or sell their rations to diversify their diet. Also, if aid agencies concentrate exclusively on the refugees and ignore the local population, this may arouse jealousy.

As a final example, some refugee assistance programmes may prove highly disruptive to the host population; for instance, a cost-recovery system for district health care is hard to maintain when high-level health care is provided free of charge on their doorstep.

Assistance programmes should therefore be planned in such a way that they support the area as a whole, always take the local population into account and cause the least possible disruption to it.

A good example of this is to be found in Guinea-Conakry, where the steadily growing influx of about 400,000 refugees from Liberia and Sierra Leone has not led to mega-camps, but to integration within local Guinean communities. The local health services have been supported by aid agencies so as to enable them to cope with the increased demands, and no parallel health services have had to be created. This integration favoured the existing cost-recovery programme as UNHCR paid for refugee health care[10]. Overall, the presence of the dynamic Liberian refugee community in Guinea has contributed significantly to the economic development of the region.

Collecting relevant information

It is important that the collection of information is conducted from the time of the initial assessment and continues throughout the course of an intervention. Not only quantitative data (number of refugees, mortality rates, etc.) are important, but also qualitative and descriptive data, related to the socio-cultural background, coping mechanisms, community structures, etc. (see also *Initial Assessment* in Part III). UNHCR has outlined a framework for programme planning that should include an analysis of 3 types of information[5].

1. First should come an analysis of the population profile and the background context of the situation. This includes demographic data, a description of the population and its sub-groups, religion, culture, economic conditions, community norms, social hierarchy, mechanisms for caring for the vulnerable, etc.

2. Second is an analysis of the different activities in which the refugees were engaged in the home country, those they are involved with in the new situation and an estimation of what more they are capable of doing. It is also important to know where and when different tasks are done, how much time they require and how they are usually divided between the sexes and between young and old, and rich and poor. This knowledge can be used to ensure that services are not scheduled when they would be inaccessible to any group involved in other activities at the same time. Consideration should be given to the possibility that traditional tasks and responsibilities may be carried out by different groups or in different ways from what was habitual previously.

3. The third type of information is an analysis of how the refugees use and control available resources, whether material resources (such as land, food and water), or skills and education. Skills and education that refugees bring with them will have to be evaluated in the light of how they can be used or adapted to the present situation. Some skills may even be redundant; for example, it is unlikely that farming skills (often the preserve of women) will be useful in a refugee situation where suitable land is unlikely to be available to the community.

Once the above and any additional information has been gathered, it should be possible to identify:
• the needs identified by the population;
• the priorities identified by the population;
• the likely acceptability of emergency assistance as proposed by the aid agency;
• the constraints to be anticipated in terms of programme acceptability;
• the constraints to be anticipated in terms of service accessibility to all groups;
• vulnerable groups and their specific needs and how programmes should cover them;
• how to encourage individual and collective initiatives by the refugees themselves.

There are 4 main methods of gathering information:

- **Key informant interviews** with an individual with particular knowledge of a specific topic. Such a person is not necessarily an 'official' from within the community but could be, for example, a traditional midwife (whose experience and close contacts with women and children may give her knowledge not otherwise available to health care personnel), a teacher (who is likely to have a better understanding of social structures) or a representative of a special and/or vulnerable group (who understands their requirements personally).

It is important to have an idea of the positions key informants occupy within the community: are they representing the view of only one 'sub-culture', or are they transmitting representative information from several sectors of the community?

- **Group discussions**: the advantage of a group discussion is that informants are able to correct each other and add information.

When information is required on a specific subject, participants in the group interview should be selected accordingly (see above, *Key informants*). In order to get a broad overview and ensure that the needs and wishes of all groups within the refugee community are taken into account, participants should be selected from all the relelevant sub-groups (young/old, male/female, ethnic/political/religious groups, etc.).

However, a word of caution: group discussions are not always appropriate. When taboo-subjects or politically sensitive issues are addressed, the discussion may be dominated by a few individuals, and social constraints may prevent some participants from expressing their views freely.

- **Observation**: whereas interviews can give information on what refugees may be thinking, observation can give information on what they actually do. It can therefore be useful to take time to walk around and have a good look at the camp in order to observe various aspects of refugee life and how it is evolving. This can help to put other information into perspective and prepare appropriate action to remedy a situation: for example, refugees in one camp seemed to approve the building of public latrines when they were interviewed on the subject prior to construction, but later observation showed these were not generally being used. It was discovered that there was a belief that a latrine previously used by a menstruating woman could make a man infertile.

- **Surveys** based on questionnaires or the measurement of specific data can be used to verify data collected by other methods. However, they take time and cannot replace the first 3 methods.

Refugee participation in programmes

The level of refugee participation will determine the success or failure of a project. If agencies fail to involve refugees, they are denying them the possibility of developing their own strategies for dealing with the situation. Time constraints during the initial emergency phase, a lack of background knowledge about the refugee population and claims that refugees cannot know what is best for them or are too traumatized to make decisions - should not be used as an excuse not to encourage refugee participation. Indeed, their involvement should start at the beginning of operations, during the initial assessment with the identification of key people for involvement in different programmes. It need not be time-consuming and will reap long-term benefits: a continous process of monitoring and evaluation by both beneficiaries and implementing partners will ensure the smooth implementation of programmes and any later adjustments that may have to be made once they are up and running.

Involvement may take different forms and may be at individual or community level with the contribution varying in terms of a material, financial, physical or administrative input. Various different types of involvement may be identified.

- Paid labour.
- Voluntary labour.
- Financial participation: cost-sharing, contributions towards services.
- Community participation: representatives of the community take an active part in setting goals, planning, implementing and evaluating programmes using the financial and material resources provided to them.
- Participation by individuals from the community: the community appoints and pays people to perform certain tasks within the aid programme.

Community activities can also be undertaken quite independently of outside agencies (e.g. religious ceremonies and all informal economic activities within the camps).

It is important to pay attention to who is actually participating and what their motives are in order to avoid the possibility of one segment of the community manipulating another (e.g. political or religious groups active in the camp).

EMERGENCY AND POST-EMERGENCY PHASES

Different levels of participation will generally correspond to the different phases of the emergency and the degree to which the population adjusts, both as individuals and as a community. The community as a whole is unlikely to have experience in dealing with large-scale emergency situations, although communities that have been uprooted on several occasions may develop their own coping mechanisms. However, even these may eventually prove inadequate if the scale and severity of the emergency increases dramatically.

In most situations, a full community-based participation cannot be expected in the emergency phase. Indeed, at this stage, when day-to-day survival is fully occupying the time, energy, and any remaining resources of the refugees, little can be expected from them. Participation is therefore generally dependent on agencies involving refugee representatives in planning and monitoring programmes, and employing them where possible.

Once the initial emergency is passed and basic needs are covered, the community will have to learn to cope, calling on its tradition and experience for help or else forced to develop entirely new structures and strategies. At this point, an outreach programme including psycho-social support will usually be necessary (see *Psycho-social and Mental Health* in Part III). As time passes, new networks and structures normally develop within the refugee community and they start to organize themselves; voluntary work can be expected and community involvement then becomes a natural asset of refugee life. However, community participation in cost-recovery programmes, such as for health care, or providing payment or material support to volunteers will only begin when the population reaches a certain level of self-sufficiency and surplus reserves are available.

CHOOSING PARTICIPANTS

As was previously indicated, in order to ensure that all groups have equal access to the services provided, that there is no discrimination between different groups and that the vulnerable are protected, participation should be divided between the different ethnic groups present, and between men and women. When choosing individuals to represent the community in planning activities, key informants must be identified who are in a position to know the needs and problems of the entire population or of specific groups within it.

Although official community leaders may seem to be the most obvious people to choose, in fact they are not always well informed about all the needs of the population and are often biased towards certain groups. Also, it often happens that individuals with strong political or military links try to take advantage of the changed situation and present themselves as appointed leaders. Their priority is not necessarily the well-being of the refugee population as a whole. In the Goma crisis, for example, aid workers have clearly been confronted with political leaders trying to dictate the way aid should be distributed without any concern for vulnerable groups.

It should therefore be a principle of planning programmes and services for refugees, that they take account of individuals, not just of the refugee community as a whole. However, it must also be acknowledged that, especially in the emergency phase, it is often difficult for aid workers to take the time to hold back, discuss and observe before immediately starting to work. This problem can be resolved by specifically assigning one person to identify key informants and core groups to participate in planning, and to ensure that they are invited to take part, wherever this is feasible, and who can then follow-up the degree and extent of refugee involvement.

Principal recommendations regarding socio-cultural aspects

- Time should be taken to observe and listen to the refugee community. Refugees should be respected as human beings and not only treated as victims.

- It is not only the essential needs of the population that should be taken into account when analysing the situation, but also the social and political consequences of their displacement.

- One person within the organization should be assigned the specific task of ensuring that planning takes account of the cultural and ethnic characteristics of the refugees.

- In order to ensure that assistance programmes are both accessible and acceptable to the refugee population as a whole, it is important to:
  - collect information in regard to demography, cultural background, religious and political beliefs, special and/or vulnerable groups through key informants and group discussions;
  - ensure that refugees are involved in the planning and implementation of activities at different levels;
  - identify vulnerable groups and their specific needs.

- The position of vulnerable groups should be strengthened by:
  - involving them in programme planning and implementation;
  - encouraging the re-building of the community so as to include them;
  - ensuring an equal distribution of jobs and opportunities among all population groups.

🕮 References

1. Slim, H, Mitchell, J. Towards community-managed relief. A case study from southern Sudan. *Disasters*, 1990, 14(3): 265-9.

2. Rivers, J P W. Woman and children last. An essay on sex discrimination in disasters. *Disasters*, 1982, 6(4): 256-67.

3. Forbes Martin S, et al. *Issues in refugee and displaced women and children*. Vienna: Expert Group Meeting on Refugee and Displaced Women and Children, 1990.

4. UNHCR. *Guidelines on the protection of refugee women*. Geneva: UNHCR, 1991.

5. Anderson, M B, et al. *A framework for people-oriented planning in refugee situations taking account of women, men and children*. Geneva: UNHCR, 1992.

6. UNHCR. *People oriented planning at work. Using POP to improve UNHCR programming. A UNHCR handbook*. Geneva: UNHCR, 1994.

7. Needham, R. *Refugee participation. A paper prepared for the PARinAC Conference*. Addis Ababa: PARinAC, 1994.

8. Martin, S F. *Refugee Women*. London: Z Books Ltd, 1995.

9.   Suetens, C, Dedeurwaerder, M. Food availability in the refugee camp of Kahindo, Goma, Zaïre, november 1994. *Medical News*, 1994, 3(5): 16-22.

10. Van Damme, W. Do refugees belong in camps? Experiences from Goma and Guinea. *The Lancet*, 1995, 346(8971): 360-2.

11. Sommers, M. Representing refugees : the role of elites in Burundi refugee society. *Disasters*, 1995, 19(1).

PART II

The emergency phase: the ten top priorities

Introduction

Refugee and population displacements over the last 20 years have mostly occurred in countries which have neither the resources nor the capacity to deal with them[1]. Countries such as Iraq, Somalia, Sudan, Ethiopia, Malawi and Rwanda have been affected by such displacements in recent years and have a gross national product per inhabitant lower than US$ 500 *per annum*, and an infant mortality rate greater than 120 deaths per 1,000 live births[1]. The economic, social and ecological costs of a massive influx of refugees create an enormous burden for the host countries. As a consequence, effective aid to refugee and displaced populations in those countries is almost always dependent on a rapid response by the international community[1].

Population movements into areas with poor resources have usually led to high mortality rates (especially in camp settings) that can be up to 60 times the expected rates for the area during the first weeks or months following displacement[1,2]. Among the displaced Dinka in El Meiram (Sudan), the death rate was so high that more than a quarter of the Dinka population died between June and October 1988. Table 1.1 illustrates the excessive mortality observed in other refugee populations during the initial emergency phase (with crude mortality rates expressed per 1,000 per month). The major causes of death are primarily common diseases that can be easily prevented or treated (see *7. Control of Communicable Diseases and Epidemics*)[2].

Table 1.1
Crude Mortality Rates (CMR - deaths per 1,000 population per month):
comparisons between refugee population and host country[1]

Host country, region	Country of origin	Period	CMR Refugees	CMR Host country
Thailand, Sakeo	Cambodia	October 1979	31.9	0.7
Sudan, West	Chad	September 1985	24.0	1.7
Ethiopia, Hartisheik	Somalia	Feb-April 1989	6.6	1.9
Kenya, Ifo camp	Somalia	March 1992	22.2	1.8
Zimbabwe, Chambuta	Mozambique	August 1992	10.5	1.5

Relief programmes must therefore be initiated promptly if excessive mortality rates are to be rapidly reduced, and priority must be given to measures likely to have a swift impact on mortality figures. Experience shows that mortality is reduced when assistance becomes well organized and coordinated[3].

Two phases may therefore be distinguished in refugee or displaced situations :

- **The emergency phase** following the arrival of refugees; this is the period during which mortality rates are higher than those experienced prior to displacement or, by convention, where the crude mortality rate (CMR) is above 1 death per 10,000 per day[1,2]. CMRs in stable populations are around 0.5 deaths per 10,000 per day (usually expressed per 1,000 per month, see table above).

- **The post-emergency phase**, or consolidation phase, starting when mortality returns to the level of the surrounding population. The CMR is under 1 per 10,000 per day and basic needs have been addressed[1,2].

The priorities of intervention

Information gathered over the last few decades has made it possible to analyse the health problems of refugee and displaced populations. As a result, the most effective strategies for controlling the mortality rate have now been properly defined, and procedures standardized. The intervention priorities in the emergency phase cover 10 sectors of activity that can be listed as follows[1]:

The ten top priorities

1. Initial assessment
2. Measles immunization
3. Water and sanitation
4. Food and nutrition
5. Shelter and site planning
6. Health care in the emergency phase
7. Control of communicable diseases and epidemics
8. Public health surveillance
9. Human resources and training
10. Coordination

Ideally, these interventions should be carried out simultaneously, which becomes feasible when different teams of relief workers are involved[3]. When several operational partners are present in the field, it is essential to rapidly assign responsibility for different programmes, as good coordination among partners is essential for their speedy implementation. It is also essential that each sector of activity is monitored, as every operating health agency needs to have a clear picture of the work being carried out in each of the different sectors.

In the emergency phase, although the emphasis is classically put on the quantity and availability of services, sufficient attention must be given to their quality as well. It is the responsibility of agencies to monitor not only the NUMBER of services available or the population that they cover, but also HOW these services are delivered. Supervision of staff plays a key role in this regard.

1. INITIAL ASSESSMENT

Health priorities are identified on the basis of a rapid collection and analysis of data, which should lead to a prompt assessment within the first few days [3]. Information is required on: the background to the displacement, the population itself, the risk factors related to the main diseases, and the requirements in terms of human and material resources[1]. This involves quantitative as well as qualitative information. Data may be gathered by sample surveys, mapping, interviews and observation. Methods will often be approximate and results may need to be corroborated later with other studies[3].

2. MEASLES IMMUNIZATION

Measles is one of the most severe health problems throughout the world, killing 1 in every 10 children affected in developing countries. Displacement, overcrowding and poor hygiene in the camps are all factors that encourage the emergence of very large-scale epidemics. In Tuareg refugee camps in Mauritania, a survey over a five-month period in 1992 showed that 40% of childhood deaths were due to measles as a result of insufficient immunization[4]. The mass vaccination of children from 6 months to 15 years old should always be an absolute priority during the first week, and can be conducted together with the distribution of vitamin A.

3. WATER AND SANITATION

A drinking water supply is a top priority. The role played by poor water supplies and inadequate sanitation in the transmission of diarrhoeal diseases is well known. During the first days of the emergency phase a minimum amount of 5 litres of water per person per day is required. During the next stage, a provision should be made for 15 to 20 litres of water per person per day. Existing water sources must be assessed and it may be necessary to ensure a temporary water supply by tanker deliveries until wells can be dug. Plastic tanks are most often used for water storage, treatment and distribution. Water quality can be checked with simple kits.

The organization of latrines and waste disposal are planned according to set standards (1 latrine or trench per 50 to 100 persons during the first days of the emergency, improved as soon as possible to one latrine per 20 persons or ideally one per family). Indicators in regard to water supply and latrines must be monitored in the same manner as disease incidence and mortality rates.

4. FOOD AND NUTRITION

Population displacements are generally either the cause - or the consequence - of food shortages. Malnutrition is frequent in refugee populations and is an important contributory cause of death. Outbreaks of disease, such as scurvy or pellagra, resulting from vitamin deficiencies are also reported among refugees[2]. Maximum attention must be given to the basic food ration during the first months after the refugees' arrival. This should be a daily minimum of 2,100 kilocalories per person. It is usually necessary to organize general food distributions. This is a major undertaking and is usually carried out by specialized agencies. Registration and a census of refugees upon arrival is essential for estimating food needs and identifying beneficiaries.

The food and nutritional assessment is an important element of the initial health assessment, providing the basis for all decisions in regard to nutritional programmes. A first quick evaluation, to get a global idea of the situation, will be followed in a second stage by quantified data collection through an assessment of the food availability and accessibility, and a nutritional survey. A survey gives information on the prevalence of protein-energy malnutrition, and makes it possible to estimate the number of children at risk who should benefit from specific programmes. For example, a nutritional survey in the Somali refugee camp of Ifo in Kenya (May 1992) showed a global malnutrition rate of more than 40%, which led to the immediate opening of several intensive feeding centres[5]. Nutritional surveys are not the only means of supervising the food needs of a population. It is also essential to monitor the basic food ration by regular, random food basket surveys of households. Health staff will often need to play an advocacy role to ensure that the food basket is adequate.

Feeding programmes for specific groups will be organized when the nutritional assessment indicates a high level of malnutrition. The most common programmes are supplementary feeding for the moderately malnourished and the most vulnerable groups, and therapeutic or intensive feeding for the severely malnourished.

5. SHELTER AND SITE PLANNING

Inadequate shelter and overcrowding are major factors in the transmission of diseases with epidemic potential (measles, meningitis, typhus, cholera, etc.), and outbreaks of disease are more frequent and more severe when the population density is high. In addition, protection against sun, rain, cold and wind is indispensable for refugee welfare, as is the provision of secure living space for families. In 1984, in Korem (Ethiopia), nearly 50,000 people lived in the highlands in tents, huts made of branches, or outdoors, at an altitude of 2,500 metres and night temperatures that went below 0°C: the mortality rate was very high, mainly due to typhus and cholera.

It is therefore important to organize the site and plan for the installation of refugees: limited number of people per site with a sufficient space per person, the necessary infrastructure for providing services (e.g. health and nutrition facilities), roads, cemeteries, etc. Construction materials should be purchased locally in order that shelter can be provided for the refugees as quickly as possible.

6. HEALTH CARE

Respiratory infections, malaria, diarrhoeal diseases and other common diseases must be dealt with in a decentralized network of health care facilities (health centres and health posts). Organizing these in situations where there are many different operating partners requires good coordination between them. Manuals and guidelines allow standardization among partners in regard to essential drugs and therapeutic policies[6,7]. Medical needs (material and drugs) should be quickly assessed in anticipation of outbreaks of diseases known to occur locally. Experience acquired over the past 20 years has led to the creation of 'kits' of essential drugs and materials. Each basic module is intended to cover the most common therapeutic needs of a population of 1,000 displaced persons over 3 months[8].

7. CONTROL OF COMMUNICABLE DISEASES AND EPIDEMICS

During the emergency phase, the four most frequent communicable diseases which together are responsible for the highest morbidity and mortality rates are: measles, diarrhoeal diseases, acute respiratory infections and malaria[1,2]. Diarrhoea is one of the main causes of death. Each incidence of disease exposes children to a high risk of death from acute dehydration. The swift installation of oral rehydration centres, spread throughout the refugee settlement, helps to decrease the mortality rates associated with diarrhoeal diseases[1].

Refugee populations are at higher risk of outbreaks of communicable diseases (measles, cholera, shigellosis, meningitis, typhus, etc.)[2]. Attention to basic living conditions is the main way of preventing epidemics, but once an outbreak occurs, decisive public health interventions are vital. Only early intervention in the initial phase can reduce mortality rates. Measures to control outbreaks vary with each type of disease. They can take the form of detection and rapid treatment for cholera or mass vaccination against meningococcal meningitis A or B, or against measles[1].

In the 80s and 90s, outbreaks of cholera and shigella have been particularly frequent, and require careful attention. Population displacement often takes place in an area where cholera is endemic. When hundreds of thousands of refugees are then concentrated in such an area, the task of coping with an epidemic requires major resources. For example: outbreaks of *Shigella dysenteria* type 1 (Sd1) have occurred in central and southern Africa after two major displacements, following the crises in Burundi in 1993 and in Rwanda in 1994[9].

8. PUBLIC HEALTH SURVEILLANCE

Epidemiological surveillance is a tool for measuring and monitoring the health status of a population. It gives quantified information to those in charge and should be established from the beginning. It is based on the daily collection of selected health data and their analysis. This surveillance should only cover diseases or other health problems that can be controlled by preventive or curative interventions. The daily crude mortality rate (CMR) is the most useful health indicator to monitor during an emergency phase; it is expressed as the number of deaths per 10,000 population per day. A CMR over 1 per 10,000 per day is the best criteria of severity and indicates an emergency situation. Calculating disease-specific mortality rates helps in determining the major killer diseases and establishing priorities. One of the objectives of epidemiological surveillance is to warn of an impending epidemic. It also makes it possible to monitor the main diseases occurring in the population and measure the impact of health programmes.

9. HUMAN RESOURCES AND TRAINING

Different types of personnel are required to implement activities in all these areas: public health doctors, sanitation specialists, nutritionists, logisticians, administrators, etc. Once the different activities and tasks have been identified, staff requirements must be determined. Staff management and the organization of work is a complex task and must not be neglected. Home-visitors are a particularly important category of staff required to ensure the link between the refugee community and assistance programmes. They should be chosen from among the refugee or displaced population. Particular attention must be paid to both their training, and to that of other local health staff.

10. COORDINATION

Good coordination among the various operational partners is the key to effective emergency relief planning. There may be multiple partners in large-scale emergencies: UN agencies, host-country authorities, local and international NGOs, and representatives from among the refugee population. UNHCR has a major role to play in the coordination of refugee work, which is especially important in complex situations where politics and diplomacy complicate logistical and technical decisions. A good coordination system, which must be organized from the outset of a programme, implies that one partner takes an overall leadership role, that a good level of communication is reached between all the partners and that overall policy is standardized.

▄ References

1. Moren, A, Rigal, J. Populations réfugiées: priorités sanitaires et conduites à tenir. *Cahiers Santé*, 1992, 2: 13-21.
2. Toole, M J, Waldman, R J. Prevention of excess mortality in refugees and displaced populations in developing countries. *JAMA*, 1990, 263(24): 3296-302.
3. Moren, A. Rapid asessment of the state of displaced populations or refugees. *Medical News*, 1992, 1(5): 5-10.
4. Paquet, C. *Réfugiés Touaregs dans le sud-est de la Mauritanie. Aspects épidémiologiques. May 1992.* [Internal report]. Paris: Epicentre, 1992.
5. Brown, V. *Somalian refugees in Kenya: Impact of emergency health relief activities in Iffo 1, Iffo 2, and Liboi refugee camps. May 1992.* [Internal report]. Paris: Epicentre, 1992.
6. Médecins Sans Frontières. *Essential drugs: Practical guidelines*. Paris: Hatier, 1993.
7. Médecins Sans Frontières. *Clinical Guidelines, diagnostic and treatment manual.* Paris: Hatier, 1993.
8. WHO/UNHCR. *The new emergency health kit.* Geneva: WHO, 1990.
9. CDD. *Guidelines for the control of epidemics due to Shigella dysenteriae type 1.* Genève: WHO, 1995. WHO/CDR/95 .4.

1. Initial assessment

Introduction

If an intervention is to be fast, effective and properly adapted to the situation, it must be based on an initial assessment conducted soon after the displaced population has arrived or the first relief effort has begun. This assessment should provide information essential to the decision-makers, allowing them to identify the intervention priorities and properly plan the programmes to be undertaken. In many cases, this information will also be made available to the international community and to donors.

This information is therefore crucial. It should cover, as objectively as possible, the qualitative and quantitative aspects of the situation in regard to the target population, the needs, major problems, local context, etc. The collection of this data should be undertaken by an experienced team, totally independent of any political or other influence.

The data to be collected and analysed can be classified into 6 categories[1]:

- the geo-political context, including the background to the displacement,
- a description of the population,
- characteristics of the environment in which the refugees have settled,
- the major health problems,
- the requirements in terms of human and material resources,
- the operating partners.

Objectives

The main objectives of the initial assessment are:

- To decide whether or not to intervene: whether an intervention is required and is feasible in view of the context.

- To define the priorities of intervention: although these priorities are mostly standardized (see *The Ten Top Priorities, Introduction*), it is frequently necessary to adapt them to the particular situation.

- To plan the implementation of these priorities: deciding strategies, determining the resources needed and working out the time frame.

- To pass on information, as well as observations of refugee living conditions and the human rights situation to the international community and donors.

An assessment in two phases

Because the collection of reliable data requires time, particularly quantified data that has to be compiled by surveys, the initial assessment may be undertaken in two steps[6].

First phase: a first rapid assessment for immediate action

This first phase should result in a rapid decision on whether or not to intervene and the type and size of intervention. It will also lead to a decision as to whether or not a second assessment phase is required and when it should take place. The second phase will be delayed or left out altogether when intervention is extremely urgent, the needs are obvious and/or resources are limited; for instance, when a major outbreak of disease is affecting the population (e.g. large-scale cholera outbreak), action will be taken immediately. This phase can be completed in the field in less than 3 days.

The information collected should indicate the severity of the situation, as well as the need and feasibility of relief intervention. It should cover:
– the geo-political context, including the reasons for the displacement,
– an estimate of population size and population movements,
– a map of the site,
– a description of the environmental conditions,
– the presence of any epidemic diseases and an estimation of the recent mortality rates,
– the availability of water and food,
– the extent to which the local authorities of the host country, and particularly the Ministry of Health (MOH) are likely to accept the intervention of relief agencies;
– the presence and activities of international or local organizations.

This data, which are covered in more detail in the next section, are obtained by fast, simple methods[6]: direct observation; interviews with refugees, agencies present in the area, the MOH and local authorities; health data from medical facilities (registers); and, if required, a rapid estimation of the population size by mapping.

Second phase: to provide a more comprehensive assessment

This second phase should allow for proper programme planning (timing priority actions and calculating the resources that are required) and for disseminating information to the international community. It should be carried out simultaneously with the implementation of relief actions; essential interventions (e.g. measles mass immunization) should not wait for the completion of the assessment. The timing would therefore normally be one to three weeks after the arrival of relief agencies, i.e. as soon as the appropriate resources and expertise are available and time allows[6].

The data to be collected also falls under the 6 categories indicated above. Quantified data will be required for calculating indicators (regarding the health and nutrition status and the availability of resources), and some will have to be assessed by sample surveys. In addition, further qualitative information is gathered in regard to the geo-political context, the socio-cultural and ethnic characteristics of the population, the existence of vulnerable groups, etc.

The time needed to complete both phases of the initial assessment will depend on the remoteness of the location, its accessibility, the security conditions, the degree to which local authorities cooperate, the resources available, and the type of survey undertaken. In most situations, valuable and complete information may be gathered during a period of 7 to 10 days[6].

Collection of data

This section covers the 6 categories of data, the reasons why they are necessary and the specific methods employed in data collection for each of these categories; the general methods of data collection are described in the next section, *Summary of methods*.

THE GEO-POLITICAL CONTEXT

Information required on the geo-political context:
- cause of displacement: war, famine, natural disaster, etc.,
- duration (in time) of displacement and conditions under which it took place: transport, access, security conditions, loss of assets,
- political situation and security conditions in the country of origin,
- military, political, security and economic situation in the host country,
- security situation on the settlement site, any human rights abuses,
- whether and to what extent the refugees are accepted by the host authorities and the local population.

Methods:
- discussions with local authorities and other relief organizations,
- interviews with refugees.

A description of the situation in the country of origin, the causes of the displacement and the circumstances (duration of journey, security, etc.) will allow a better understanding and interpretation of the data collected during the initial assessment. It may also help to foresee the outcome of the refugee problem (whether repatriation is likely in the near future or not), and the number of newcomers to expect.

A description of the situation in the host country (security, acceptability of international organizations, obtaining authorizations, etc.) is also essential for assessing the feasibility of interventions, and whether refugees will have access to the local infrastructure (e.g. any existing health facilities), etc.

Security conditions must be clearly described since they can have a limiting effect on the presence of intervention teams, and affect the implementation of programmes (e.g. whether or not it will be possible to provide night shifts for nutritional centres, in-patient wards, etc.).

DESCRIPTION OF THE REFUGEE POPULATION

Information required on the refugee population:
- demography: estimate of total population and distribution by age-group and sex,
- origins of the refugee population, ethnic background, clan membership, etc.,
- socio-cultural characteristics (including type of leadership and community organization, religion, particular customs, etc.),
- vulnerable groups (unaccompanied children, female-headed households, the elderly, disabled and minority groups): the importance of these groups and their specific problems.

Methods:

Estimation of population size:
- mapping,
- aerial or satellite photographs,
- sample survey to assess the average number of persons per shelter,
- extrapolating vaccine coverage data onto the general population,
- census (rarely).

Qualitative information on the population:
- observation of the refugee setting,
- interviews with key informants, focus group discussions.

Estimating the population size is a major element of an assessment. It is necessary for determining the target population, quantifying the needs, and calculating indicators (population size is used as the denominator). Even rough estimates of population figures may be used. Information on different age groups (and possibly gender distribution) within the refugee population permits the identification of any under-represented age groups and assists in planning activities (e.g. mass immunization of children under 15 years). This estimation needs to be repeated and updated regularly as part of overall surveillance. The figures provided usually differ depending on the methods used and the sources providing them (e.g. UNHCR, local authorities, etc.). The final figure will most often be decided on the basis of a compromise between those provided by the different sources. Nevertheless, it is imperative that all operational partners use the same population figures for planning and evaluating programmes.

However, the description of the population should be more than the compilation of population figures. Other essential information on social patterns, cultural beliefs, etc. must be known if programmes are to be planned so that they reach all individuals and respond adequately to their specific needs; for instance, in many Islamic countries, women may not use health services if separate departments are not provided for men and women. The assessment of vulnerable groups is particularly important; high numbers of unaccompanied children have been reported in recent refugee emergencies, such as among Rwandan refugees in eastern Zaire (1994)[6]. (See also *Socio-cultural Aspects* in Part I.)

About the methods

A/ Several methods may be used to estimate population size:
- A census conducted upon arrival remains the most accurate method, but

is time-consuming and rarely feasible when there are large influxes of new arrivals. If it is to remain accurate, it must be regularly updated by keeping count of births, deaths and new arrivals.

- A good estimate may be obtained by calculating the number of shelters in the settlement and the average number of refugees per shelter. The number of shelters can be assessed by several methods: the most convenient one is to count them on an aerial photograph (taken from a plane or satellite). If such a photograph is not available, a precise map of the settlement should be drawn. The map is then divided into squares. A sample of these squares is selected at random and the number of shelters within them is counted making it possible to calculate the average number of shelters per square. An estimate for the whole settlement is then reached by extrapolation. A description of this method, known as 'mapping', is available[2]. The next step is to determine the average number of persons per shelter by sample survey (see below *Summary of methods*).

- Data from a mass vaccination campaign (e.g. measles or meningitis) may be used if a vaccine coverage survey has been conducted. The size of the population is estimated by extrapolating the results of vaccine coverage based on the number of doses administered. However this method is not very accurate and it is in any case rare that a mass campaign AND a coverage survey have already been conducted in the early days of an intervention.

B/ Qualitative information on the population can be collected by interviewing key informants and/or focus group discussion with persons belonging to several ethnic and social groups, including minority groups. Direct observation of the camp itself also provides valuable information on what people are doing.

THE ENVIRONMENT IN WHICH THE REFUGEES HAVE SETTLED

Information required on the refugee environment:

- water supply: quantity (litres per person per day), availability and quality,
- physical characteristics of the site and surroundings (map of the site), and information related to climate (rainy season),
- accessibility, state of the roads, road map,
- types of shelter in use, proportion of refugees with proper shelters,
- total surface and shelter surface available per refugee,
- disposal of excreta: defecation areas, type and number of latrines (number of persons per latrine),
- general hygiene on the site,
- presence of vectors transmitting communicable diseases (e.g. lice for typhus fever).

Methods:

- direct observation (of shelters, water, length of queues at the water points, latrines, hygiene, etc.),
- interviews with key informants,
- sample surveys (percentage of refugees with shelters, number of refugees per latrine, availability of water containers, etc.).

The quantity of water available per person and per day is a crucial piece of information; it should be compared with the standard recommendations (5 litres per person per day in the acute stage of the emergency, then 15 to 20 litres per person per day).

One of the priorities is to find or make a map of the site, on which all the physical characteristics and existing facilities may be indicated. A precise road map must be drawn up if one is not already available. The time and duration of the rainy season and the state of the roads must be known in advance in order to plan general distributions and eventual evacuation.

In regard to shelters, it is important to know the proportion of refugees sleeping in protected shelters in order to arrange distributions of plastic sheeting. The surface available for each person (total or shelter surface) will determine the degree of crowding; overcrowding is an important risk factor for numerous communicable diseases.

The arrangements for the disposal of excreta (including the number of persons per latrine, existence of defecation fields) and other sanitation characteristics must be assessed.

About the methods

Most information will be obtained by direct observation and in discussion with refugees. The percentage of refugees sleeping in protected shelters can be obtained by a sample survey. The quantity of water available is based on the capacity and out-flow of the water sources (sources already present on the spot or installed upon the arrival of the refugees); when these are unknown or cannot be calculated, it is assessed on the basis of a sample of households, calculating the capacity of water containers and the number of times these containers are filled each day. The number of persons per latrine is calculated by dividing the population by the number of latrines, or by conducting a sample survey of the population[2].

THE MAJOR HEALTH PROBLEMS

Information needs on the major health problems:
- mortality: rates and causes of mortality,
- morbidity data on the most common diseases (measles, diarrhoeal diseases, ARI, malaria),
- presence of diseases with epidemic potential (cholera, shigellosis, measles, meningitis, hepatitis, etc.),
- prevalence of acute malnutrition,
- data on vaccine coverage (e.g. meningitis vaccine).

Methods:
- locating any community burial place, and counting graves,
- interviews with health workers,
- health surveillance system, if already existing,
- retrospective sample survey for mortality and morbidity,
- nutritional survey.

In most refugee or displaced populations, the priority health problems include: measles, diarrhoeal diseases (including cholera and shigellosis), acute respiratory infections (ARI), malnutrition, malaria and, in some cases, meningitis (see *7. Control of Communicable Diseases and Epidemics*).

The crude mortality rate is the best indicator for assessing the severity of the situation and must be estimated in order to establish a baseline for evaluating the ongoing effectiveness of assistance programmes[6]. The mortality rate is expressed by the total number of deaths per 10,000 persons and per day (see also *8. Public Health Surveillance*).

Data concerning the causes of death make it possible to identify the most common killer diseases. Disease patterns, and particularly the occurrence of diseases with epidemic potential, should be assessed; the information should cover diseases which may occur in the area of origin, the host area, and those currently present in the population. Early information on which diseases are present, or potentially present, makes it possible to undertake appropriate curative and preventive measures urgently (e.g. screening and early treatment of cholera and shigellosis cases, mass vaccination against meningitis etc.).

The prevalence of acute malnutrition should be assessed when nutritional problems are expected, and is a factor in deciding whether or not to set up selective feeding programmes (see *4. Food and Nutrition*).

Vaccine coverage can be measured for measles vaccine, but it is rarely necessary to do this at the beginning of a programme, since mass measles immunization of children remains a priority even in a population known to have had a previous high coverage. In some cases, it may be useful to know the meningitis vaccine coverage.

About the methods

- The recent mortality rate may be assessed using 3 main methods:
    - by counting the number of graves, although this is not always feasible (e.g. impossible in settings where corpses are incinerated) and this method cannot be used to assess the mortality rate prior to refugees settling on the site, or
    - by gathering data on death registrations, if available, from lists or registers that are held by refugee leaders or other authorities, or from hospitals, or
    - by a retrospective mortality survey, when time allows (see below *Summary of methods*).
    As this indicator is difficult to estimate, it is useful to compare mortality information from different sources.
- Disease patterns are assessed by:
    - discussions with health workers from the refugee population and host health care services; this may be a way of getting qualitative information,
    - direct observation by medical staff; this is useful for assessing the presence of certain health problems, such as measles,
    - retrospective sample surveys when quantitative data is needed on the incidence of diseases in the period before the refugee arrival or since

their arrival; however, these are not routinely recommended because they are costly, use up time and energy and, above all, have minimal influence on the planning and management of interventions[4].

- The prevalence of acute malnutrition should be measured by a nutritional survey (using the weight-for-height index). Information on food availability (see below) is required in order to interpret survey data. The decisional aspects of nutritional assessment are described in *4. Food and Nutrition*, and the methodology is explained in guidelines[5].

- Vaccine coverage data, if required, could also be measured by a sample survey in children (using the WHO/EPI method)[12].

- An epidemiological surveillance system must be established at the time of the initial assessment to allow the calculation of mortality and morbidity indicators from the very first days. It will thus include a system for collecting data on mortality (counting the number of daily burials or registrations by home visitors) and a system for detecting diseases. Unfortunately, it may take one to two weeks before such systems are properly functioning and providing reliable data.

REQUIREMENTS IN TERMS OF HUMAN AND MATERIAL RESOURCES

Information needs:

Human resources:
- qualified staff from the refugee and host populations,
- a certain level of training, especially for medical staff.

Material resources:
- food available: existing food reserves, food rations distributed, if any, etc.,
- cooking utensils (percentage of families possessing these),
- water containers (percentage of families possessing these),
- soap, blankets, clothes, etc.,
- existing health facilities,
- types of energy sources available.

Methods:
- interviews with health staff, local health authorities and key refugee informants,
- direct observation of the site and surroundings (health facilities),
- information on food distributions from agencies or local authorities,
- sample survey of population (for non-food items).

Each aid programme requires qualified staff, local and expatriate. The expatriate staff requirements depend on the availability of qualified medical staff and their level of training.

The availability and accessibility of food, particularly of any food ration already being distributed, must be roughly assessed in the early days in order to plan for food needs.

The availability of non-food items (cooking utensils, cooking fuel, water containers, soap, material for shelters, etc.) should be evaluated because they have an important impact on other sectors; for instance, if they are not available, part of the food ration will probably be exchanged or sold so as to procure them. The availability of water containers determines access to water.

The existing health services of the host area must be identified and their capacity to treat refugees assessed. This includes existing health facilities (particularly referral hospitals) and access to them, a referral laboratory for analysing specimens (for epidemic preparedness) and an organization chart of the host country's health care services (who is in charge of immunization, nutrition, whether or not health care is free of charge, etc.).

About the methods

An assessment of food availability requires information on any food distributions that may have been carried out or are planned: agencies and local authorities should be asked who is in charge of distributions and what is the food ration already distributed or planned for future distributions (including an estimate of the number of kilocalories distributed per person and per day). A rough idea of the food reserves (including livestock) should be obtained, and food availability in any local markets should also be assessed (see *4. Food and Nutrition*).

The availability of non-food items is assessed by direct observation on site, information on any general distribution of non-food items and, possibly, sample surveys to estimate the percentage of families with essential non-food items such as cooking utensils and water containers.

THE OPERATING PARTNERS

Information on which organization is doing what and when, is essential for planning the intervention and distributing tasks among the partners. Administrative procedures and host country regulations, such as policies in regard to visas, travel permits, authorization to operate in the area, recruitment of human resources, etc., should also be properly assessed. Contacts must be made with the MOH, the local authorities, the local and international organizations that are involved in refugee assistance, etc. to obtain this information. A system of coordination among partners, if not yet existing, should be rapidly initiated.

SUMMARY OF METHODS

- **Systematic observation** of the site and the population is essential for assessing many qualitative aspects, but this is often overlooked. A lot of information can be gathered simply by walking through different parts of the site, observing the state of the population, looking at food sources and refugee assets, etc. This should be a systematic observation which may, for instance, follow a prepared check-list of what to look out for[6]; several models for such check-lists are available in guidelines[7,8,9].

- **Interviews with key persons** from the refugee community (key informants) can be a means for collecting qualitative information on the conditions prior to displacement and the reasons behind it, any assets they may have brought with them, traditional beliefs and behaviour, etc.[6] These key informants may be official or unofficial leaders, community elders, teachers, health workers, religious leaders, etc.

- **Focus group discussions** offer the advantage that informants are able to correct each other and add information to each others' statements. The selection of participants depends on the objective of the discussion: when information is required on a specific subject, participants should be selected according to their expected knowledge; when more general information is assessed, such as population needs and traditional beliefs, participants should be chosen from among all relevant sub-groups of the population: young and old, male and female, different ethnic, social and religious groups etc. (see *Socio-cultural Aspects* in Part I). Any discussions with refugees should take into account the fear and suspicion that are usually present in crisis situations[10].

- **Discussions with representatives** of the local health authorities, staff of local health facilities, and other organizations working on the site (UN agencies, NGOs, local churches, etc.) are essential and a quick way to gather information on many subjects (e.g. the main health risks, available resources, actions already carried out and by whom, etc.).

- **A survey of a representative sample** of the population may be carried out in the second phase of the assessment allowing various indicators to be calculated.

Table 1.2
Information to be gathered in an initial sample survey

Priority information	Information that can be collected if required
– retrospective mortality – number of refugees per shelter (estimate population size when number of shelters is known) – litres of water available per person per day – number of persons per latrine – age distribution of the population – nutritional status of under five's	– proportion of protected shelters – non-food items available (blankets, utensils, etc.) – vaccine coverage (meningitis, possibly measles) – recent major diseases

The second column of the table presents other indicators that could be obtained if the information they provide would be useful for implementing programmes.

The two sampling methods most often used are:

- *A systematic sampling procedure:* this can be used when the refugee site is well organized in clearly defined rows, and is the easiest of the two to implement (it reduces the necessary sample size by half - no cluster effect).

- *A cluster sampling procedure:* this is the only possible method when the site is not organized.

These two techniques are described in epidemiological guides[11].

When mortality and morbidity rates are being assessed retrospectively, the period over which they are measured must be defined by recent significant events (e.g. arrival in the camp, beginning of a civil war, etc.).

The duration of a survey varies from 2 to 15 days, depending on the density of the population (scattered or not), the means available (human resources and transport), the subject matter and the methodology used; for instance, a survey to assess mortality rates properly would require a sample of 3,000 people. (A survey of 30 clusters of 30 families would generally collect information on 5,000 people including more than 900 children aged 6-9 months and about 200 children aged 12-23 months.)

Whatever methods are used, it is important to verify the information gathered by cross checking the results obtained by different methodologies[10]. For instance, an estimation of population figures is frequently made by comparing figures received from different sources; the needs expressed by refugees during interviews should be checked by direct observation of households wherever possible, etc.

The information gathered must be analysed and compiled in an assessment report. A model form for this is given in the appendix; it shows how to present the quantified data obtained, but this must be complemented by an analysis of the results and a written report covering the qualitative information obtained.

Principal recommendations regarding the initial assessment

- The initial assessment is aimed at allowing decision-makers to decide whether or not to intervene, to identify intervention priorities, to plan the implementation of these priorities and to pass on information to the international community and donors. The initial assessment should be undertaken by an independent and experienced team.

- The data collected should cover the geo-political context (including security conditions), a description of the refugee population (including vulnerable groups), the characteristics of the environment (including a map of the site), the major health problems, the requirements in human and material resources, and the operating partners.

- The first rapid assessment, which must be completed within three days, should use fast, simple straightforward methods to obtain information and result in a quick decision on whether to intervene or not, and the type and size of intervention.

- In a second phase, one to three weeks after the arrival of the relief agencies, quantitative and qualitative data should be collected in order to make proper programme planning possible.

- The mortality rate is the best indicator for assessing the severity of the situation and must be established as a base-line for evaluating the effectiveness of assistance programmes.

- The information gathered must be verified by cross-checking the results obtained by different methodologies.

References

1. Moren, A, Rigal, J. Populations réfugiées: priorités sanitaires et conduites à tenir. *Cahiers Santé*, 1992, 2: 13-21.

2. Moren A. Rapid assessment of the state of health of displaced populations or refugees. *Medical News*, 1992, 1(5): 5-10.

3. Médecins Sans Frontières. *Evaluation rapide de l'état de santé d'une population déplacée ou réfugiée*. Paris: Médecins Sans Frontières, 1996.

4. Boss, L P, Toole, M, Yip, R. Assessments of mortality, morbidity and nutritional status in Somalia during the 1991-1992 famine. *JAMA*, 1994, 272(5): 371-6.

5. Médecins Sans Frontières. *Nutrition guidelines*. Paris: Médecins Sans Frontières, 1995.

6. Toole, M J. The rapid assessment of health problems in refugee and displaced populations. *Medicine and Global Survival*, 1994, 1(4): 200-7.

7. Mears, C, Chowdhury, S. *Health care for refugees and displaced people*. Oxford: Oxfam Practical Health Guide No. 9, 1994.

8. Simmonds, S, Vaughan, P, William Gunn, S. *Refugee community health care*. Oxford: Oxford University Press, 1983.

9. Médecins Sans Frontières. *Mission exploratoire - Mission d'évaluation.. Situation avec déplacement de populations*. Paris: Médecins Sans Frontières, 1989.

10. Scrimshaw, S, Hurtado, E. *Rapid assesment procedures for nutrition and primary health care*. Tokyo: United Nations University, UNICEF, UCLA Latin America Centre, 1987.

11. Dabis, F, Drucker, J, Moren, A. *Epidémiologie d'intervention*. Paris: Arnette, 1992.

12. WHO. *Training mid-level managers : the EPI coverage survey*. Geneva: WHO, 1991. WHO/EPI/MLM/91.10.

2. Measles immunization

Introduction

Measles remains a major cause of childhood mortality throughout the world, especially in developing countries. However, the disease can be prevented by the administration of measles vaccine, which is one of the most cost-effective public health tools [20]. Measles immunization has been included in the Expanded Programme on Immunization (EPI) since the 70s and has significantly contributed to reducing both measles morbidity and mortality in most countries. Despite a high level of global vaccination coverage in 1993 (according to WHO, a coverage of 78% was reached in the under-two age group, all countries taken together), there were an estimated 45 million cases and 1.2 million deaths throughout the world [20]. One of the explanations for this is the fact that vaccine coverage figures vary widely between regions: 19 countries, most of them in Africa, report vaccine coverage below 50% [5,20].

Measles is one of the most serious health problems encountered in refugee situations and has been reported as the leading cause of mortality in children in several refugee emergencies. Outbreaks of measles are frequent, especially in camp settings; an important risk factor for measles transmission is overcrowding [3]. For instance, a severe epidemic occurring in the Wad Kowli refugee camp (Sudan, 1985) resulted in over 2,000 measles deaths over a four-month period [2]. Complications (such as pneumonia, diarrhoea and croup) are very common in refugee settings where measles fatality rates can reach particularly high levels, exceeding 10% [2,3]. See *7. Control of Communicable Diseases and Epidemics*. It is for this reason that WHO has included refugee children among the groups at high risk from measles [2,22].

However the high mortality due to measles is preventable, and mass immunization against measles, coupled with vitamin A distribution, is one of the top priorities in the initial phase of a refugee influx, even if no cases are reported and even if the refugees are coming from areas with a high level of vaccination coverage, as measles outbreaks can still occur in populations with a high level of coverage [2,3]. The current vaccine appears to provide excellent but not perfect protection: under normal conditions, it protects 85% of children when administered at 9 months of age [22]. This means that a high level of coverage still leaves a significant number of people susceptible to measles and therefore vulnerable to further outbreaks given the extreme infectiousness of the virus [5,22]. It is therefore essential to aim for a coverage level close to 100%. (For instance, in a camp of 100,000 people, there would normally be around 15,000 from 9 months to 5 years of age (about 15%). If the vaccination coverage is 80% in the age group from 9 months to 5 years and vaccine efficacy is 85%, it may be estimated that 4,800 children in this age group will be susceptible to developing measles - 3,000 unvaccinated and 1,800 non-immune due to vaccine inefficacy.)

Although this chapter focuses on the initial mass campaign, it is essential to maintain immunization activities afterwards in order to vaccinate new arrivals and those who have been missed in the campaign.

Objectives

The major objective of mass measles immunization is to prevent measles outbreaks. To achieve this, it is necessary to aim for a vaccination coverage level close to 100% (90% to 100%) in the age group from 6 months to 12 or 15 years. If a measles outbreak occurs before mass immunization has taken place, the objectives are to reduce the number of cases and help prevent measles deaths; it should be remembered that, even among already exposed individuals, measles vaccine may reduce the severity of the disease if administered within 3 days of exposure[21].

The target population

In developing countries, the target age group for measles immunization is a complex issue:

- On the one hand, measles represents an important threat to young children: in developing countries, over 25% of all measles cases are reported among children under 9 months, and case-fatality rates are highest among the youngest[2,20].

- On the other hand, the vaccine must be administered when there is no longer a risk of interfering with maternal antibodies in order to achieve an optimal response. The recommended age of vaccination in developing countries is currently from 9 months to 2 to 5 years of age, according to EPI strategy. When the age of immunization is reduced below 9 months, the vaccine efficacy rapidly diminishes: 85% at 9 months, 50% at 6 months[7,8].

In refugee emergencies, overcrowding and other factors increase the risk of infection in young children and the severity of the disease in all age groups[3]. The target age group must be extended: all children aged between 6 months and 12-15 years should be immunized during the emergency phase. In open situations, where the refugees are hosted by the local community, these groups among the resident population should also be vaccinated.

- Immunization of children from 6 months of age is recommended as infection at an early age is particularly frequent in high-density populations such as refugee settlements and is associated with high fatality rates[2,3]. However, because of low vaccine efficacy at that age, any child who has been vaccinated between the ages of 6 and 9 months must receive a second dose as soon as possible after 9 months of age[7].

- Children should be vaccinated up till 12-15 years of age as this age group is increasingly susceptible to measles: there is a shift in age-specific incidences from younger to older age groups, and cases of children up to 14 years have been on the uprise[26]. For instance, in Malawi, from March

1988 to December 1989, 45% of the 1,540 reported cases of measles occurred in children aged 5 years and over (MSF unpublished data).

Measles-related morbidity and mortality can also be high in this group. The upper age limit should be decided after taking into account the possibility that women may become pregnant at an early age. If an outbreak occurs, and if age groups older than 15 years are affected, the target population can be expanded further, in line with the age-specific attack rates observed[3].

Measles vaccination is only contra-indicated in pregnant women because the vaccine contains live attenuated virus. Malnutrition, HIV and AIDS, previous measles vaccination or infection, and common health problems (such as fever, diarrhoea, etc.) are not contraindications[2,3,5,9]. In fact, measles vaccination is a top priority for malnourished children, especially in feeding centres[1,5] (see *4. Food and Nutrition*). A second dose given to children previously immunized provides an even better protection[6].

Planning an immunization programme

The resources required to implement mass immunization should be available as soon as refugees begin to gather on sites. One agency should take overall responsibility for the programme and coordinate the various efforts involved. Responsibility for each component of the programme needs to be clearly assigned to the different partners involved (health agencies, Ministry of Health and local EPI representatives and refugee leaders). The national EPI programme of the host country should be involved from the beginning[3].

1. ESTIMATE THE SIZE OF THE TARGET POPULATION

The size of the total population must be known in order to estimate the number of children to be vaccinated; it is assumed that children between 6 months and 15 years of age represent 35% to 45% of the total population. If the actual population figures are not known when planning mass immunization, they should quickly be estimated. These figures are normally calculated during the first phase of the initial assessment (see description of methods in the section *Initial Assessment* above).

2. OBTAIN A MAP OF THE SITE

A map of the site or area is required in order to identify the different sections and facilities in the camp. Access roads, reception area for new arrivals, health structures and other gathering places (markets, school, etc.) should all be indicated.

3. DEFINING VACCINATION STRATEGIES

Because of the high risk of measles infection, eligible children should be immunized as soon as possible, ideally at the time they enter a camp or settlement[3]; vaccination strategy should aim at vaccinating the maximum number of children in the shortest possible time.

In most situations, the organization of a first and rapid mass campaign followed by routine immunization in fixed facilities is the preferred strategy for achieving a high vaccination coverage quickly and then maintaining it[3,24].

The initial mass immunization campaign

Two strategies are possible for implementing mass immunization[3]:

- Mass vaccination is carried out by outreach teams on dispersed immunization sites. Immunization sites are established in the different sections of the camp and the refugees gather there to be vaccinated. Such intervention is indicated when the population has already settled on the site before immunization could be organized, or when a sudden influx of refugees has occurred; these are the situations most frequently encountered.

- Immunization can also be carried out at refugee arrival (screening centre), ensuring that newcomers are immunized as soon as they arrive. This can only be implemented when a screening facility has been set up, and when the influx of refugees is steady and moderate[3]. When applicable, this strategy is generally used in conjunction with the first one: a rapid mass campaign is organized over the whole site to immunize those who are already settled and new arrivals are then immunized as they enter the site.

Another strategy involves mobile teams, which go from shelter to shelter to administer the vaccines. However, this is generally discouraged as organization is difficult (handling the vaccines is complicated: ensuring sterile material and a cold chain, etc.) and the level of effectiveness is low. It is also slow and not easily supervised.

A measles vaccination campaign should be accompanied by simultaneous vitamin A supplementation to children (see below 'Nutrient deficiencies' in *4. Food and Nutrition*), as recommended by the WHO. Although some studies have suggested that giving simultaneous high doses of vitamin A interferes with seroconversion in children around 6 months, it should remain the recommended policy in refugee camps. Indeed, due to the higher risk of vitamin A deficiency in such a setting, it is much more likely that the benefits outweigh the risks[25].

In some situations, the association of polio to measles immunization has been advised. However, this is not recommended in refugee settings, where polio is not a major killer.

Traditional beliefs and customs, and how the refugee community has organized itself, must also be considered when planning a mass campaign, to ensure that it will be both acceptable and feasible[3].

Fixed immunization strategies

The measles immunization programme must never be suspended. Once the target population has been adequately covered in the initial campaign, a system for maintaining immunization should be established. Measles immunization then becomes an integral part of health care activities[3].

On-going immunization is required to cover:
- children who might have missed the initial vaccination campaign,
- new arrivals,
- children vaccinated at the age of 6 to 9 months who must receive a second dose at 9 months,
- new groups of children reaching the age of 6 months.

In addition, every child admitted to an in-patient department should imperatively be checked for measles vaccine status, and immunized if required.

The preferred strategy is to establish fixed vaccination points in existing health services and the screening centre. The availability of vaccine storage facilities on the site or close by will determine how many fixed immunization points can be established, and how they should be organized (see below, 'Fixed immunization strategy'). If vaccine stores are remote from the refugee site, immunization days could be planned at convenient intervals (e.g. every month), providing the population is relatively stable in size[3].

Selective and non-selective vaccination

- Selective vaccination implies that the vaccination status of the child is checked (on the basis of a vaccination card) before giving the vaccine: the vaccine will be administered to anybody who cannot produce an official document to prove that they have already been vaccinated.

- In the case of non-selective vaccination, vaccination status is not verified and all children will be vaccinated regardless of their immune status. It must be remembered that a second dose of vaccine has no adverse effect, but provides better protection (however, a repeated dose of vitamin A should be avoided).

Non-selective vaccination is preferred, especially during mass vaccination campaign, because it is not only much more rapid, it also leaves little chance for error[5].

4. ASSESSMENT OF NEEDS

Vaccines

The quantity of vaccines required is estimated in line with the size of the target population, the coverage aimed at (ideally 100%), the number of doses required, the proportion of vaccine lost during a mass campaign (15%) and the reserves to be held in stock (25%). Vaccines can either be ordered from UNICEF or through UNHCR or will be supplied by the implementing agency; they may initially be provided by the national EPI, and replaced later after ordered vaccines arrive.

Equipment

Emergency immunization kits, including cold chain equipment, are available from different organizations. For example, MSF kits are available, equipped with disposable material, that are designed to allow 5 teams to vaccinate

10,000 people. In mass campaigns targeting refugee populations, only disposable injection material should be used [10]. The use of Immojet, which is again recommended by WHO, is not advised in emergency refugee situations because of its fragility. Registration material must be prepared, including individual vaccination cards and tally sheets.

The measles vaccine is very sensitive to heat. It must be kept refrigerated or frozen in central vaccine stores[3,11]. It is therefore crucial to ensure a good cold chain, which must be assessed before vaccines are ordered[12]. The use of national vaccine storage facilities should be requested from local health authorities where these exist, but refugee settlements are often located in areas that lack cold stores so such facilities usually have to be installed. Ideally, each main site should have a vaccine storage facility (see below, *Organization of immunization activities*)[3].

Staff

Immunization teams (see below) should be set up. Since there are usually only a few qualified staff available, teams will mostly be composed of people without any specific qualification or experience, recruited to perform specific tasks for which they will be given a specific training. Training manuals are available from the national EPI or WHO[15]. A written job description should be provided for each person[13].

Supervision of vaccination teams is crucial; qualified health staff (e.g. nurses) should be recruited for this whenever possible, 1 supervisor for ideally 1 or several teams.

> **One immunization team = 20 people**
> *(in a refugee camp context)*
>
> 1 supervisor (for one or more teams)
> 1 logistics officer (for one or more teams)
> 4 staff members to prepare the vaccines
> 2 staff members to administer the vaccines
> 6 staff members to register and tally
> 6 staff members to maintain order (crowd control)

Organization of immunization activities

THE MASS IMMUNIZATION CAMPAIGN

The campaign will start once all the material has been assembled and the personnel trained. It should be completed as quickly as possible, dependent on the number of teams involved and the target population to be immunized: for instance, one immunization team that includes 2 vaccinators can vaccinate 500-700 people per hour.

Practical organization is described in guidelines[9]. The main aspects are:

- A training session which should take place 2 to 3 days before the start of the campaign and include a dress rehearsal to ensure that all team members understand their roles[13].

- Information about the campaign should be disseminated among the population (e.g. the previous day) by community and religious leaders, home-visitors, health staff, etc. This information should cover the need for vaccination, the absence of side effects, which age groups are to be vaccinated, the dates, times and place of vaccinations, etc. This is crucial for the success of the campaign, as it raises awareness among the population and facilitates organization. Local authorities and other organizations should also be informed[3].

- Immunization sites should be selected and organized. The number of sites depends on the size of the population to be vaccinated (e.g. one or two sites for every 10,000 refugees) and how it is spread out over the site. They should be easily accessible, with separate entrances and exits, and large enough to exclude the risk of overcrowding. Details of immunization sites and how to organize them are fully described in reference documents[9]. Well-organized sites are the key to the success of the campaign with well-trained teams operating on each site.

- Individual vaccination cards are issued to each child. The importance of keeping the card so that it can be presented to health services at a later date should be clearly explained to the accompanying person. If children are vaccinated before the age of 9 months, this must be specified on the card and it must be made clear that they have to be brought back for the second dose at the age of 9 months.

- A daily record should be made of the numbers vaccinated per day (and per site) and the number of doses used (see below, *Evaluation*).

FIXED IMMUNIZATION STRATEGY

As was previously indicated, where fixed vaccination points are set up, these must be integrated into the existing health services:

- health centre and hospital: systematic checking of vaccination status, and vaccination sessions;
- health posts: checking vaccination status, vaccination on the spot or referral to an immunization point;
- feeding centre: regular vaccination sessions (e.g. twice a week);
- screening centre: systematic vaccination of new arrivals or referral to immunization point;
- home-visitors: checking of vaccination status and referral to immunization point.

The availability of immunization services in these facilities will depend primarily on the vaccine cold storage facilities; these should be made available in all health centres (refrigerator or 7-day cool box) whenever feasible[3]. Health posts and screening centres are either equipped with vaccine storage facilities, or if not available, children are referred to the nearest vaccination facility. It is particularly crucial to monitor and record the cold chain temperatures daily. In health centres, immunization may be given daily or weekly; when there is a continual influx of large numbers of new arrivals, it should be done on a daily basis[3]. Home-visitors should carry out checks on the vaccination status of people in the area they are responsible for.

A particularly difficult issue is how to pick up those children that need to be revaccinated at nine months. Experience in refugee situations shows a very low rate of second doses given after 9 months. It is essential that every possible means are used to trace them: active screening by home-visitors, information sessions in health care facilities, etc.

In the post-emergency phase, measles immunization will be integrated within the EPI, provided the necessary conditions are met (see *Child Health Care in the Post-emergency Phase* in Part III).

Evaluation

An evaluation of the immunization programme should be based on routinely collected data and, if necessary, on a survey of vaccination coverage.

ROUTINELY COLLECTED DATA

Immunization coverage data is obtained by comparing the numbers vaccinated with the size of the estimated target population. The validity of this method depends on the accuracy of the target population estimate and of the collected data. Routine monitoring takes the form of daily and weekly summary sheets, based on tally sheets[9]. Data from each team is collected daily by the team supervisor, and the results for each site are calculated daily by the person responsible for the programme. A weekly report should be issued, providing information on the numbers vaccinated and the estimated coverage level.

At the end of the campaign:
- all the collected data is compiled,
- the monitoring of morbidity and case fatality rates is continued (see below, *8. Public Health Surveillance*),
- if necessary, a vaccination coverage survey is undertaken (see page 63).

Future action is planned according to the results obtained; a further mass vaccination campaign should be implemented if the coverage results are not satisfactory.

VACCINATION COVERAGE SURVEY

This survey allows confirmation of the results obtained from routinely collected data. It need not be undertaken systematically after each campaign, but only when the accuracy of results is questionable as, for example, in the case of large population movements or when there are numerous cases of measles despite an estimated vaccination coverage level exceeding 90%. The survey indicates, at a given point in time, the proportion of the target population that has been vaccinated. It does not give information on vaccine efficacy. The classical method uses a two-stage cluster sample (sample size of 210 children, in 30 clusters of 7 children), and is described in WHO/EPI documents[15]. This vaccination coverage survey may be coupled with a nutritional survey.

VACCINE EFFICACY

A study of vaccine efficacy should be undertaken if vaccine failures are suspected: for instance, if a measles outbreak should occur or continue, despite a high level of vaccination coverage (over 90%), and in the absence of any significant population movement[14]. This study should assess the field vaccine efficacy, i.e. the vaccine efficacy under field conditions, and compare it to the theoretical vaccine efficacy of 85% when administered at 9 months of age. If the field vaccine efficacy is well below the theoretical one, possible causes should be investigated (inadequate cold chain, poorly respected vaccine schedule etc.).

Several methods exist for measuring vaccine efficacy and are described in WHO/EPI documents[23]. A first estimate may be obtained from routine data and is handy for using in emergency situations. It provides a fair estimate of vaccine efficacy and can indicate whether a more detailed study is necessary. In practice, if this rapid estimate shows a vaccine efficacy greater than 80%, it is probably unnecessary to proceed with further investigations. However, if it gives a vaccine efficacy below 80%, a more detailed evaluation will be required. Other methods, using more complex epidemiological methods (cohort study or case-control study), require specific expertise.

The validity of vaccine efficacy studies depends on diverse factors[14,23]:
– the measles case definition used (see below, *Measles control* in section 7B.)
– whether there is an active case detection effort being made among the immunized and unimmunized
– how accurately vaccination status is determined from cards or vaccination history (as reported by parents).
– the risk of measles exposure (should be similar for immunized and unimmunized populations).

Rapid estimate of field vaccine efficacy[23]

1. The vaccine efficacy (VE) is estimated as the difference in attack rates (AR) between the vaccinated and unvaccinated groups, expressed as a percentage of the attack rate in the unvaccinated group:

$$VE\ (\%) = \frac{AR\ unvaccinated - AR\ vaccinated \times 100}{AR\ unvaccinated}$$

2. When attack rates are unknown, vaccine efficacy can be estimated from the proportion of cases occurring in immunized individuals, per vaccination coverage level (or percentage of immunized population). This estimation is facilitated by using curves: values are plotted and vaccine efficacy is deducted. Accuracy depends on the validity of the estimated vaccination coverage.

Principal recommendations regarding measles immunization

- Mass immunization against measles is always one of the top priorities in the initial phase of a refugee influx, even if no cases are reported or refugees are coming from areas with a high level of vaccination coverage.

- All children aged between 6 months and 12-15 years should be vaccinated during the emergency phase. All children immunized between the age of 6 and 9 months have to be revaccinated from 9 months on. There are no contraindications for measles vaccination, except in pregnancy.

- A vaccination coverage of close to 100% in the target age group should be aimed for in order to prevent measles outbreaks.

- The recommended strategy is the organization of a first and rapid mass campaign coupled with vitamin A supplementation, to be followed by a routine immunization programme integrated within existing health facilities.

- An evaluation of the vaccination programme, based on routinely collected data, should be carried out. A vaccination coverage survey does not have to be undertaken systematically after each campaign (this is only necessary when the accuracy of the results is questionable).

References

1. Hussey, G. *A discussion document presented at WHO clinical research meeting.* Banjul, Gambia: 1993.

2. CDC. Famine-affected, refugee, and displaced populations: Recommendations for public health issues. *MMWR,* 1992, 41(RR-13): 1-76.

3. Toole, M J, Steketee, R W, Waldman, R J, Nieburg, P. Measles prevention and control in emergency settings. *Bull WHO,* 1989, 67(4): 381-8.

4. Cutts, F T, Dabis, F. Contrôle de la rougeole dans les pays en développement. *Cahiers Santé,* 1994, 4(3): 163-71.

5. Expanded programme on immunization: accelerated measles strategies. *Wkly Epidemiol Rec,* 1994, 69(31): 229-34.

6. WHO. *Immunization Policy.* Geneva: WHO, 1986. WHO/EPI/GEN/86.7 Rev 1.

7. WHO. *The Immunological Basis for Immunization: measles.* Geneva: WHO, 1993. WHO/EPI/ GEN/93.17.

8. Preblud S R, Katz S L. *Vaccines.* Philadelphia: Eds Plotkin and Mortimer, 1988: 182-222.

9. Médecins Sans Frontières. *Conduite à tenir en cas d'épidémie de rougeole.* Paris: Médecins Sans Frontières, 1996.

10. Médecins Sans Frontières. *Guide of kits and emergency items. Decision-maker guide.* Paris: Médecins Sans Frontières, 1996.

11. WHO. *Stabilité des vaccins.* Geneva: WHO, 1989. WHO/EPI/GEN/89.8.

12. WHO. *Product information sheets 1993/1994.* Geneva: WHO, 1994. WHO/UNICEF/ EPI.TS/93.1.

13. Médecins Sans Frontières. *Guide pratique pour la formation des personnels de santé.* Paris: Médecins Sans Frontières, 1994.

14. Paquet, C. *Réfugiés touaregs dans le sud-est de la Mauritanie. Aspects épidémiologiques.* [Internal report]. Paris: Epicentre, Médecins Sans Frontières, 1992.

15. WHO.*Training mid-level managers.* Geneva: WHO, 1991, WHO/EPI/MLM/91.10.

16. Dabis, F, Drucker, J, Moren, A. *Epidémiologie d'intervention.* Paris: Arnette, 1992.

17. Faillet, A, Fermont, F. Estimation of vaccine coverage using different sampling methods: Rohingya refugees, Bangladesh. *Medical News*, 1994, 3(1): 13-9.

18. UNHCR/MSF/PAM. *Enquêtes anthropométriques rapides au sein des populations en situation précaire.* [Draft]. Paris: Médecins Sans Frontières, 1991.

19. EPI. *Measles outbreak response.* A background document prepared for the Global Advisery Group Meeting. Washington D C: EPI/WHO, 1993.

20. WHO. *Measles control in the 1990s: revised plan of action for global measles control.* Geneva: WHO, 1994. WHO/EPI/GEN/94.2.

21. WHO. *Efficacy of measles immunization shortly after exposure in preventing disease transmission.* Geneva: WHO, 1989. EPI/RD/PROTOCOL/89.1.

22. Clements, C J, Strassbourg, M, Cutts, F T, Torel, C. The epidemiology of measles. *World Health Stat Q*, 1992, 45(2-3): 285-91.

23. Field evaluation of vaccine efficacy. *Wkly Epidemiol Rec*, 1985, 60: 133-40.

24. Children Vaccine Initiative. Doubt over measles targets prompts new vaccination strategy. *CVI Forum.. Special report*, 1994, No 7.

25. Semba, R D, Munasir, Z, Beeler, J, et al. Reduced seroconversion to measles in infants given vitamin A with measles vaccination. *The Lancet*, 1995, 345(8961): 1330-2.

26. Measles - Recents trends and futur prospects. *Wkly Epidemiol Rec*, 1994, 69(33): 245-52.

3. Water and sanitation

Introduction

Water and the environment play an essential role in the spread of many communicable diseases and epidemics. Diarrhoeal diseases, mostly caused by poor hygiene and a lack of safe water, are a major cause of morbidity and mortality among refugee and displaced populations. Large-scale and severe outbreaks have occurred frequently, particularly in the initial phase of a refugee crisis situation. The most striking example is that reported among Rwandan refugees in Goma (Zaire) in 1994, where extremely high mortality rates were associated with explosive epidemics of cholera and shigellosis; a household survey reported that more than 85% of deaths during the first weeks following the initial massive influx were associated with diarrhoeal diseases.

The goal of a water, hygiene and sanitation programme is therefore to plan for and maintain a minimum risk threshold in regard to water and environment-related morbidity and mortality. Such a programme must be considered as an integral part of preventive health activities in the same way as, for example, measles immunization. The techniques used in the emergency phase should be adapted later on to the post-emergency phase; these techniques should be simple but effective.

In the emergency phase, priority should be given to the following:
- the water supply to the population, focusing on providing sufficient quantities of water; the quality should be improved as quickly as possible, but improvements must not affect the quantity actually distributed,
- the control of excreta disposal and general hygiene on the site,
- increasing public awareness of the basic rules of hygiene.

Water supply activities

Like any other population, refugees require immediate access to an adequate water supply in order to maintain life and health and this becomes even more vital in refugee camps where overcrowding increases the risks of pollution and epidemics of water-borne diseases. Attention must therefore be paid to water provision from the outset of any attempt to deal with a refugee emergency[2].

1. FIRST STEP: ENSURING A SUFFICIENT QUANTITY OF WATER

It is essential that water is supplied in sufficient quantities. Extreme water shortages can lead to dehydration and death. Lack of water also leads to poor hygiene and increases the incidence of hygiene-related diseases such as faeco-orally transmitted diseases (diarrhoeal diseases), diseases transmitted by lice (e.g. typhus) and other milder diseases such as scabies and conjunctivitis[1,2,3].

The first objective is therefore to supply a sufficient quantity of water; its quality is a later consideration. A large amount of poorer quality water is preferable to a small amount of good quality drinking water.

Requirements

Any water-supply programme is based on the needs of the population; the population size must therefore be determined in order to plan appropriate logistical means (see *1.Initial Assessment*). It is essential that programme planners bear in mind that huge amounts of water are required in refugee emergencies, involving considerable logistical requirements and transport problems. In comparative terms, a human being's daily water requirement in terms of quantity is ten times greater than the food requirement.

> During the first days of the emergency phase,
> a minimum amount of water is required for survival[3]:
> **5 litres of water per person per day (source: WHO)**

But this ration does not reduce the risk of epidemics in the population; it is meant mainly for drinking and cooking, and permits only a very low level of hygiene. Quantity must therefore be increased as quickly as possible.

Some of the problems associated with providing sufficient amounts of water in the first days can come from poor management and unequal distribution, with some groups favoured over others, and refugees may have to fight to obtain it in order to survive.

> In the next stage of the emergency phase, the amount of available
> water must rapidly be increased to a sufficient quantity[2]:
> **15 to 20 litres of water per person per day**

This amount includes water for drinking, food preparation, personal hygiene and dish/clothes washing. If this threshold is not reached very quickly, risks from the transmission of water-borne diseases will obviously increase (see above).

Although water requirement standards have been set, the quantity of water consumed varies from one country or region to another, depending on the climate and the habits of the population. However, for health reasons it is recommended not to put any limit on water consumption. The quantities of water recommended in health facilities are described (below page 78).

Measures for meeting the requirements

Local constraints and conditions dictate the means required to supply water.

- When water is available on site, it can come from various sources: surface water (e.g. rivers or lakes), wells, bore-holes, springs, etc. The first thing to do is to protect water sources from pollution using fairly basic measures in the emergency phase (e.g. fencing off), then technically more sophisticated ones in the post-emergency phase. The different types of water source and the methods of supplying it to the refugee population are described below in Table 3.1. A description of techniques and detailed information are provided in several guidelines [2,3].

- When water is available nearby (e.g. within a maximum radius of 30 kilometres), the temporary solution is to transport water in tankers. For instance, in Goma (Zaire) in 1994, 200,000 refugees in the Kibumba camp received a daily ration of 2,000,000 litres of water brought in by tankers. This costly method should only be carried out on a short-term basis during the time required for relief teams to plan and prepare for other alternatives, such as moving the population, sinking wells or piping in water. Transport by tankers usually requires a careful organization of all aspects of road transport (road improvements, vehicle maintenance, scheduling and monitoring tanker rotation, etc.).

- When a sufficient quantity of water is not available near the refugee site, consideration must be given to moving the population closer to a water source (see *5. Shelters and Site Planning*).

  - *Surface water: rivers or lakes:* Surface water is rarely an ideal source for although it may be easily accessible and provide an acceptable yield, it is always regarded as contaminated. Sources such as protected wells might therefore be preferable. But, since priority must begiven to quantity, surface water is generally the solution that responds the fastest to the needs of an emergency phase.

    In 1988, in Meiram in southern Sudan, the water situation was so critical that the water distributed to displaced populations was pumped from a swamp. Pumping has to be organized for surface water, and water quality will have to be taken into account [1,3]: very polluted water should be pre-treated with appropriate techniques prior to chlorination (see below *Improving water quality*).

  - *Well or bore-hole:* A well must be protected and fitted with a pump to prevent direct contamination. The choice and installation of pump should be decided by experts. A shallow well can be equipped with a hand pump (average yield of 1,000 litres/hour) [1,2,3,9,11]. In emergencies, surface motorized pumps are most commonly used to obtain a greater flow [1,2,3]. A bore-hole or a deep well can be equipped with a special electric submersible pump, adapted to the yield required and to the nature of the hole. Electric submersible pumps can produce a considerable amount of water.

  - *Spring* [1,3,8,10]: The spring must be protected and other measures taken to limit water contamination. A springbox must be built, and supervised by experts.

Table 3.1
Water supply methods in refugee settlements

Sources	Measures for water supply	Human resources
Surface water[2,5]	Organize pumping (keep pumping areas distant or upstream from human activities) and prevent the population from coming directly to the water source. Keep pumping areas distant from human/animal activity. Treat the water (see *Improving water quality*).	Sanitation officer or logistician with experience in sanitation programmes.
Well[1,2,3,9,11]	Protect the well and fix drain-off for surplus water. Cover it and install pump (hand, motorized or electric).	Sanitation officer expert in the specific field.
Bore-hole	Protect and fix drain-off for surplus water. Install electric pump, and keep pumping areas distant or upstream from human activities.	Expert in this field.
Spring	Catch the water where it emerges. Build springbox and install direct distribution. Fix run-off drain for surplus water. Protect by setting up a surrounding clean area.	Expert in this field.

Water availability

It is not enough to supply large amounts of water to a refugee site. Water must be immediately available to the population, and easily accessible; for instance, long queues at water points should be avoided (waiting time should be less than 2 hours). To ensure adequate availability, it is essential to adhere as closely as possible to the criteria listed below.

- Location of water points and accessibility[2,3]

  Immediate arrangements should be made to store water and to distribute it at water points away from the water sources; for example, 'bladder tanks' (with volume capacities of $2m^3$ or $15m^3$) or flexible water tanks with metal frames ($30m^3$) enable water to be transported or stored and clarified (by sedimentation/flocculation) as well as treated prior to distribution, and avoid direct contamination. It is important to provide all refugee sites with appropriate material for water storage.

  The water points should be set up so as to ensure accessibility in regard to both distance and waiting time, and the following provisions should be foreseen:

  - 1 hand-pump for 500 to 750 persons,
  - 1 tap for 200-250 persons,
  - a maximum of 6 to 8 taps per distribution unit.

It is essential to ensure that water is available to the whole population: for example, the lack of water points among Kurdish refugees in Iraq in 1991 in the first stages of intervention, caused disputes around water installations and refugees cut into the main supply pipes to get at water faster. Care should be taken that water points are installed at a reasonable distance from shelters for safety reasons (minimum of 30 metres).

- Water point yields
  Tap flows must be monitored. The number of water points should be increased if the out-flow is insufficient (under 5 litres/minute/tap) in order to speed up the water distribution.

- Water containers
  It is important to ensure that the population has enough water containers for storing and carrying water (minimum overall capacity of 40 litres per family). If this is not the case, a distribution of water containers should be organized urgently. The containers should adhere to health standards and be easy to carry. Water in buckets may be quickly contaminated by dirty hands; jerrycans reduce water contamination but are not so easy to carry and difficult to clean properly inside.

2. SECOND STEP: IMPROVING WATER QUALITY

Requirements

Water should not pose a health risk and should have an appearance and taste acceptable to the population. Ideally, the water supplied should meet WHO quality standards. However, in emergencies it is generally very difficult or even impossible to adhere to these standards[3]. The main goal is to provide water which is clean enough to restrict water-borne diseases, i.e. containing the fewest possible pathogenic germs. The presence or absence of pathogenic organisms is the only criteria of real importance to health.

The bacteriological quality of untreated water should be assessed. This is based on detection of the presence and number of organisms which are indicators of faecal pollution, i.e. faecal coliforms (always present in large numbers in the faeces of humans and other animals). This bacteriological analysis can be performed by using field testing kits (e.g. Del Agua/Oxfam kit), which provide results within 24 hours but are expensive and require experienced or specially trained sanitation officers[3].

> **Water for consumption should contain
> less than 10 faecal coliforms /100 ml.**

Note: In urban settings, water may have specific constituents such as heavy metals or toxic chemicals, etc., which would require the involvement of experts.

Measures for meeting the requirements

The following principles must be respected in order to ensure good quality water:

- water from deep wells, protected springs and deep drilling may be considered safe and used without treatment;
- surface and near-surface water are considered to be contaminated, and this water must be treated;
- prior to treatment (usually chlorination), water should be checked for its turbidity and pre-treated if necessary;
- priority should be given to the selection and protection of water points.

• Chlorination

Water disinfection with chlorine compounds (mostly calcium hypochlorite) is the most effective treatment method in emergencies[1,3,5,6]. Chlorine reacts in water and immediately neutralizes pathogenic germs. A residual effect is obtained by disinfecting storage containers: distributed water should always contain residual chlorine (between 0.3 and 0.5mg/litre). However, chlorination is relatively difficult to implement, and needs to be supervised constantly. Each batch of water to be treated requires a specific amount of chlorine. Indeed, chlorination is only partially effective due to the suspended matter in water (turbidity) which protects the pathogenic agents (shield effect). As a result, when turbidity is too high, pre-treatment is required before chlorination. Turbidity often increases in the rainy season.

• Pre-treatment

Water turbidity can be measured simply by looking through the water (in a transparent container), or with special equipment[3]. If the water turbidity is greater than 20 NTU units (nephelometric turbidity unit), pre-treatment is required, i.e. eliminating suspended matter before chlorination. The pre-treatment techniques selected depend on water turbidity and may consist of natural sedimentation or accelerated sedimentation by the addition of chemical compounds (flocculation techniques)[1,8,9]. Both of these techniques require supervision by experienced staff.

• Water quality control

Throughout the water distribution chain, quality checks should be made regularly.

- *At the beginning of the chain*: untreated water may undergo a bacteriological control, but a visual check of the site may be enough to assess the presence of polluted water. Water turbidity should be checked, to decide whether pre-treatment is required. The pH content should also be tested because water disinfection requires more processing when the pH is very high (higher than 8.5). Residual chlorine is assessed and should be twice as high as the standard for water distributed at the end of the chain (i.e. 0.6 - 1mg/litre).
- *In the middle of the chain* (water distributed at water points): water should always be tested for its free residual chlorine content.

– *At the end of the chain* (households): there should be a final check of the water containers. If there is no longer any free residual chlorine in the remaining water, the concentration of faecal coliforms must be checked.

Tests should be carried out at a regular frequency:
– several times per day for free residual chlorine (at the beginning and in the middle of the chain);
– weekly or with each climate change for turbidity and pH content;
– weekly for detecting faecal coliforms in epidemic and emergency periods;
– monthly for detecting faecal coliforms in stable, post-emergency situations.

Sanitation and hygiene

Sanitation and hygiene programmes aim at ensuring a safe environment and reducing the incidence of environment-related diseases. In order to achieve these aims, attention must be paid to the disposal of excreta, the disposal and treatment of waste water, and the collection and disposal of solid waste. In refugee settings, social disruption, the concentration of people used to a different standard of hygiene and the lack of sanitation facilities, such as latrines, can lead to major health risks. Excreta and waste are often disposed of indiscriminately around a refugee site in the first stages of an emergency and there are many transmission mechanisms for communicable diseases, i.e. hands, water, animals, food, etc.; pathogenic agents are transmitted much more easily under such precarious conditions, and sanitation measures are therefore required urgently.

A refugee sanitation programme relies on simple techniques at first, with improvements added later on. As it is essential that the refugees cooperate, they should be properly informed about the measures that are being implemented. This aspect of health awareness should be dealt with in close collaboration with refugee representatives and under the supervision of teams of local staff.

EXCRETA CONTROL

Human excreta (mainly faecal matter) are responsible for the spread of many infectious diseases[1,2]. It is therefore crucial to organize a proper disposal of excreta from the beginning of the programme. In large-scale refugee emergencies it is recommended that two teams be set up; one to take care of the water supply and one for hygiene and sanitation (see *9. Human Resources and Training*).

There are many excreta disposal techniques, but in each situation, even in the emergency phase, a certain understanding of the habits of the population is necessary in order to decide which one to employ. Any excreta disposal system should be adapted to their habits and customs in order to ensure they will be used correctly. If this principle is ignored, the system may either not be used or may be damaged, eventually even becoming a health hazard in itself[1,2,3,8].

- At the start of operations, during the first days of the emergency phase, community facilities for excreta disposal, adapted for a large number of users, should be organized. The simplest and most quickly prepared are:
  - defecation areas or fields,
  - shallow trench latrines,
  - collective latrines.

Refugees who have already settled on the site before the start of the operation will already be using certain ('wild') areas for defecation. These areas must be identified and, depending on the environmental characteristics, improved and/or sanitized. At this stage, the target should be:

> **One latrine or trench per 50 to 100 persons.**

If they are not maintained on a regular basis, these communal facilities will pose an acute risk for the spread of infectious agents. Maintenance teams should therefore be organized to clean and disinfect them (e.g. using quick lime).

- During the next days of the emergency phase, in conjunction with these simple procedures, further hygienic measures should be taken with a view to providing more durable installations. The construction of family latrines is preferable and must be rapidly scheduled. UNHCR recommends 1 latrine for every 20 persons but such collective latrines are often poorly maintained.

> **One latrine per 20 persons (UNHCR)**
> **One latrine per family (ideally)**

A rapid distribution of tools should then be organized in order to allow refugees to build their own latrines.

The amount of space available must also be taken into account. It may be necessary to extend the site in order to find space for building additional latrines (see *10. Coordination: Camp management* and *5. Shelter and Site Planning*). In exceptional situations, where space is totally insufficient, moving the refugees to another site might be indicated.

There are no ideal technical solutions to the problem of excreta disposal. However, the following factors should be taken into account:
  - the social, cultural and religious customs, and habits of the refugee population,
  - the water-table level and its seasonal variations,
  - soil composition,
  - locally available material,
  - population size and how it is concentrated on the site

WASTE WATER CONTROL

There are two categories of waste water:

- Run-off rain-water and waste water from water points are not a direct health risk for the population, but must be carefully controlled.
  - Site planning must take drainage for rain-water into account from the outset in order to avoid soil erosion and flooding during heavy rains. Drainage trenches are usually located along the access roads.
  - Waste water disposal at water points is ensured by trenches connected to main drainage or a soak-away pit. When this is not undertaken, stagnant water may become breeding sites for mosquitoes and may infiltrate and contaminate water sources.

- Waste water collected from washing areas and from health facilities may be significantly contaminated; for instance, sewage water may contain millions of faecal coliforms. Waste water should be evacuated by infiltration into the soil whenever possible. A safe distance of at least two metres between the underground water source and the infiltration system should be respected. Since this water usually contains a lot of matter and soap, evacuation requires a clarification process (in grease traps) before evacuation; if this is not done, the evacuation system will be rapidly obstructed.

SOLID WASTE CONTROL

Solid waste in a refugee setting is usually composed of waste produced by the community as a whole, and waste resulting from medical activities.

Waste produced by the refugee population

This includes organic refuse such food waste, market refuse, sweepings, etc, and is an especially acute problem in urban-like situations, such as refugee camps, because of their high population density. Markets in refugee camps are particularly sensitive areas and should ideally be located on the outskirts of a camp for sanitary reasons. In Malawi, poor hygiene in the refugee camps was an important risk factor for numerous epidemics of cholera, and the market-place was reported to be the starting point of at least one outbreak[13]. Emergency measures must be employed to prevent a large accumulation of waste:

- organizing waste collection by cleaning teams with transport by trucks,
- creating a landfill system, i.e. trenches or individual pits, where waste is safely disposed of and daily covered with a layer of soil[1,3,8].

When the amount of waste is of limited volume and spread throughout the settlement, community or family refuse pits should be dug beside the shelters with tools distributed to families early on. A close collaboration should be maintained with refugee representatives and volunteer teams in regard to the organization of this task.

Contaminated medical waste

This includes contaminated medical waste from health centres (dressing materials, syringes, needles, etc.) which should first be incinerated and then disposed of in a pit on site. Other anatomical waste should be buried deeply or disposed of in a pit dug on site[3,4,7].

DISPOSAL OF THE DEAD

Dead bodies may be a major source of contamination in a time of cholera outbreak; they may also be a health hazard when the cause of death was typhus or plague (because of infestation by infected lice or fleas). The following measures should be implemented:

- In all situations, corpses must be protected from animals. The best method is that which is acceptable to the population and is physically possible. Burial is generally the simplest method, and a cemetery or burial place should be planned on the site, ideally at the outskirts (see *10. Coordination: Camp management*).
- When there is a very high mortality rate, priority must be given to the collection of corpses and the digging of communal graves; corpses should be disinfected with quicklime.
- In a cholera outbreak, corpses are highly contagious. They must be disinfected in the cholera treatment unit and buried as quickly as possible. Returning bodies to the families should be avoided if possible.

PERSONAL HYGIENE

Poor personal hygiene, such as neglecting to wash hands after using toilets, is often the cause of communicable diseases being spread through the faecal-oral route.

In addition to water, a detergent such as soap is also necessary. Personal body and clothes hygiene should be possible if there are sufficient quantities of water combined with adequate sanitation methods.

In emergencies, a large-scale distribution of soap should be planned early on with a minimum target of 250 to 500 grams of soap per person per month.

VECTOR CONTROL

The presence of vectors such as insects and rats is directly linked to the physical and climatic conditions of the settlement's environment. They are likely to be a hazard in emergency refugee settings, where overcrowding, poor refuse and excreta disposal, inadequate personal and food hygiene provide favourable conditions for them to live and breed[14]. Reducing the number of vectors in an emergency situation is not easy. Knowledge of the biology of each vector, even a rudimentary knowledge, is always essential for implementating effective control measures. It is vital to know how, where and when to act against a particular vector. All vector-control activities should follow these general principles[3]:

- the site should be made unfavourable to the development and survival of vectors (environmental hygiene);

– control is generally more effective if it focuses on forms that have not yet attained sexual maturity (eggs, larvae, etc.);
– complete eradication is frequently unattainable; the goal should be to maintain a vector population beneath a fixed threshold; beyond that threshold, the risk of epidemic would be too great.

The general measures for vector control are described below; specific measures for controlling vectors that pose a significant health risk are described in Table 3.2.

Preventive measures (environmental hygiene)

The first and the most effective measures in regard to vector control are general sanitation measures aimed at providing a cleaner site[3,14]. These will limit the risks of vector proliferation and thus of vector-related diseases. It is obvious that these measures should always be undertaken, whether or not vectors are present.

They include:
– the construction of a sufficient number of adequate latrines to prevent dissemination into the environment of pathogenic agents carried by various insects (with or without using intermediary hosts);
– the elimination of stagnant water and protection of water containers to prevent the proliferation of mosquitoes (see above);
– the collection and disposal of solid waste to prevent rats and flies assembling;
– improvements in personal hygiene (provision of water and soap) and reduction of overcrowding (site planning).

The measures listed above should be complemented by monitoring the refugee population and the environment for the early detection of parasites (e.g. lice) as part of the surveillance activities.

Control of existing vectors

Once disease vectors become a significant problem among the population or on the site, other measures may be required, such as chemical controls. However, these should always be planned alongside measures to achieve improvement in environmental and personal hygiene as described above.

The selection of an insecticide is a complex decision. Since the appearance of DDT (dichloro-diphenyl-trichloroethane) 40 years ago, numerous chemical products have been created to destroy disease vector agents and insects harmful to agriculture. Two major problems have arisen: disease vector insects have developed resistance to these products, and their toxic effect on humankind has created a public health problem that is sometimes considerable. The choice of insecticide must be recommended by an environmental health expert and should take into consideration[15,16]:
– national recommendations for vector control,
– the type of vector,
– the residual effect sought,
– vector resistance to the available products,
– product toxicity.

As it may be risky to use old stocks of insecticide available locally, these must be verified by an expert before use.

• The mass use of insecticide is never without risk, and is not always effective. It may be indicated in a few situations, such as when there is a severe outbreak of a disease transmitted by vectors (e.g. relapsing fever or dengue) or when it is difficult to control breeding sites. It always requires specialist advice and close supervision. All use of chemical compounds must follow very strict rules (wearing gloves, paying attention to the proximity of any water source, etc.); this is in the safety interests both of the sanitation teams and the refugee population.

• Impregnating mosquito nets with chemical compounds (with repellent effects) has shown good results in protecting against mosquitoes. Pilot projects are being studied in order to determine whether or not it is feasible to carry out large-scale distributions of mosquito nets and whether or not they are used by refugees. This would mainly be indicated in the post-emergency phase, where malaria is a major health problem (see section *Malaria control*) and would require former study of the vector biting habits (e.g. inside/outside). The impregnation of shelters has been the most widely used method up till now.

Table 3.2
Vectors representing significant health risks and the main control measures [3,14]

Vector	Health risks	Environmental hygiene	Chemical control
Mosquitoes: **– Anopheles** **– Culex** **– Aedes**	– Malaria – Japanese encephalitis – Yellow fever, dengue	Destroy breeding sites for all types: – Eliminate stagnant water – Idem and protect latrines – Protect water containers	Insecticide or larvicide If epidemic, individual protection by mosquito-net
Lice	Epidemic typhus (LBTF), relapsing fever (LBRF)	Reduce overcrowding, improve hygiene, educate population	Insecticide powdering for individuals and clothes
Fleas	Plague, endemic typhus	Clean shelters and surrounds	Insecticide powdering for clothes and bedding If plague, first destroy fleas, then rats
Flies	Eye infections (trachoma), diarrhoeal diseases such as shigellosis	Hygiene is the most essential Refuse disposal, clean spilled food, waste water disposal, etc.	To be avoided as much as possible! Pour used oil into latrines In a large-scale epidemic, at least treat health facilities
Ticks	Relapsing fever (TBRF)	Household hygiene	Ether or insecticide to kill ticks
Mites	Scabies, scrub typhus	Personal hygiene	Benzyl benzoate on patients

Vector control measures specific to individual diseases are covered in 7. *Control of Communicable Diseases and Epidemics.*

In plague epidemics, it is essential to destroy the flea population without harming the host species (rodents) otherwise there will be a greater risk of fleas infesting (and infecting) humans.

Water, sanitation and hygiene in health facilities

A health facility not only represents a concentrated area of patients but also a concentrated area of germs.

The most stringent measures possible should therefore be taken in regard to water, hygiene and sanitation: a supply of good quality water, latrines, solid waste control and the hygienic disposal of waste water from showers, hand washing, kitchens, etc.

However, these requirements may have to be realistically adapted in emergency situations[4,6,7]. The standard requirements are described in Table 3.3.

Table 3.3
Water/sanitation standards in health facilities

	Health facility or item	**Standards**
Water requirements	Hospitalization ward	50 litres /person /day
	Surgery/maternity	100 litres /person /day
	Per dressing/consultation	5 litres /dressing
	Feeding centre	20-30 litres /person /day
	Kitchen	10 litres /person /day
Cleaning interval	Showers/toilets	once a day
	Floors	once a week
	Walls/ceiling	once every 6 months
	Beds/sheets	after each patient
	Floors/operating table/delivery bed	after each operation /delivery
Refuse	Excreta	one pit ($0.04m^3$) filled/person /year
	Waste	volume produced = 3 dm^3/ person/day, plan 100 litres waste-bin /25 patients

Human resources

A water, hygiene and sanitation programme in emergency situations requires the necessary human resources to carry it out. It is therefore essential to draw up job descriptions early on, defining the role of each participant in detail.

Water and sanitation programmes should be organized and supervised by an environmental health technician. In large-scale emergencies, two head technicians may be needed, working in close coordination, i.e. one for the water programme and one for hygiene and sanitation (see above). The environmental health technician should define the different tasks and organize teams to carry them out:

- surveillance of the various links in the water-supply chain (pumping, storing and treating),
- maintaining water distribution points,
- building collective latrines and maintaining them,
- preparing slabs for family latrines,
- collecting and disposing of waste,
- hygiene in health facilities: cleaning latrines, waste disposal, spraying, preparing chlorine solutions, etc.,
- public education on basic rules of hygiene,
- monitoring environmental health indicators.

Principal recommendations regarding water and sanitation

- In an emergency refugee situation, priority must be given to meeting water needs. The amount provided in the early stage should be enough to meet drinking and cooking requirements and should then be increased as quickly as possible in order to ensure a satisfactory level of hygiene. In addition to a sufficient water supply, soap must be provided as soon as possible. Improving water quality and ensuring access to water should also be tackled quickly.

- Human excreta, medical wastes, etc. are always contaminated; arrangements for their control and disposal in well-defined areas should be instituted as quickly as possible, using simple techniques.

- The site should be cleaned in order to prevent intermediate carriers (vectors) from developing and spreading diseases.

- Health facilities such as feeding centres, health centres, etc. should respect the hygiene principles mentioned above as early as possible.

- These preventive measures should be very quickly linked to disease surveillance. Monitoring morbidity and mortality data will highlight any weak points in a water, hygiene and sanitation programme.

✎ References

1. Cairncross, S, Feachem, R G. *Environmental health engineering in the tropics: An introductory text.* John Wiley, 1993.

2. UNHCR. *Water manual for refugee situations.* Geneva: UNHCR, 1992.

3. Médecins Sans Frontières. *Public health engineering in emergency situations.* Paris: Médecins Sans Frontières, 1994.

4. Médecins Sans Frontières. *L'hygiène dans les soins de santé en situation précaire.* Paris: Médecins Sans Frontières, 1992.

5. Thomson, M C. *Disease prevention through vector control.* Oxford: OXFAM Practical Health Guide No 10, 1995.

6. Renchon, B. *Manuel d'utilisation des désinfectants. dans les situations de réfugiés - Principes directeurs du HCR pour le choix et l'utilisation des désinfectants.* Geneva: UNHCR, 1994.

7. Médecins Sans Frontières. *Guide pour la mise en place ou reconstruction d'hôpitaux ruraux en milieu isolé.* Paris: Médecins Sans Frontières, 1987.

8. Ockwell, R, and al. *Assisting in emergencies : a resource handbook for UNICEF field staff.* Geneva: UNICEF, 1986.

9. *Water for the world* - Technical notes. Washington, DC: USAID.

10. Thomas D., Jordan Jnr. *A handbook of gravity-flow water systems.* London: Intermediate Technology Publications Ltd, 1984.

11. Watt, S B, Wood, W E. *Hand dug wells and their construction.* London: Intermediate Technology Publications Ltd, 1985.

12. The Goma Epidemiological Group. Public health impact of Rwandan refugee crisis: What happened in Goma, Zaire, in July, 1994? *The Lancet*, 1995, 345: 339-44.

13. Moren, A, Stefanaggi, S. Practical field epidemiology to investigate a cholera outbreak in a Mozambican refugee camp in Malawi, 1988. *J Trop Med Hyg*, 1991, 94: 1-7.

14. UNHCR. *Handbook for Emergencies.* Geneva: UNHCR, 1982.

15. WHO. *Matériel de lutte contre les vecteurs.* Geneva: WHO, 1991.

16. WHO. *Specification for pesticides used in public health.* Geneva: WHO, 1985.

4. Food and nutrition

Introduction

Food shortages and nutritional problems are frequent in refugees or displaced populations, and have led to high prevalence rates of acute malnutrition, when compared to rates commonly found in non-refugee populations[16]. Indeed, rates higher than 20% have been reported among refugees in Somalia (1980), Ethiopia (1988-89) and Kenya (1991), and among displaced persons in Ethiopia (1985), Sudan (1988) and Liberia (1990)[3]. Protein-energy malnutrition (PEM) is known to be a major contributory cause of death in refugee populations, mostly because malnutrition increases vulnerability to disease and thus its severity, especially in regard to measles[3,13,16]. The analysis of data collected in 42 camps in Asia and Africa, indicates a clear association between the prevalence of malnutrition and high mortality rates in refugee camps in the emergency phase[13]. In addition to PEM, nutrient deficiencies such as avitaminosis A or scurvy play a key role in nutrition-related morbidity and mortality[3].

Two main factors explain why the risk of malnutrition is higher in a population which has been displaced (and whose environment has suddenly changed):

- The sudden and massive reduction in food availability (due to a real lack of food or an inadequate distribution of rations) and in food accessibility (no means of buying food or inequities in the food distribution). This severely affects the food security of a household - i.e. the ability of a household to feed its members[1].
- The impaired health environment, i.e. higher exposure to communicable disease, lower standard of health services, lack of water, poor hygiene, etc.

This justifies placing food supply and nutritional programmes high on the priority list of refugee programmes[3]. These programmes also have positive consequences for the health status of refugees - by improving their resistance to disease - and on their psycho-social well-being; however, they may also complicate the overall political situation because food may be used as a tool by dominant groups.

A broad range of actions may be taken to improve food security[1]. However, in the emergency phase of a refugee situation, the choice of intervention programme is limited and the highest priority is to ensure the distribution of adequate food rations to the whole population, through general food distributions. In addition, selective feeding programmes will be set up as required in order to respond to the increased needs of specific groups, particularly malnourished children. Measures may also be required to prevent or control possible nutrient deficiencies (see below *Nutrient deficiencies*).

Objectives

OBJECTIVES OF FOOD INTERVENTION PROGRAMMES

The general objectives are to meet the basic food needs of all refugees and to decrease the mortality and morbidity resulting from malnutrition.

Therefore, the operational objectives are:

– To ensure a minimum average food ration of 2,100 Kcal/person/day containing an adequate nutrient content;

– To reduce the prevalence of malnutrition and mortality from malnutrition by the treatment of acutely malnourished individuals and the prevention of malnutrition in other groups at risk.

THE ROLE OF THE HEALTH AGENCIES

Health agencies have an important role to play in nutritional interventions because they have an obvious responsibility in the treatment of nutritional diseases (PEM and nutrient deficiencies). According to their field of activity, expertise and capacity, these agencies will decide with which kind of nutritional intervention they want to be involved.

• They usually carry out selective feeding programmes for acutely malnourished children (and possibly for other vulnerable groups).

• It is their responsibility to monitor the regularity and adequacy of food rations.

• They generally leave general food distributions to organizations with more specific experience and capacity, but in some situations they may also take charge of this (either temporarily or over a longer period)[1].

Assessment

An assessment of the food and nutritional situation should always be part of the initial health assessment; it can be covered in two stages (see *1. Initial Assessment*).

1. A quick evaluation should be carried out as early as possible, to provide a global picture showing the severity of the situation, indicate whether a rapid intervention is necessary and facilitate in planning the necessary resources (food quantities and staff required). This evaluation is based on observation, interviews with key informants and discussions with organizations already operating.

At this stage, the assessment should gather information on the general status of the population, any existing food distributions and how they are organized, rough estimates of household food reserves, whether or not there is a market, etc. Although a number of visibly malnourished individuals may be present, it should not automatically be presumed that there is a large-scale problem; further evaluation will be needed.

2. At the second stage, quantified data should be gathered on the nutritional situation in order to decide the type and size of nutritional programmes (e.g. selective feeding). Data should be collected to cover the prevalence of malnutrition, food availability and accessibility, and other factors affecting the nutritional status. The prevalence of malnutrition is a key indicator and must be assessed by a nutritional survey.

However, conducting a survey is expensive and time-consuming, and there are a few situations in which it may not be conducted:

– when the need for nutritional assistance is obvious and very urgent (e.g. very poor overall health status or high mortality among children); for instance, in Somalia in 1991-92, the nutritional situation among the displaced was so critical that immediate action was required and took priority over gathering nutritional data;

– when agencies do not have the capacity to act even after identifying the size of the problem;

– when the survey is not feasible, for example, due to security problems or a lack of resources (logistics and human resources).

FOOD AVAILABILITY AND ACCESSIBILITY

The quantity and quality of the food available to refugees is insufficient in most situations unless distributions are carried out. The initial data to be gathered include:

– information relating to food distributions that may already have taken place: theoretical food ration, ration actually distributed, distributing agency, target group, frequency of distributions, etc.;

– assessment of local market: type and price of food available;

– the food basket of individual households may be estimated by a sample survey, but this is rarely carried out in the emergency phase.

It may be particularly difficult to make such assessments in open situations where refugees are integrated into the local population, because food sources may be diverse: food aid, food shared with locals, food that is purchased, bartered for, or gathered (wild fruit, etc.).

THE NUTRITIONAL STATUS OF THE REFUGEE POPULATION

The prevalence of acute malnutrition in children under 5 years of age is generally used as an indicator of this condition in the entire population, since this group is more sensitive to changes in the nutritional situation and international reference values may be used[1,3]. It makes it possible to know whether there is a nutritional problem, and, if so, how significant it is.

How to measure malnutrition

The nutritional status of each individual child is generally measured by the weight-for-height index (W/H) which is recommended as the most reliable indicator in emergencies because it reflects the current situation and is sensitive to rapid change[1,2]. In addition, bilateral oedema in children indicates severe malnutrition, irrespective of their W/H[1,3]. Another indicator of nutritional status is the measure of the mid-upper arm circumference (MUAC). Although the MUAC measure is quickly taken, it is not a reliable indicator because the risk of measurement error is high (considerable variability between the results reached by different observers), there is not complete agreement on which cut-off values should be used, and there is no clear correlation with the W/H index (MUAC cut-off values are available in guidelines[1,3]). MUAC is therefore only used for rapid assessment when a classical survey is not possible, or for quick identification of malnourished children (see section *Selective feeding programmes*, page 92)[1].

Implementation of the nutritional survey

The survey is performed on a representative sample of children aged between six months and five years, using the W/H index. Sampling procedures and survey techniques are discussed in nutritional guidelines[1]. It is important to plan the survey properly in order to minimize the impact on other activities. The time needed depends on the resources available (human and material), the distances involved and the accuracy required. For instance, a survey in a camp situation can be conducted within one week, including training staff.

How to express malnutrition rates

W/H indices are interpreted by comparison with a 'reference population'. Survey results should preferably be expressed in Z-Scores (number of standard deviations above or below the median value in the reference population) to allow international comparisons and for statistical reasons[2,3].

Three indicators may be calculated:

- the prevalence of global malnutrition (% of children with W/H under -2 Z-Scores and/or oedema); global malnutrition consists of moderate and severe malnutrition;
- the prevalence of moderate malnutrition (% of children with W/H <-2 and ≥-3 Z-Scores);
- the prevalence of severe malnutrition (% of children with W/H under -3 Z-Scores and/or oedema).

However, results are sometimes expressed as a percentage of the median of the reference value (i.e. median weight of the reference population with the same height) [1,2]. Results are roughly similar, but will show a lower prevalence than results expressed in a Z-Score.

OTHER INFORMATION

Information regarding contextual factors is essential for interpreting the results of the nutritional survey. These include: mortality figures, major outbreaks of disease, micronutrient deficiencies, housing conditions, water supply and sanitation, climate, customary diet of the population, security situation, provision of health services, etc[1].

INTERPRETATION OF THE RESULTS

The essential indicators for decision-making are the global acute malnutrition rate and the severe acute malnutrition rate. A global malnutrition rate below 5% is considered common in major parts of Africa and Asia; a rate between 5% and 10% should act as a warning.

Such survey data may quantify the severity of a situation but are not sufficient to make a complete interpretation of the nutritional situation; other factors have to be considered[1].

- The estimate of severity may be biased as a result of:
  - a very high mortality rate among the most vulnerable, which may lead to under-estimating the malnutrition problem (because some of the severely malnourished have disappeared);
  - the timing and season of the year.

- It is useful to know the distribution of malnutrition in the population, per age group, date of arrival, ethnic groups, camp section, etc., as severely affected sub-groups may be masked by the average result (e.g. newcomers). Identifying them can help to target programmes more effectively.

- Three main contextual factors should be taken into account when interpreting the results:
  - mortality figures;
  - general food rations and food accessibility: quantity and quality of the rations distributed and the equity of the distribution system (see below)[3]. Food reserves in refugee households, or money available for purchasing food, also have to be considered;
  - major outbreaks of disease, which may contribute significantly to high malnutrition levels, or the presence of nutritional deficiencies.

Interventions

Based on the results of the assessment and on local conditions (security or availability of resources), a sound intervention strategy must be worked out.

The classical emergency food interventions are[1]:

1. General food distributions to ensure adequate food rations for all.

2. Selective feeding programmes:
   - Supplementary feeding programmes (SFPs) providing food supplements and medical follow-up for the moderately malnourished in targeted SFPs and food supplements to vulnerable groups (e.g. pregnant women) in blanket SFPs, and
   - Therapeutic feeding programmes (TFP) for the treatment of the severely malnourished.

HOW TO DECIDE ON THE INTERVENTIONS

A flow chart can be used to help interpret the seriousness of a situation and select the appropriate type of intervention; it is based on several factors[1].

- **General food ration available**: a minimum daily average food ration of 2,100 Kcal/person/day should be assured for all refugees. When the ration is inadequate, the food supply must be improved. Low rations are also a factor in deciding on feeding programmes (see below).

- **Malnutrition rate**: the rate of malnutrition generally indicates the level of intervention required.

- **Aggravating factors** which influence the nutritional situation: their presence indicates that a higher level of intervention is required. Included among such factors are:
  - a crude mortality rate (CMR) > 1/10,000/day (i.e. emergency phase),
  - an inadequate food ration (below 2,100 Kcal/person/day),
  - epidemics of measles, shigella, or other important communicable diseases,
  - severe cold and inadequate shelter,
  - an unstable situation, e.g. caused by a new influx of refugees.

Figure 4.1
Flow chart for nutritional interventions

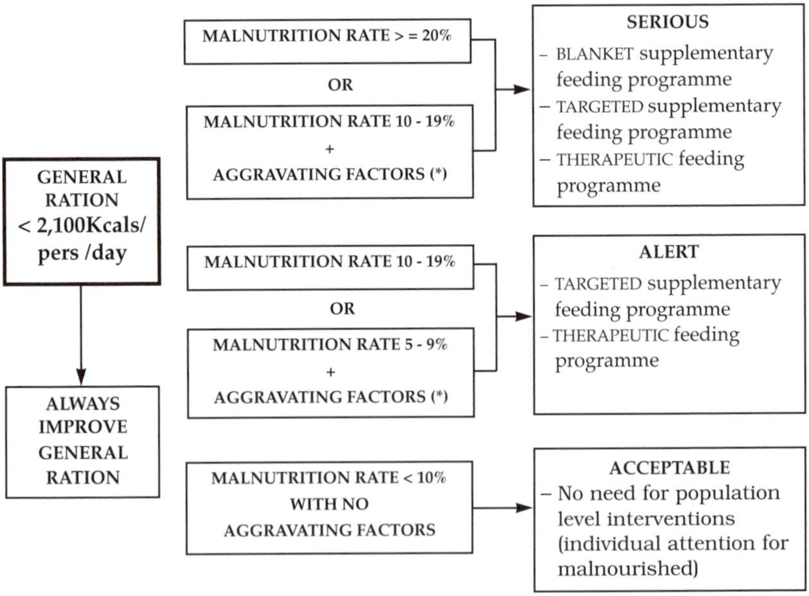

This flow chart is meant as a supportive guide and not as a set of rules. Other considerations, such as the vulnerability of specific groups, logistical constraints, the capacity of the agencies involved in nutritional programmes and the distribution of tasks among them, can also play an important role.

RESPONSIBILITIES AND COORDINATION

From the start, the responsibilities of each of the partners involved have to be clearly defined: host country authorities, refugees, UNHCR, WFP, health agencies and other NGOs, etc. (see Table 4.2).

Table 4.2
Agencies involved in providing food relief for refugee or displaced populations

Agencies involved	Role and responsibilities
WFP	Supplies basic commodities for the general ration (cereals, pulses, salt, sugar and blended food). Provides funds for internal transport, storage and food handling. Donates food to NGOs for in-patients (hospitals), 'Food for Work' for staff. May donate food for feeding programmes (e.g. oil, sugar and corn soya blend - CSB).
UNHCR	Coordinates food aid to refugees (and all relief assistance). Coordinates food transport and distribution or subcontracts these tasks to agencies. Supplies complementary food items if necessary (e.g. fish, meat, milk, biscuits and vegetables). Supplies food items to supplementary and therapeutic feeding programmes.
UNICEF	May supply food for selective feeding programmes. May (rarely) provide food assistance to internally displaced persons.
Food aid agencies	May provide food assistance independently (ICRC). May implement food distribution when sub-contracted by UNHCR (Care, CRS, etc.).
Health agencies	May implement selective feeding programmes (blanket or targeted). Must monitor regularity and adequacy of general rations and nutritional status.

In regard to refugee situations, UNHCR and WFP have agreed on how to share responsibility for ensuring the general food supply to the population in a 'Memorandum of Understanding' [11]. Internally displaced persons do not usually fall under the mandate of UNHCR, although UNHCR may provide some resources. In such situations, WFP, ICRC or NGOs could provide food assistance.

In addition to their implementing role, the health agencies, which may be the only operatives with a full-time presence in the field and therefore the only witnesses on hand, should monitor the general ration supplied, pass information on to the coordinating body and the agencies concerned and advocate the provision of adequate rations. The health and nutrition status of the population and the impact of selective feeding programmes are dependent on this monitoring (see below under *Surveillance and monitoring*).

Good coordination between partners is vital for ensuring that programmes are implemented in a coherent manner. This coordination is usually assured by UNHCR (in refugee situations) and can be facilitated by the use of internationally agreed guidelines.

GENERAL FOOD DISTRIBUTION

Most refugee or displaced populations are largely dependent upon food aid for survival, at least in the short term. The aim is to ensure that food is available and accessible to the whole population through the distribution of an adequate food ration[1,10,13]. Such intervention is required whatever the level of malnutrition.

Assessment of needs

The assessment of refugee food needs is usually the responsibility of UNHCR and WFP. Local governments should be involved, and NGOs occasionally participate. Three specific aspects must be assessed in order to organize the food supply.

- Population figures

  The number of beneficiaries must be known in order to plan food needs (see *1. Initial Assessment*). This is closely linked to the registration process that determines who is entitled to food aid (see below).

- Quantity of general food ration

  An average general ration has to be set in order to meet minimum nutritional needs. Different agencies have different ration standards.

  - *Several agencies (MSF, SCF, OXFAM, etc.)* recommend a minimum average ration of 2,100 Kcal/person/day[1,5].
  - *ICRC* sets a target ration of 2,400 Kcal/person/day to take into account factors that increase nutritional needs (see below)[1].
  - *UNHCR and WFP* are currently working out methods for assessing different levels of requirements for different regions, i.e. the basic level of energy requirements will vary in line with the presence of factors influencing nutritional needs[5].

  Factors that require an increase in the general ration include:[1]
  - bad general health and nutrition status (general malnutrition or epidemics);
  - low temperatures, inadequate shelter or lack of blankets;
  - increased activity level (e.g. farming);
  - age and sex composition of the population (e.g. a higher proportion of adult males);
  - where non-food needs are not met because part of the general ration is being bartered or sold in exchange for non-food items (see below under *Food diversion*, page 91);
  - wastage caused through grinding process if unmilled cereals are distributed, poor food storage and other wastage that may decrease the nutritional value of the ration;
  - losses attributable to the distribution system itself.

Other factors affecting food aid requirements:[1]
- where the food items distributed are unfamiliar to the refugees or poorly accepted by them, their real nutritional intake may be reduced. This requires the distribution of other commodities, or an increased ration to allow refugees to exchange part of it to buy preferred goods on the local market, e.g. local staples, vegetables, etc. (see below);
- in open situations (i.e. where refugees are living among the local population), and if populations have reached a stage where they are not entirely dependent on food aid, the ration only has to cover part of their nutritional needs.

- Quality of the general food ration

Food rations must have adequate protein, fat, mineral and vitamin contents [1]:
- the minimum ration of 2,100 Kcal/person/day should contain at least 10% protein energy and 10% fat energy;
- the classic food basket should contain 6 basic ingredients: a cereal, a pulse, oil/fat, and, in principle, a fortified cereal blend, sugar and salt according to a joint UNHCR and WFP decision; it may sometimes include fish or meat. Grinding facilities are needed if whole grain is distributed[11];
- complementary food items (e.g. fortified blended food or staple foods) are often crucial for nutrient intake and ensuring acceptability of the food ration, and may be distributed (e.g. to vulnerable groups). If refugees have access to these items in a local market and can afford to purchase them, this will also help complement the food ration[3];
- UNHCR and WFP have banned the distribution of dried milk powder in refugee rations, and it is only used in therapeutic feeding; bottle-feeding should be avoided, and breast-feeding promoted;
- it is important to distribute culturally acceptable and familiar food. For example, Somalis in the 1980s were given food but were not familiar with its preparation process.

Implementation of general food distributions

The distribution process and its implementation are described in *10. Coordination: Camp management.*

The main factors required for successful food distributions are:
- political willingness on the part of food donors to supply food;
- adequate planning of the food supply system and good logistical organization (purchase, storage, transport of food to the distribution site, etc.). This is a cumbersome task which requires expertise in the field;
- registration of individuals or families entitled to a food ration, with the distribution of ration cards, usually under the responsibility of UNHCR (for refugees);
- a distribution system ensuring that everybody receives the same ration (equity). A distribution committee, in which women should be well represented, should be set up to represent the refugees in discussions concerning the distribution system. The family is the natural unit targeted for distribution, and one of the most equitable systems is to distribute to heads of households (men or women), based on registration. This can also be done effectively

through groups of families or other community structures[21]. The system of distribution through community leaders is quicker (no need for registration) and gives more responsibility to the refugee communities, but it frequently results in distribution inequities and food diversion; it is therefore usually limited to the early phase (before registration) or situations where registration is not possible. It is currently suggested that women should be the distributors of food (or at least choose representatives who will be involved) because they are fairer in their allocations and more vulnerable to distribution inequities[21];

– good organization, ensuring regularity of distributions: distributions (e.g. every two weeks) from a well-planned site permitting an orderly, unhampered flow of people and the presence of staff with clearly-defined responsibilities. In camps, there should be at least one distribution site per 20,000 to 30,000 refugees[21];

– regular monitoring of the ration actually received (see below *Surveillance and monitoring*);

– clear definition of the agreed responsibilities of the different partners and an effective coordination.

Figure 4.3
Food flow from donor to beneficiary[1]

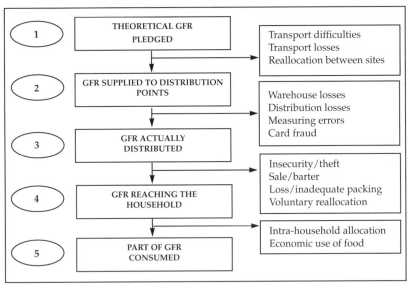

However, food distributions have often met problems in trying to cover the basic needs of the target population. There are several factors or obstacles which hamper the provision of adequate rations.

• **Problems with the food supply**: gaps in food delivery are frequent and can be due to several factors: lack of funds from donors, supplies based on donor country surpluses can lead to insufficient quantities of essential items like oil and legumes, poor management, etc.[10,12]

- **Food losses which may occur at different points in the system** (see Figure 4.3): during transport, warehousing, distributions, etc. The storage of large quantities of food frequently leads to severe security problems.

- **Inadequate nutrient content of the ration**, particularly over the longer term: for instance, the type of food aid supplied by donors and the logistical problems of distribution make it difficult to provide the six basic ingredients regularly and in sufficient quantities.

- **Food diversion**: food aid is highly sought after because of its value and the quantities involved. Food diversion is therefore common, but two different types of diversion should be distinguished, the first having positive effects but the second having very adverse effects:
  - food diversion by households which exchange part of the ration for non-food items or complementary food items is common because food aid may be the only form of capital for refugees. Food aid sold on the local market does not suggest excessive rations. On the contrary, it can reveal that households are obliged to find alternative ways to get hold of essential items such as shelter, firewood, etc. and to diversify their diet[8];
  - food diversion by powerful groups (armed groups, refugee leaders etc.), especially if these groups are in control of distributions, leads to inequities in access to food and is especially detrimental to weaker households (e.g. female-headed households).

- **Poor organization of distribution and logistical problems**, sometimes leading to security problems.

- **Lack of coordination among partners**, which may make it difficult to supply all items regularly.

- **Problems with food preparation** in households: lack of cooking utensils or firewood, or a lack of knowledge to prepare the items distributed, etc.

In spite of these obstacles, it is important that all efforts focus on providing an adequate food ration to all refugees to cover their basic food needs. This highlights the necessity to closely monitor the food rations actually received by the population.

Alternatives to general food distributions

- Providing opportunities for refugees to acquire food by themselves may sometimes be envisaged. Such programmes can take the form of[8]:
  - cash distributions to the population (e.g. refugees in European countries);
  - distributions of food items with a high economic value and high local demand (e.g. oil), which are cheap to transport and which can be bartered for other food items;
  - income-generating programmes and support for individual efforts to grow certain foodstuffs (e.g. vegetable gardens).

However, these programmes require a thorough analysis of the situation and certain economic conditions must be in place. In addition, they are more complex to manage, and up till now have not been proven to work.

For all these reasons, it is rarely possible to develop such programmes during the emergency phase. Their feasibility depends on the size of the local economy, local agricultural potential, the presence of sufficient food supplies in the local market and the extent to which refugees have access to a market[8].

• Food-for-work programmes: the use of this incentive to pay refugee workers is discussed in *9. Human Resources and Training.*

• In certain rare situations - where there is great insecurity or where utensils are not available for individual food preparation (e.g. among the displaced in Somalia in 1992), the mass preparation of cooked meals is the only way to ensure access to food. Such programmes should only be undertaken as a temporary last resort because of the heavy logistical requirements and the negative psycho-social consequences for the population.

SELECTIVE FEEDING PROGRAMMES

Even if the overall food needs of refugees are adequately met, inequities in the distribution system, disease and various social factors may contribute to a high degree of malnutrition among certain groups. These groups may be targeted to receive food supplements in order to upgrade their diet to a level that responds to their increased needs. Those that are already acutely malnourished must receive medical and nutritional attention.

Children under five are considered a priority because of their greater vulnerability (although older malnourished children may also be admitted)[1].

Special feeding programmes are usually necessary to avoid the health services being overwhelmed by large numbers of malnourished refugees[1].

The three main types of feeding programmes are see Table 4.4:

– therapeutic feeding programmes (TFP),
– targeted supplementary feeding programmes,
– blanket supplementary feeding programmes.

They differ in their objectives and the target group at which they are directed[1]:

Table 4.4
Feeding programmes

Progamme	Objectives	Target group
TFP	Reduction of mortality	Severely malnourished children
Targeted SFP	Reduction of acute PEM rates Reduction of mortality	Moderately malnourished children Children discharged from a TFP
Blanket SFP	Prevention of further deterioration in the nutritional situation Reduction of mortality	Children under 5 years Pregnant and lactating women Socially and/or medically needy individuals Elderly people

Criteria for admission and discharge

Clearly defined criteria are needed to establish who should receive which level of treatment and to set firm criteria for referral. Admission into and discharge from feeding programmes should be based on anthropometric criteria (generally based on the weight-for-height index), and maintain a coherence in the entry and exit criteria between SFPs and TFPs. Some guidelines for such criteria are available, but several factors should be taken into consideration to fix cut-off points: programme objectives, available resources, the possibilities for follow-up, any national relief policies that may exist, general food availability, etc. The criteria can be changed in the course of a programme in order to reflect changing circumstances.

In general, admission criteria are based on nutritional status and age, while discharge criteria are based on nutritional status, ongoing increase of weight and general health status [1].

Screening and selection

Once the implementation of targeted feeding programmes has been decided, eligible malnourished children should be identified by a mass screening of under-five's (see *10. Coordination: Camp management*). This can be done at the reception area for new arrivals and through the network of home visitors. MUAC is generally used for rapid screening (with MUAC cut-off points for referral to SFP and TFP), but the admission of children selected by MUAC for feeding programmes should be based on the W/H index.

THERAPEUTIC FEEDING PROGRAMMES

Therapeutic feeding centres should provide the severely malnourished with their full nutritional requirements and medical care. They may be comprised of two units, offering two levels of care[1]:
– an intensive 24-hour care unit ensuring the first phase of treatment: management of medical complications and initiation of nutritional treatment. When complications are brought under control (1-7 days), the child is transferred to the day-care unit;
– a day-care unit ensuring the second phase of the treatment: nutritional treatment and medical follow-up.

Some circumstances make it impossible to organize a 24-hour unit (e.g. poor security, lack of staff or the large number of severely malnourished), and only day-care will be provided.

The principles for treatment in Therapeutic Feeding Programmes

• *In the first phase* [1]:
  – diagnosis and treatment of complications with special attention to dehydration and infections,
  – routine treatment of intestinal parasites and other infections (in many cases antibiotic and routine malaria treatment will be required),
  – systematic measles immunization on admission, and a therapeutic dose of vitamin A,

- careful initiation of nutritional therapy through 6 to 12 daily meals of special milk preparation (High Energy Milk),
- continued breast-feeding for infants,
- if needed, supplements of other vitamins (e.g. vitamin C).

- *In the second phase* [1]:
  - nutritional rehabilitation through fewer meals but with a higher caloric content (high energy milk, porridge or meals consisting of local food),
  - standard treatment and prophylaxis of anaemia with ferrous salt and folic acid (but iron supplements are only given after 14 days),
  - vitamin supplement if needed,
  - psycho-social stimulation.

Organization of TFPs

A TFP centre should be located where it is accessible to the population, and near to a central health facility (health centre or hospital). The intensive care unit requires a separate area, and standards of care similar to a paediatric intensive care unit.

A TFP requires a sufficient number of medically-trained staff, all of whom must be given clear job descriptions and specific training and should be supervised by a doctor or a medical assistant (see *9. Human Resources and Training*). A centre usually caters for 60-100 children. A kitchen, clean water supply, latrines and a washing area must be provided.

SUPPLEMENTARY FEEDING PROGRAMMES

In supplementary feeding programmes, a high quality of food is provided to supplement the daily diet. The SFP approach aims at providing standard attention to large groups, in contrast to the individual attention provided in a therapeutic feeding centre. As previously stated, there are two main types of SFP:

- **Targeted Supplementary Feeding Programmes** where a nutritional supplement and medical follow-up are provided to those who are already moderately malnourished in order to prevent them from becoming severely malnourished. The principle target group is the under-fives, but older severely malnourished may sometimes be admitted.

- **Blanket Supplementary Feeding Programmes** which provide all members of vulnerable groups (i.e. all under-fives, pregnant and lactating women, and the elderly) with a food supplement.

  Such action may be decided in situations where the general food supply is grossly inadequate, or when it is suspected that food rations do not reach all refugees.

  The objective is to prevent an increase in malnutrition and mortality rates. In this case, the programme may include up to 40% of the total population. However, it should be a temporary measure with the first priority given to restoring the general food supply.

Wet ration or dry ration

Blanket and targeted supplementary feeding can take two forms:
– wet rations, i.e. prepared meals consumed 'on-site' (the child is brought to the feeding centre every day),
– dry rations, i.e. food rations issued weekly to take home for preparation and consumption.

The advantages and disadvantages of both of these are listed in Table 4.5.

Table 4.5
Comparison between wet and dry supplementary feeding programmes

	WET **SFP**	DRY **SFP**
ADVANTAGES	– targets beneficiaries more effectively – better individual medical follow-up – easier where there is a lack of firewood/utensils – smaller quantities of food needed	– requires fewer resources easier to organize – requires less time for mothers and encourages better attendance – better coverage by serving more children – family remains responsible for feeding – lower transmission of communicable diseases
DISADVANTAGES	– irregular attendance due to distance or insecurity – high level of requirements in logistics, staff and time – risk of poor acceptability by families – risk of skipping meals at home	– problems of inadequate preparation of unfamiliar foods – when security is bad, risk of thefts of rations – risk of ration diversion to adults

Although there is no evidence that one design is more effective than the other, in emergency situations dry rations are preferred in order to provide rapid cover for a maximum of beneficiaries[15]. However, some circumstances may require wet feeding programmes; for instance, where there is a lack of firewood and water.

Main principles of the Supplementary Feeding Programmes

• The food ration must be sufficient and consideration given to the fact that part of the ration will be shared with family members (dry ration), or will substitute for a regular meal at home (wet ration): around 500-700 Kcal for wet feeding, and around 1,000-1,200 Kcal for dry rations (double or triple the wet rations to compensate for sharing).

• Dry rations should contain a cereal or blended food as a base, with a high-protein source and high-energy source (oil), preferably distributed as a mixture (premix). The actual composition depends on the availability of items and local food habits.

- Admission and exit criteria may vary according to changing conditions (general status, capacity, etc.). For instance, when general food rations are too low, it might be possible to retain children on a SFP until the food situation has improved[1].

- In targeted SFPs, new admissions should undergo medical screening, receive basic treatment (in the SFP centre or in a nearby health facility), and medical follow-up. An oral rehydration treatment (ORT) area should be established in the centre.

  It is essential to check for measles immunization status and give vaccination if necessary. A prophylactic dose of vitamin A could be given, vitamin deficiencies should be treated, and vitamin C given if scurvy is a risk in that area.

Organization of SFPs

The number of centres to be set up should be calculated on the basis of 1 wet SFP centre for every 250 beneficiaries and 1 dry SFP centre for 750-1,000 beneficiaries per week (150-200/day).

The location should be planned to ensure accessibility for the population (a wet SFP should be more accessible than a dry SFP) and should ideally be near a health facility. Wet feeding centres require kitchens.

THE DECISION TO CLOSE A SELECTIVE FEEDING PROGRAMME

Feeding programmes are interventions undertaken to respond to emergency nutritional needs. When the emergency is over (post-emergency phase), the closure of such programmes should always be considered, and must certainly be decided when the following conditions are present:

- the number of beneficiaries has fallen to such a low level that it is no longer efficient to run separate feeding units, and

- a nutritional survey has clearly shown a significant decrease of the global acute malnutrition rate in the refugee population, and

- conditions are stable and basic needs are met, as should be the case in a post-emergency phase (see *Part III, The Post-emergency Phase*), i.e.:

  - adequate and reliable food distributions,

  - effective public health measures in place,

  - stable population and no major influx expected.

Supplementary feeding programmes should be closed down when the above conditions are met; therapeutic feeding programmes may be transferred to the in-patient service where care for the severely malnourished can be ensured.

Surveillance and monitoring

Nutritional surveillance and monitoring covers 3 sectors:

1. Food availability and accessibility
2. Health and nutritional status
3. Feeding programmes

Indicators, sources of information and methodology differ in part between the emergency phase and the post-emergency phase due to the obvious differences as regards situation stability, time constraints and, possibly, food sources.

IN THE EMERGENCY PHASE

1. Food availability and accessibility

In the emergency phase, monitoring the general food distribution is essential as it is generally the main source of food in households. A necessary piece of information is the actual amount and quality of food that reaches the family. Losses in the food chain may occur at several levels, and result in substantial differences between the theoretical general food ration and the average ration actually received *per capita* (see Figure 4.3). Furthermore, there may be inequities in the actual food distribution, i.e. considerable variation in access to food rations between and within population groups, due to over- and under-registration of beneficiaries, diversion during the distribution process, etc.[1] This monitoring should be carried out by an independent agency (preferably a health agency) which has the confidence of all parties involved. Data should be gathered at the different levels of the food chain and from various sources in order to locate possible failures in the system.

- Information from distributing agencies

  Data on the target (or theoretical) food ration are available from the relief coordinating agency (usually UNHCR) and the agencies supplying the food (WFP, EC, etc.). Data on the food ration reaching the distribution spot and intended for distribution can be requested from the distributing agencies (ICRC, Care, etc.). A first estimate of the food rations actually distributed can be based on the distribution reports of the distributing agencies, but the best sources of information will be the beneficiaries themselves (see below *Food basket monitoring*). For example in Malawi (1988) a compilation of distribution records helped to prove that the pellagra outbreak among Mozambican refugees was due to the very low amount of niacin in general rations [19].

- Food basket monitoring at distribution points[1]

  The purpose of 'Food Basket Monitoring' (also called 'On site distribution monitoring' [21]) is to check food distributions regularly in order to advocate for a better quantity and quality of rations when required. A random sample of beneficiaries is selected during a distribution, and the amount of food they receive is weighed. This monitoring is particularly good at revealing inequities in food distribution. However, this method has two limits: it only assesses households actually receiving food aid and is only applicable when food is handed out to heads of household and at central distribution points.

- Household survey

It makes it possible to assess whether there are households which are entitled to food aid but are actually not receiving any. However, this method is a heavy undertaking and will generally not be carried out in the emergency phase (see *Part III, The Post-emergency Phase*).

2. Health and nutritional status

- Nutritional status

Nutritional surveys are useful in the emergency phase to follow up the nutritional status and possibly deciding to redirect nutritional programmes. These surveys should be repeated regularly in the emergency phase (i.e. every 3 months) when there is a higher risk of an inadequate food supply and a higher number of newcomers. It makes it possible to monitor the trends of malnutrition rates over time (if population, areas surveyed and methodologies are comparable over time)[1].

- Morbidity and mortality

Crude mortality rates, under-five mortality rates and morbidity reports (particularly reports on outbreak) must also be monitored to help interpret nutritional data.

3. Feeding programmes

- Monitoring feeding centres

This monitoring requires a proper registration system in every feeding centre and is based on the monthly collection of data on programmes. They should preferably be expressed as a proportion of the total number of exits from a programme, and not the number of new admissions (which may greatly vary over time)[1].

Indicators to be monitored monthly are:
- proportion of recoveries: the most important indicator as it reflects the ultimate objective;
- proportion of deaths: reflects the quality of care;
- proportion of defaulters: reflects the level of programme compliance;
- attendance rate: reflects acceptability and accessibility of programme;
- coverage of the target group: reflects acceptability and accessibility of programme;
- average weight gain per kilo in TFP: very good indicator of the quality of the programme.

Objectives or target figures should be defined for every programme and compared with results actually obtained. Some indicative cut-off points are given in nutritional guidelines[1].

- Monitoring programme effectiveness
  The impact of the programme on the health status of the population is difficult to measure as there are many other factors which may influence malnutrition and mortality rates in the population.

IN THE POST-EMERGENCY PHASE

1. Food availability and accessibility

- Monitoring of the general food distribution should continue, based on information provided by the agencies concerned and food basket monitoring at distribution points.

- Other sources of food often complement the general ration distributed: food provided directly (e.g. farming), or indirectly by income-generating activities (jobs or small businesses). Food availability should be monitored in several ways:
  - by monitoring market availability and prices: especially for main staple foods, food with an important cultural value, protein-rich foods, etc.;
  - by information culled directly from the refugees themselves;
  - by a household food availability survey i.e. the formal weighing of available items in selected households in order to calculate the food availability per person. This method is useful for assessing other food sources, but is time-consuming and not completely reliable because it cannot account for several unknown factors (e.g. proportion of food that will be bartered, etc.). It may be a proper tool in some situations: where there is a considerable number of other sources than food distributions or where it is suspected that a large number of entitled households do not receive general rations[20].

2. Health and nutritional status

According to how the situation evolves and what resources are available, there are several options for monitoring the nutritional status:
  - nutritional surveys may still be conducted regularly (e.g. every 6 months in the post-emergency phase);
  - a set of indicators may be monitored, which could include the number of malnutrition cases (information from out-patient department records and hospital admissions), market prices, general food ration, etc. When such data reflect a degradation in the nutritional situation, a nutritional survey may be conducted to confirm this.

3. Food and nutritional situation of the local population

This should be assessed and monitored to assist decision-making in food and nutritional interventions, and provide a better understanding of the overall food system in the area.

4. Feeding programmes

If feeding programmes are still being implemented, monitoring should continue until it is decided to close them down.

✎ Key references

1. Médecins Sans Frontières. *Nutrition guidelines*. Paris: Médecins Sans Frontières, 1995.

Other references

2. Boss, L P, Toole, M, Yip, R. Assessment of mortality, morbidity and nutritional status in Somalia during the 1991-1992 famine. Recommendations for standardization of methods. *JAMA*, 1994, 272(5): 371-6.

3. CDC. Famine-affected, refugee, and displaced populations: Recommendations for public health issues. *MMWR*, 1992, 41(RR-13): 1-76.

4. Young, H, Jaspars, S. *Nutrition matters - people, food and famine*. London: Intermediate Technology Publications Ltd, 1995.

5. Jaspers, S. *Workshop on improving nutrition in refugees and displaced people in Africa*. December 1994. [draft]. Machakos, Kenya: 1995.

6. Norton, R, Nathanial, L. Quantity and quality of general ration. Workshop on the improvement of the nutrition of refugee and displaced people in Africa. Machakos, Kenya, December 1994. *ACC/SCN*, 1994.

7. WFP. *Food aid in emergencies - Book A: Policies and principles*. Rome: WFP, 1991.

8. Wilson K.B. Enhancing refugees own food acquisition strategies. *J. Ref. Studies*, 1992, 5(3/4): 226-46.

9. Toole, M J. Micronutrient deficiencies in refugees. *The Lancet*, 1992, 339(8803): 1214-6.

10. Seaman, J. Management of nutrition relief for famine affected and displaced populations. *Trop Doct*, 1991, 21(suppl 1): 38-42.

11. WFP. UNHCR. *Memorandum of understanding on the joint working arrangements for refugee, returnee and internally displaced persons feeding operations*. [s.l.]. Geneva: UNHCR, 1994.

12. *Access to food assistance: Strategies for improvement*. Washington D C: Refugee Policy Group. Centre for policy analysis and research on refugee issues. 1992.

13. Toole, M J, Nieburg, P, Waldman R J. The association between inadequate rations, undernutrition prevalence, and mortality in refugee camps: Case studies of refugee populations in Eastern Thailand, 1979-1980 and Eastern Sudan, 1984-1985. *J Trop Ped*, 1988, 24: 218-23.

14. Golden, M H, Briend, A. Treatment of malnutrition in refugee camps. *The Lancet*, 1993, 342(8867): 360.

15. Shoham, J. *Emergency supplementary feeding programmes*. London: ODI. Good Practice Review 2, 1994.

16. Toole, M J, Waldman, R J. Prevention of excess mortality in refugees and displaced populations in developing countries. *JAMA*, 1990, 263(24): 3296-302.

17. Briend, A. Treatment of severe child malnutrition in refugee camps. *Eur J Clin Nutr*, 1993, 47(10): 750-4.

18. Waterlow, J C. *Protein energy malnutrition*. Londres: Edward Arnold, 1992.

19. Malfait, P, Moren, A, Malenga, G, Stuckey, J, Jonkman, A, Gastellu-Etchegorry, M. Outbreak of pellagra among Mozambican refugees - Malawi, 1990. *MMWR* 1991, 40(13): 209-13.

20. Suetens, S, Dedeurdewaerder, M. Food availability in the refugee camp of Kahindo, Goma, Zaïre, November 1994. *Medical News*, 1994, 3(5): 16-22.

21. UNHCR. *Commodity distribution. A practical guide for field staff*. [draft]. Geneva: UNHCR, 1996.

Nutrient deficiencies

Introduction

Vitamin and other nutrient deficiencies can cause significant problems in many refugee and displaced populations dependent on food aid, especially when they flee to areas where they do not find the variety of food to which they are accustomed. Such deficiencies may result in outbreaks of scurvy (vitamin C), pellagra (niacin), beriberi (vitamin B1) and other diseases related to the vitamin B complex (vitamins B2 and B5). Deficiencies in other nutrients have also been reported, although these have not caused large-scale problems: vitamin A deficiency, iron (anaemia) and, less commonly, iodine deficiency (goitre) [1,2,3]

These deficiencies and the subsequent outbreaks of disease resulting from them are predictable and can be avoided by a good surveillance system and the prompt implementation of preventive measures. As they are clearly related to the limited nutrient content of the general food rations which are distributed, it is therefore essential to monitor the quality of the food ration and detect cases of any deficiency in the population (see Table 4.6).

The best possible preventive measure is to ensure food diversification (provision of varied items and fresh food) but this is rarely possible in emergencies. The alternatives are food fortification, the provision of fortified blended food (corn soya blend - CSB, and wheat soya blend - WSB) or vitamin supplementation (mass distribution of tablets, e.g. vitamin A)[1,2]. The latter strategy is not feasible in the long run for water-soluble vitamins (vitamins B and C) as these would have to be distributed frequently (weekly or more) because of low body storage capacity.

The general measures required to control outbreaks of disease are described in *7. Control of Communicable Diseases and Epidemics.*

Table 4.6
Major nutrient deficiencies

NUTRIENT	DEFICIENCY	RISK FACTORS
Vitamin A[5,11]	Xerophthalmia	Low vitamin A content of the general food ration, poor health and nutritional status, and measles.
Vitamin B1 *(thiamin)*	Beriberi	Ration based on polished rice.
Vitamin B2 *(riboflavin)*	Ariboflavinosis	Ration based on cereal flour unfortified with B2 (local cereal usually).
Vitamin PP or B3 *(niacin)*[5]	Pellagra	Ration based on maize with limited amount of groundnuts, fish or meat.
Vitamin C	Scurvy	Semi-desert area with limited provision of animal products (milk), fresh fruits and vegetables.
Iron[5]	Anaemia	Ration limited in meat content.
Iodine	Goitre, cretinism	Population living in area with low iodine soil content and with no iodine salt fortification of food.

Vitamin deficiencies

VITAMIN A DEFICIENCY

Cases of vitamin A deficiency have been regularly reported among refugee and displaced populations (Eastern Sudan, 1985[10], Ethiopia 1984-85[2] and 1993-94) and are mainly caused by:

– an inadequate vitamin A content in general food rations (except if red palm oil is distributed), and/or

– a poor health and nutritional status in a population, and especially the occurrence of measles, which is frequently the case in the emergency phase. Body reserves of vitamin A can be rapidly depleted under such circumstances.

This implies that general preventive measures should always be undertaken in any refugee situation (before the occurrence of any deficiency).

The clinical manifestations of vitamin A deficiency are night blindness and ocular lesions (e.g. Bitot's spots), mostly xerophthalmia, which can ultimately lead to blindness if untreated[7]. As these lesions are not easy to identify and differentiate from other ocular lesions, detection requires experienced health staff.

The prevention of vitamin A deficiency is essential to avert xerophthalmia; it also decreases the severity of other infectious diseases. It is proven that vitamin A supplementation reduces under-five mortality rates and decreases the measles case fatality rate[8].

Assessment and surveillance

In the first place, a crude estimate should be made of the vitamin A content of the general food ration as well as an assessment of food items with a high vitamin A content available on the local market that refugees can afford to buy. Any case of xerophthalmia should be recorded and notified to the health coordinating agency. In any given population, a few cases of xerophthalmia generally indicate that the vitamin A reserves of most people are depleted.

Prevention

As previously stated, efforts must be made to prevent vitamin A deficiency in any refugee population, but the presence of a general vitamin A deficiency demands especially urgent action. Intervention must be considered in both the emergency phase and the post-emergency phase.

• In the emergency phase, the recommended strategy is supplementation through a mass distribution of vitamin A to children aged from 6 months to 15 years. This is usually carried out in tandem with the measles immunization campaign (see *2. Measles Immunization*).

• In the post-emergency phase, preventive measures include mass distribution of vitamin A, drug supplementation, food fortification and food diversification. The choice of strategy is based on the vitamin A content of the general ration.

Preventive strategies in the post-emergency phase:

- Vitamin A supplementation: (see Table 4.7)
  - When the food ration contains less than 50% of the recommended daily allowance, it is recommended to undertake a mass vitamin A distribution every 4 to 6 months[1].
  - When the general ration content in vitamin A is over 50% of the recommended allowance but still inefficient, there are two possible strategies for vitamin A distribution: either through regular mass campaigns or through the child health services. Distributions through the latter channel can face two problems: strict regulation is required to avoid repeated doses, and it is likely that children aged over one year would not be properly covered because experience shows that the preventive activities of child health services are mostly attended by infants under 12 months.

Table 4.7

Vitamin A supplementation to specific groups (see appendix for doses)

SPECIFIC GROUPS	DOSE	COMMENTS
Measles cases	Two doses (400,000IU)	Decreases risk of mortality
Severe malnutrition	Treatment dose	Should not be given if therapeutic milk is used (e.g. Nutriset)
Moderate malnutrition	Preventive dose	Should not be given if red palm oil is part of the ration
Women at delivery	Preventive dose	Only given at delivery or within four weeks after delivery
Pregnant women	No supplement	Risk of teratogenic effect on foetus
Infants < 6 months	No supplement	Breast-feeding is the best source of vitamin A

There is a risk that some children may receive an excessive intake of vitamin A as a result of repeated doses, particularly in supplementary feeding programmes: they may receive doses of vitamin A during the mass campaign, at first admission in the feeding programmes or during regular readmission. This risk is higher in large feeding programmes during the emergency phase, when supervision is more difficult.

- Food fortification[1]
  Providing blended foods fortified with vitamin A in the general food ration can be a solution; however, as there is a considerable variation in the micronutrient composition of commercially blended food, it is important to verify the composition of the blended food distributed. In addition, vitamin A is quickly destroyed by heat.

- Food diversification[1]
  This is the best solution although the most difficult one to achieve in practice. Red palm oil and other food rich in vitamin A, if available, should be included in the general ration. The availability of fresh fruit (e.g. mangoes) and vegetables on the local market will also help to alleviate the problem.

- Case management

    All individuals with clinical signs of xerophthalmia should immediately receive an oral treatment of vitamin A[11]. However, the risk of vitamin A over-dosage (intra-cranial hypertension) resulting from overprescription by untrained staff must be borne in mind. Spontaneous recovery without sequelae usually takes place once the vitamin A intake is stopped.

VITAMIN B DEFICIENCIES

The vitamin B group is composed of several water-soluble vitamins. The most common deficiencies are related to vitamin B1 and result in beriberi and to niacin (vitamin PP) which can lead to pellagra. Diseases resulting from deficiencies related to other vitamin Bs, such as vitamins B2, B5 and B6, may also occur.

Vitamin B1 (thiamin) deficiency

Beriberi outbreaks have been reported regularly among refugee populations (e.g. Cambodian refugees in Thailand in 1985, Liberian refugees in Guinea in 1990)[1]. Outbreaks of beriberi are likely to occur in any population dependent on a general food ration based on polished rice with a limited quantity of legumes (nuts or beans)[1]. High case fatality rates occur among infants affected by beriberi if no prompt treatment is administered. However, these outbreaks are entirely preventable, although sporadic cases of beriberi can also occur in severely malnourished children[4].

- Assessment and surveillance

    When the general food ration is based on rice, information should be collected on the quality of the rice (degree of milling/polishing) and the amount and quality of beans or nuts distributed. If the thiamin content of the general ration is below the UNHCR recommended daily allowance (1.1 milligrammes/person/day), immediate action should be undertaken.

    Any case of beriberi should be recorded and notified to the coordinating agency. Diagnosis of beriberi should be based on a clear case definition and distinction should be made between sporadic cases occurring in a few severely malnourished children and an outbreak of beriberi reaching other groups of the population[18].

- Interventions

    1. Preventive measures should be implemented when the thiamin content of the general ration is insufficient. There are two alternatives:
        - food diversification: provision of adequate amounts of groundnuts or beans in the general food ration is the best strategy[1]; or
        - food fortification: the addition of blended food fortified with thiamin (e.g. 60 grammes/person/day of CSB) to the general food ration.

    2. When there is a confirmed outbreak of beriberi, control measures can take the form of:
        - weekly mass drug supplements to the entire population: this can be a solution for a limited period until there is an improvement in the general ration content. However, such distributions are very time-

consuming, require numerous staff, are difficult to monitor and there is a frequent problem with compliance;

– the two preventive measures previously described (provision of blended food or provision of groundnuts or beans) should also be undertaken.

In addition, a contingency stock of thiamin can be prepared to respond rapidly to any eventual outbreak of beriberi.

• Case management

Moderate beriberi cases can be treated with oral doses of thiamin (or sometimes intra-muscular); severe cases may require intravenous thiamin[4]. Patients with 'wet beriberi' respond very quickly to treatment, while peripheral neuropathy in 'dry beriberi' can prove more resistant[4].

Deficiency in niacin (Vitamin PP or B3)

Niacin deficiency leads to pellagra which can be fatal and is often associated with other vitamin B deficiencies[18]. The clinical picture is characterized by a dry dermatitis, followed by diarrhoea and dementia as the disease progresses. Pellagra outbreaks can occur in refugee and displaced populations dependent on food rations based on maize and containing insufficient quantities of groundnuts. A large-scale pellagra outbreak occurred among Mozambican refugees in Malawi (1989 and 1990)[16,17] and pellagra cases have been reported in several refugee camps (Zimbabwe, Angola and Nepal in 1993)[1]. It affects principally adults, particularly women[16,17].

• Assessment and surveillance

In a population dependent on a general food ration based on maize, the niacin content must be monitored and immediate action taken if it is below the recommended allowance (15mg /person /day). Any suspected case of pellagra must be monitored. Suspected cases should be confirmed and a clear case definition established.

• Intervention

1. When the niacin content of the general ration is insufficient, preventive measures should be taken before any case of pellagra appears. These may take the form of:

– food fortification, which is the most practical and effective strategy for preventing pellagra in emergency situations via the provision of niacin-fortified food, generally blended cereals. In the post-emergency phase, the fortification of maize flour can be also effective, as was seen in Malawi in 1991[1]; or

– food diversification, which can be achieved by providing groundnuts, dried fish or meat in the food ration[1]. In practice, the provision of groundnuts is feasible but the provision of dried fish or meat will be very difficult to achieve. Another alternative is to include fortified blended food (CSB) into the general ration. However, the inclusion of 60g of standard CSB in the general ration will only provide between 30% to 40% of the recommended daily allowance[1].

2. In case of an outbreak of pellagra, a weekly mass drug supplementation of niacin and vitamin B complex could be given to the entire population,

but this can only be recommended when a large confirmed outbreak occurs and then only for a limited period of time (until an improvement in the general ration composition) [1]; supplementation is generally not feasible in the long term because of similar problems to those mentioned in regard to vitamin B1 interventions (large resources required, time-consuming, difficult to monitor and poor compliance).

- Case management

It is recommended that patients receive a simultaneous oral treatment of niacin and vitamin B complex because of the common association of a niacin deficiency with other vitamin B deficiencies [18]. Patients usually respond to treatment within 10 to 14 days.

Other Vitamin B deficiencies

Outbreaks of other vitamin B deficiencies have been reported in refugee populations: vitamin B2 (ariboflavinosis) in Afghanistan, 1994, and vitamin B5 (nutritional neuropathy) in Afghanistan, 1993[15]. As these deficiencies are often found in association, the clinical picture may cover a large spectrum of signs: neuropathy with burning feet syndrome, glossitis, conjunctivitis, angular stomatitis, etc. However, one of these symptoms will generally be dominant. These outbreaks are probably under-reported because the symptoms are non-specific and may be masked by other deficiencies, or the clinical signs are assumed to be due to other causes.

The main recommendation in regard to these deficiencies is to be aware that a sudden increase in the number of cases of stomatitis, conjunctivitis, glossitis, burning feet syndrome and other signs of neuropathy could be linked to vitamin B deficiencies. Confirmation of the deficiency is required before any intervention is undertaken.

Vitamin B2 deficiency is likely to occur in a population dependent on a food ration based on refined cereal - if this is not fortified with riboflavin and - if it contains only a small amount of beans or nuts[6]. Related mortality seems very rare. The population groups at higher risk are schoolchildren and pregnant or lactating women. The specific symptom associated with vitamin B2 deficiency is a type of glossitis (purplish red tongue)[6]. Patients usually respond well to an oral administration of vitamin B complex[18].

Outbreaks of vitamin B5 and B6 deficiencies can occur in a population dependent on well-refined and unfortified cereal containing a high proportion of carbohydrate compared to fat and proteins. The group most at risk seems to be women[15].

- Intervention

In case of outbreak:
- treatment of individual cases and mass supplementation of vitamin B complex are only temporary responses;
- food fortification is the most convenient solution either through fortification of the cereal flour or provision of fortified blended food;
- in the longer term: well-refined or polished cereals should be avoided and the quality of the ration improved with respect to the proportion of carbohydrates, fats and proteins.

VITAMIN C DEFICIENCY

Vitamin C is a water-soluble and very unstable vitamin, quickly destroyed by heat and air. Deficiency of vitamin C leads to scurvy. Outbreaks of scurvy have occurred in several refugee populations: Somalia (1982, 1985, 1989), Ethiopia (1988, 1993), Sudan (1984, 1989), Kenya (1992 to 94), etc.

Risk factors: scurvy outbreaks are likely to occur in arid areas, especially during the dry season, when refugees have been settled for a few months and have only limited access to fresh fruits, vegetable or milk on the local market[19,20,21]. Clinical cases of scurvy will usually be observed when the daily intake of vitamin C is below 10 to 15mg and this is likely to occur when people are entirely dependent on general food distributions[1,20]. The main groups at risk seem to be women of child-bearing age (especially during pregnancy) and the elderly [1,19,20].

Assessment and surveillance

A clear case definition of scurvy should be established for an area at risk: for instance, bleeding gums and painful joints. Scurvy should be included in the routine surveillance system, and must be notified to the health coordinating agency. A general vitamin C deficiency can be assumed where a few scurvy cases occur in a population in a high risk situation, e.g. in arid areas (Horn of Africa), where the diet contains few fresh products, etc.

Preventive measures

Vitamin C outbreaks are predictable, but efficient preventive measures remain a complex issue, because of the instability of the vitamin and the low body storage capacities.

- In situations where there is risk of a vitamin C deficiency, the following options are available:
  - Drug supplementation to vulnerable groups (women, children and the elderly): this can be effected through existing feeding programmes, if in place. Another strategy is through the weekly distribution to women via ante and post-natal consultations, but compliance is usually limited.
  - Food fortification[1]: fortification of cereal is not effective because most of the vitamin C is destroyed by cooking. Fortified blended food (with a high vitamin C content) can be a solution if not cooked to the extent that it no longer retains a sufficient residual amount of vitamin C. It cannot be stored for lengthy periods. More research is needed to measure the real impact and feasibility of this solution.
  - Food diversification: the provision of fresh fruit, vegetables or milk is the best solution to the problem. Scurvy outbreaks may be avoided where refugees are able to obtain fresh food on the local market. In arid areas, where the availability of these products is limited, the agencies in charge of the food supply are rarely able to provide them. The provision of longer-lasting vegetables would however be of interest as a research option. Promotion of vegetable cultivation is also recommended as a long-term solution but is not easy to implement (e.g. arid areas or a nomadic population). A few experimental programmes, involving the

distribution of vegetable seeds, have been reported: for instance, in the Sarahoui camps in Algeria, collective gardens have been set up, requiring water desalination and an irrigation system.

- In case of a scurvy outbreak:
    - Mass vitamin C drug supplementation may be considered. However, such distributions have to be carried out on a daily basis to be effective, which is unpractical on a large scale. Weekly or bi-weekly distributions can be considered, but in Somalia (1985-87) and Kenya (1992), these had a limited impact mainly due to poor compliance[1,3,20].

Case management

Scurvy can be fatal if untreated but cases usually respond well to oral treatment. After recovery, a weekly preventive dose can be given for a few weeks. It should be borne in mind that vitamin C deficiency increases the risk of anaemia.

Mineral deficiencies

IRON DEFICIENCY

Iron deficiency is probably the most prevalent nutrient deficiency occurring in refugee populations all over the world. The lack of animal products in the usual refugee food ration is also a risk factor[1].

Iron deficiency, frequently associated with folate deficiency, leads to nutritional anaemia and is responsible for well over half the total number of all anaemia cases (worldwide prevalence of about 30%)[18,22].

Two other major causes of anaemia are malaria and hookworm, however, a good differential diagnosis of the causes of anaemia is rarely possible in the field[26]. Nutritional anaemia can be exacerbated as a result of parasitic infections, food taboos and the practice of other traditional beliefs[23].

Pregnant and lactating women, and children aged between 9 and 36 months are at most risk as they have higher iron needs[24].

Assessment and surveillance

When high number of cases of clinical anaemia are observed in health facilities, additional information has to be collected on the diet available[1]. However, iron deficiency is considered an important problem in any refugee population and action should always be taken to alleviate it.

Intervention

In any situation, high risk groups should receive iron supplementation.

- Pregnant and lactating women should be given iron supplements (and folic acid) from the fourth month of pregnancy on via supplementary rations or ante and post-natal care. The frequent problems of poor compliance can be reduced through education and follow-up by home-visitors or traditional birth attendants (TBAs)[11,22].

- Severely malnourished children should not receive iron supplements during the first two weeks of admission to a therapeutic feeding centre because of the increased risk of infections. Folic acid, however, should be given from the first day of admission[12].
- Regarding the moderately malnourished, the administration of iron supplements is still under discussion.

When larger target groups are considered, the choice of strategy to be employed depends on disease patterns (i.e. other causes of anaemia) and the resources available.

- Fortification: fortified blended food (e.g. CSB CSM) can be included in the general rations. The recommended daily allowance may be provided by 60g of blended food (except for pregnant and lactating women who require additional amounts) [1].
- Mass supplementation: mass distributions of iron supplements are usually not recommended because of practical problems resulting from the size of the population and the side effects [25].
- Diversification: this can be achieved via the routine provision of meat in food rations. However, this is rarely feasible on a large scale [1].

Case management

The management of clinical anaemia requires first of all the identification of its probable cause[26].

- In anaemia due to iron deficiency, the most effective treatment is the oral administration of ferrous sulphate for at least two months (ideally two months after normalization of the haemoglobin). Supplements of vitamin C also improve iron absorption. Parenteral iron therapy is not indicated[18]. Folate and iron supplements are usually given in association due to the frequent simultaneous presence of both deficiencies. Other associated parasitic infections should be treated at the same time.
- In anaemia due to malaria, antimalarial drugs will be administrated as a priority; folate should be given, but iron is generally not recommended (unless an associated iron deficiency is confirmed)[26]. Blood transfusion should be limited to life saving measures, because of difficulties of organizing safe transfusions in refugee settings. It is imperative to restrict its use to strict indications, and systematically perform HIV testing (see also *HIV, AIDS and STD* in Part III).

IODINE DEFICIENCY

Iodine deficiency disorders (IDD) exist in many regions of the world, especially in mountains and river deltas where levels of soil iodine are low. Nearly 30% of the world's population lives in such iodine-deficient environments[27]. Goitrogens in local diets (such as thiocyanate in cassava) contribute to and reinforce the IDD problem but they are generally not the primary cause. IDD presents a broad clinical spectrum: cretinism, retarded psycho-motor development in children and goitre.

IDD is rarely reported in refugee and displaced populations, probably because of its low priority in emergencies, but this health problem may be underestimated[24]. IDD is likely to be a problem when refugees settle in an iodine-deficient area. The refugee situation is not an additional risk factor in itself unless the food basket has a limited iodine content. An IDD control programme will not appear on the priority list in the emergency phase.

Assessment and surveillance

When refugees are in an area at risk, an assessment of the problem in the host population may be undertaken in the post-emergency phase. The information gathered should cover any national control programmes, the prevalence of IDD in the population, the availability of iodine (seafood or iodized salt)[28] and the presence of goitrogens in the local food basket. This data will be used for deciding whether or not there are potential IDD problems among the refugee population.

If a longer stay in an area at risk is expected, an evaluation of the IDD prevalence in the refugee population may be carried out through the interpretation of two main indicators[28].

1. The goitre prevalence rate, estimated via clinical examination, is a sensitive indicator. Surveys are commonly carried out in schoolchildren, as they represent one of the most vulnerable groups.
2. Urinary iodine is a useful indicator for confirming the problem as it is the most practical and sensitive biochemical test although difficult to organize and not essential for decision-making[29].

Intervention

According to IDD/WHO guidelines, once the goitre prevalence exceeds 5% in children of school age, the population can be considered to have an iodine deficiency and intervention should be considered[28].

- Periodic administration of iodized oil (oral or by injection) to the most vulnerable groups (children under five, school pupils and women of child-bearing age) is the best choice as a short-term strategy and can be included in MCH activities[30,31].

- The iodization of salt is the least expensive and the safest programme for the prevention and control of IDD[27,28]. The absence of a national salt iodization programme complicates this, but the presence of a general food distribution network may facilitate it. A key issue is the availability of iodized salt, and health agencies have a role to play in lobbying WFP and other agencies in charge of food supply to ensure that it is included in food rations.

Case management

Cretinism can be prevented, but not treated, by giving prophylaxis to pregnant women. Goitres can be treated by the oral administration of iodine. Surgery should not be considered, except in rare cases with severe complications or where malignancy is suspected[26].

Principal recommendations regarding nutrition

- Food and nutritional assessment should always be part of the initial assessment.

- The objectives of nutritional interventions are to ensure an adequate food ration for all; to treat severely and moderately malnourished persons; to prevent malnutrition in vulnerable groups.

- The general food ration should be adequate in quantity and in quality (nutrient content). The main factors required for successful and regular distribution are: political willingness, adequate planning of the food supply, registration of population, good organization of the distribution, regular monitoring.

- Vitamin and other nutrient deficiencies can cause significant problems in populations dependent in food aid. The outbreaks of nutrient deficiencies are predictable and can be avoided. The monitoring of the quality of food rations and the prompt detection of cases of any deficiency are essential. The best preventive measure is food diversification, alternatives are food fortification and mass suplementation.

- The selective nutritional interventions involve 3 main types of programmes:
  - therapeutic feeding programmes to treat the severely malnourished,
  - targeted supplementary feeding programmes to treat the moderately malnourished,
  - blanket supplementary feeding programmes to prevent malnutrition in vulnerable groups (under-five population, pregnant and lactating women, social and medical cases, etc.).
  These programmes require clear definition of the criteria for admission and discharge, a logical coherence between the different selective feeding programmes, and an effective screening method.

- The choice of selective nutritional interventions is based on the quantity and quality of the general food ration, the prevalence of malnutrition and aggravating factors such as high mortality, outbreaks, climate, population instability.

- Nutritional surveillance and monitoring of programmes are essential to evaluate and adapt the interventions. This surveillance will cover 3 sectors: food availability and accessibility, health and nutritional status, effectiveness of the selective feeding programme.

🔖 Key references

1. Toole, M J. *Preventing micronutrient deficiency diseases. Workshop on the improvement of the nutrition of refugees and displaced people in Africa, Machakos, Kenya,* Kenya: 1994.

2. Rigal, J. Actualité de carences vitaminiques historiques parmi les populations réfugiées ou deplacées. *Santé Développement,* 1993, 106: 4-7.

Other references

3. Toole, M J. Micronutrient deficiencies in refugees. *The Lancet*, 1992, 339(8803): 1214-6.

4. Garrow, J S, James, W P T. *Human nutrition and diet. Fat-soluble vitamins and water-soluble vitamins*. London: Churchill Livingstone, 1993. 208-38.

5. UNHCR. *Food aid and nutrition 'briefing kit'*. Working document, update, October 1993. Geneva: UNHCR, Division of Programmes and Operational Support, 1993.

6. Warren, K S, Mahmoud, A A F. *Tropical and geographical medicine*. New York: McGraw-Hill Inc, 1990.

7. WHO. *La lutte contre la carence en vitamin A et la xérophtalmie*. Proposal of WHO/FISE/USAID/IVACG/Helen Keller. Geneva: WHO, 1982. Série de rapports techniques No. 672.

8. Beaton, G, Martorell, R, et al. *Effectiveness of vitamin A supplementation in the control of young child morbidity and mortality in developing countries*. ACC/SCN. Nutrition Policy Discussion Paper No. 13, 1993.

9. Hathcock, J N, Hattan, D G, Jenkins M Y, McDonald J T, Sundaresan, P R, Wilkening, V L. Evaluation of vitamin A toxicity. *Am J Clin Nutr*, 1990, 52: 183-202.

10. Nieburg, P, Waldmann, R J, Leavell, R, Sommer, A, DeMaeyer E M. Vitamin A supplementation for refugees and famine victims. *WHO Bull*, 1988, 66(6):689-97.

11. WHO/FISE/IVACG. *Suppléments en vitamine A. Guide pour leur emploi dans le traitement et la prévention de la carence en vitamin A et de la xérophtamie*. Geneva: WHO, 1989.

12. Médecins Sans Frontières. *Nutrition guidelines*. Paris: Médecins Sans Frontières, 1995.

13. Briend, A. A personal communication.

14. Médecins Sans Frontières. *Essential drugs - Practical guidelines*. Paris: Médecins Sans Frontières, 1993.

15. Bigot, A, Chauvin, P, Moren, A. *Epidemic of nutritional neuropathy in Afganistan, April 1994*. Internal report. Paris:Epicentre, 1994.

16. Malfait, P, Moren, A, Malenga, G, Stuckey, J, Jonkman, A, Etchegorry, M. Outbreak of pellagra among Mozambican refugees, Malawi 1990. *MMWR*, 1991, 40(13): 209-13.

17. Malfait, P. *Pellagra outbreak among Mozambican refugees, Malawi 1990*. [Internal report]. Paris: Epicentre, 1990.

18. Cook, G. *Manson's tropical diseases*. 19th edition. London: Saunders, 1996.

19. Nutrition - Scurvy and food aid among refugees in the Horn of Africa. *Wkly Epidemiol Rec*, 1989, 64(12): 85-92.

20. Desenclos, J C, Berry, A M, Padt, R, Farah, B, Segala, C, Nabil, A M. Epidemiological patterns of scurvy among Ethiopian refugees. *WHO Bull*, 1989, 67(3): 309-16.

21. Philips, M P. *Investigation of a scurvy outbreak among displaced Dinka population in South Darfur, Sudan, July-August 1989*. Dissertation for the Diploma in Epidemiology. London: Faculty of Public Health Medicine, 1993.

22. International Nutritional Anemia Consultative Group. *Guidelines on maternal nutritional anaemia*. INACG, 1989.

23. WHO. *Iron supplementation during pregnancy: Why aren't women complying? A review of available information*. Geneva: WHO, 1990. WHO/MCH/90.5.

24. CDC. Famine-affected, refugee, and displaced populations: Recommendations for public health issues. *MMWR*, 1992, 41(RR-13): 1-76.

25. Idjradinata, P, Watkins, W E, Pollitt, E. Adverse effects of iron supplementation on weight gain of iron-replete young children. *The Lancet*, 1994, 343: 1252-54.

26. Médecins Sans Frontières. *Clinical guidelines, diagnostic and treatment manual*. Paris: Hatier, 1993.

27. Underwood, B. Current status of iodine deficiency disorders: A global perspective. *NU News on Health Care in Developing countries*, 1994, 8: 4-7.

28.   ICCIDD. Indicators for tracking progress in IDD elimination. *IDD Newsletter*, 1994, 10(4):37-40.

29.   Dunn, J T, ICCIDD. Techniques for measuring urinary iodine - An update. *IDD Newsletter*, 1993, 9(4):40-3.

30.   Eltom, M, Karlsson, F A, et al. The effectiveness of oral iodized oil in the treatment and prophylaxis of endemic goitre. *J Clin Endocrinol Metab*, 1985, 61(6): 1112-7.

31.   Moreno Reyes, R, Tibin, S H, Elbadawi, S A, Boelaert, M, et al. Iodine deficiency control by the health area management team of Wadi Saleh district, Western Sudan. *IDD Newsletter*, 1990, 6(3).

5. Shelter and site planning

Introduction

Refugees arriving in any specific area tend to settle down in different ways: often, they concentrate on an unoccupied site and create a 'camp'; at other times, they spread out over a wide area and establish rural settlements; and sometimes they are hosted by local communities (rural or urban). The latter two situations, also called 'open situations', occur less frequently than the first (see below and the *Introduction* to Part II).

A poorly planned refugee settlement is one of the most pathogenic environments possible. Overcrowding and poor hygiene are major factors in the transmission of diseases with epidemic potential (measles, meningitis, cholera, etc.). The lack of adequate shelter means that the population is deprived of all privacy and constantly exposed to the elements (rain, cold, wind, etc.). In addition, the surrounding environment may have a pronounced effect on refugee health, particularly if it is very different from the environment from which they have come (e.g. presence of vectors carrying diseases not previously encountered)[4].

Camps usually present a higher risk than refugee settlements in open situations as there is more severe overcrowding, and less likelihood that basic facilities, such as water supply and health care services, will be available when refugees first arrive[2,7]. Relief work is more difficult to organize for very large camp populations, such as some of the Rwandan refugee camps in Zaire (Goma, 1994) which contained more than 100,000 refugees.

In order to reduce health risks, it is essential that site planning and organization takes place as early as possible so that overcrowding is minimized and efficient relief services are provided. Shelters must be provided as rapidly as possible to protect refugees from the environment, and infrastructure installed for the necessary health and nutrition facilities, water supply installations, latrines, etc. All this must be initiated within the first week of intervention[3].

Relief agencies are usually faced with one of two possible situations: either the camp is already established with a refugee population that has spontaneously settled on a site prior to the arrival of relief agencies, or site planning is possible prior to their arrival, for example, when they are being transferred to a new camp.

Whichever is the case, prompt action must be undertaken to improve the site and its facilities; poor organization in the early stages may lead to a chaotic and potentially irreversible situation in regard to camp infrastructure, with consequent health risks. For example, lateral expansion of a site must be accounted for from the beginning in order to avoid overcrowding if refugee numbers increase.

Two possibilities: a refugee camp or integration into the host population

There is always a lot of discussion as to whether the formation of a refugee camp is acceptable, or whether resources would be better directed to supporting local communities who host refugees. The two main types of refugee settlement - camp or integration into the local population - each offer both advantages and disadvantages as laid out in Table 5.1:

Table 5.1
Camp or integration into the local population:
advantages and disadvantages[7,8]

	CAMP	INTEGRATION
ADVANTAGES	– provides asylum and protection – more suitable for temporary situation – easier to estimate population numbers, to assess needs and monitor health status – some basic services are easier to organize (e.g. distributions, mass vaccinations) – allows visibility and advocacy – repatriation will be easier to plan	– favours refugee mobility, easy access to alternative food, jobs, etc. – encourages refugee survival strategies – possibility of refugee access to existing facilities (water, health etc.) – enhances reconstruction of social/ economic life and better integration in the future
DISADVANTAGES	– overcrowding increases risk of outbreaks of communicable diseases – dependence on external aid, lack of autonomy – social isolation – little possibility of realizing farming initiatives – degradation of the surrounding environment – security problems within the camp – not a durable solution	– population more difficult to reach, leading to difficulties in monitoring health needs – implementation of relief programmes more complex, requires knowledge of local situation – risks destabilizing the local community, risk of tensions between local community and refugees

Health agencies are generally not involved in deciding between the two options. Every refugee situation is specific to itself. The main factors influencing the way in which they eventually settle are the number of refugees, the capacity for the local community to absorb them, the ethnic and cultural links between the refugee and local communities and the political and military situation. In practice, the predominant factor is the relationship between refugees and the local population.

It should, however, be pointed out that relief programmes, particularly food aid, may well play a role in attracting refugees into a camp situation even when integration would probably be a better option for them.

It is camp situations that are dealt with more specifically here, because camp populations are exposed to greater health risks. However, most of the principles described below may also be applied to open situations.

Site planning

Site planning must ensure the most rational organization of space, shelters and the facilities required for the provision of essential goods and services. This requires supervision by experts (e.g. in sanitation, geology, construction, etc.) which must be integrated into the planning of other sectors, especially water and sanitation[2]. It is therefore essential that there is coordination from the beginning between all the agencies involved and between the different sectors of activity, especially in an emergency situation when time is generally in short supply.

Site planning in refugee situations is normally the responsibility of UNHCR (or an agency delegated by UNHCR). As UNHCR is usually not present where there is an internally displaced settlement, another agency will have to take charge. Although health agencies will not always be involved in organizing a site, they should nevertheless make sure that this is undertaken correctly because of its direct influence on the subsequent health situation; it is therefore necessary to have an understanding of the basic principles of site planning.

As stated above, the possibilities in regard to site planning depend largely on which of the two refugee situations described will be encountered.

1. In most cases refugees have already settled on a site and planners may well be faced with chaotic conditions. The immediate priority must be to improve or reorganize the existing site, and in rare instances it may even be advisable to move the refugee population to another site (see below, page 120).

2. The ideal but far less frequently encountered situation is that where site planning can be carried out before the arrival of refugees on a new site. The most appropriate site layout may then be worked out in advance and in accordance with guidelines.

In both situations, the following principles must be respected as far as possible.

- Sufficient space must be provided for everybody: space for every family to settle with the provision of amenities (water and latrines) and other services, and access to every sector. High density camps should be avoided because they present a higher risk for disease transmission, fire and security problems[2].

- Short-term site planning should be avoided as so-called temporary camps may well have to remain much longer than expected (e.g. some Palestinian refugee camps have been in existence since 1947)[2]. This means that consideration must be given to the possibilities for expansion should the population increase[1].

- A few small camps (ideally *circa* 10,000 people) are preferable to one large camp because they are easier to manage and because they favour a return to self-sufficiency[2]. Unfortunately, this is rarely possible when there is a massive influx of refugees (e.g. the refugee movements in Rwanda and Burundi, 1993-94).
- Refugees should be involved and consulted. Their social organization and their opinions should be taken into account wherever possible.
- Local resources (human and material) and local standards should be employed whenever feasible. Seasonal changes (e.g. the rainy season) must also be taken into consideration.

SITE SELECTION

The ideal site, responding to all requirements, is rarely available. The choice is generally limited, as the most appropriate areas will already be inhabited by local communities or given over to farming. In any case, relief agencies are seldom on the spot to select a site before refugees arrive.

However, there are certain criteria in regard to site selection which must still be taken into account[1,9].

- Security and protection: the settlement must be in a safe area (e.g. free of mines), at a reasonable distance from the border, and from any war zones.
- Water: water must be available either on the site or close by (see *3. Water and Sanitation*).
- Space: the area must be large enough to ensure 30m[2] per person (see Table 5.2).
- Accessibility: access to the site must be possible during all the seasons (e.g. for trucks).
- Environmental health risks: the proximity of vector breeding sites transmitting killer diseases should be avoided as far as possible (e.g. tsetse fly for trypanosomiasis). Where such areas cannot be avoided, they must be treated (see *3. Water and Sanitation*).
- Local population: every effort should be made to avoid tensions arising between local and refugee communities; for instance, legal and traditional land rights must be respected.
- It is important that the terrain should slope in order to provide natural drainage for rain water off the site[4].

Energy sources should also be considered when selecting a site, particularly as deforestation resulting from using wood for cooking fuel entails politico-ecological problems.

SITE ORGANIZATION

Once the site has been secured, the planning and location of the required infrastructure must be worked out. A map should be used and the road network drawn onto it. The area should then be divided into sections and locations decided for the different facilities. Good access by road to every section and each installation is essential for the transport of staff and materials (e.g. food and drugs) in order to ensure the different services are able to function.

Several factors should be taken into account in deciding the spatial organization of facilities and shelters (location and layout):

– space required per person and for each installation,
– accessibility of services,
– minimum distance required between facilities and shelters(see Table 5.2),
– cultural habits and social organization of the refugee population (clans and extended families),
– ethnic and security factors, relationships among different sections/ members of the community, etc.

Cultural and social traditions are a determining factor in ensuring refugee acceptance of the infrastructure and services provided, particularly in regard to housing, sanitation, burial places, etc. However, as the layout that might be preferred by the refugees is not always the one that would allow the most efficient delivery of aid, site planning generally requires compromise solutions that take into account the different points of view[2].

Table 5.2
Some quantified norms for site planning[1,2]

Area available per person	30m²
Shelter space per person	3.5m²
Number of people per water point	250
Number of people per latrine	20
Distance to water-point	150m max.
Distance to latrine	30m
Distance between water-point and latrine	100m
Firebreaks	75m every 300m
Distance between two shelters	2m min.

ESSENTIAL INSTALLATIONS

(see *10. Coordination: Camp management*)

Essential installations are described in Table 5.3. Some are likely to be centralized:

– reception centre,
– health centre,
– hospital,
– meeting place for home-visitors, etc.

Other facilities, such as health posts, latrines, washing areas, etc., should be decentralized. Care must be taken to ensure that there is sufficient space for such decentralized services in all the camp sub-divisions.

Table 5.3
Main installations required on refugee sites
(see *10. Coordination: Camp management*)

- Roads and firebreaks.

- Water supply and sanitation facilities (defecation areas, latrines, waste disposal pits, washing places, etc.).

- Health facilities: health centre, health posts, hospital, pharmacy and site for cholera camp.

- Meeting place for home-visitors.

- Nutritional facilities: therapeutic and supplementary feeding centres.

- Distribution site and storage facilities (in separate locations).

- Administrative centre, reception area.

- Other community facilities: market, schools, cemetery, meeting places, etc.

The location of health facilities must be carefully determined (see *6. Health Care in the Emergency Phase*).

• The central health facility should be located in a safe and accessible place, preferably on the periphery of the site in order to avoid overcrowding and allow for future expansion. The space required depends on the type and desired capacity of the medical services to be provided.

• The hospital, if one is necessary, is usually an expansion of the in-patient service of the central facility. The criteria are thus similar but more space is required (in line with the number of beds). It is particularly important to plan space for water and sanitation facilities, as well as room for eventual expansion (e.g. outbreaks of disease).

• The peripheral health facilities should be centrally located within the areas they are to serve so as to ensure easy access. The number required depends mainly on the size of the population (e.g. 1 health post per 3,000-5,000 refugees).

• A site for a cholera camp must be identified in advance, separate from other health facilities. It must be large enough to ensure sufficient capacity for potential needs and be provided with adequate water and sanitation facilities[6].

THE LAYOUT OF SHELTERS

The way shelters are grouped has an important influence on the re-establishment of social life, on the use of latrines and water-points, and on security.

In general, the site should be divided into smaller units for management purposes. For example, it could be divided into sectors of 5,000 and sections of 1,000 people. However, the formation of such units must take into account the existence of any groups within the population which may be mutually hostile.

Two main ways of grouping shelters are described:

1. The preferred method is to organize the site into basic community units, constituted by a number of shelters and community facilities (latrines, water-points and washing areas)[1,3]. These basic units should correspond in design as closely as possible to that with which the refugees are most familiar. Examples for designing such community units are available in several reference books[2,4,9].

2. Laying out shelters in lines and rows is another possibility, but is usually not recommended because this deprives families of personal space, and increases the distances to latrines and water-points. On the other hand, such a layout can be implemented quickly and is often preferred when there is a sudden and massive influx of refugees to cope with.

Since in most cases the population will have settled on a site before any site planning can be carried out, solutions will have to be sought for improving the situation.

• Usually, the site may be improved without moving all the shelters. A better organization of facilities, improving access to all sections of the camp, and carefully planning sections for new arrivals will decrease health risks and improve camp management.

• A thorough reorganization of the site (and most shelters) may sometimes be necessary, although radical change is usually not advised. Such reorganization should be considered when there is a real threat to refugee health from overcrowding or a danger of fire, etc. For example, it was decided to move and reorganize all shelters in the Rwandan camps for refugees from Burundi in 1993, in order to counter the high fire risk and to facilitate the management of relief assistance.

• Critical problems, such as a lack of water in the area, insecurity or potential danger resulting from the camp's proximity to the border, may present major obstacles to the camp remaining where it is. A move to a new site could then be considered, but the operational problems involved in a move and the social and psychological consequences for the population must be carefully weighed up in advance.

Shelter provision

The objectives of providing shelters are: protection against the elements and against vectors, provision of sufficient housing space for families, and restoring a sense of privacy and security. Shelters are required in every refugee emergency; but the type and design of shelter, who constructs it and how long it should last will vary in every situation[2].

However, some general principles may be concluded[2]:

- Shelters that have already been built by refugees or buildings occupied by them (e.g. schools) must be assessed. It is important that consideration is given to the amount of space available for each person, to ventilation (e.g. risk of respiratory infection) and for protection against rain, as these factors may entail signficiant health risks.

- Wherever possible, refugees should construct their own shelters and should receive material (including appropriate tools) and technical support to assist them in doing so.

- It is best to use suitable local materials where available. Special emergency shelters (e.g. tents) and pre-fabricated units have not yet proven practical because of their high cost and the problems of transporting them. It is also difficult to persuade refugees to accept something which is not within their cultural traditions. However, some types of prefabricated shelter are still being tested and may be suitable for use in the first weeks of an emergency.

- A minimum sheltering space of 3.5m[2] per person is recommended in an emergency. However, different cultures have different needs.

- Single-family shelters are preferable (unless multi-family units are traditional).

WHEN REFUGEES FIRST ARRIVE

The provision of shelter is a high priority. Immediate action should be taken to assess the arrangements already made and provide material for temporary shelters[2].

There are several common solutions for temporary shelters:

- shelters built by the refugees themselves, with material found locally or distributed by agencies, is the most common solution;

- tents may be useful when local material is not available and as very short term accommodation, but they are expensive and do not last long;

- plastic sheeting may be used for constructing temporary shelters or to protect them. Methods for setting up plastic temporary shelters are described in guidelines[5];

- local public buildings, such as schools, may provide shelter initially but are not usually suitable for large numbers. They are a very temporary solution.

THE POST-EMERGENCY PHASE

Temporary shelters should no longer be used after the emergency stage has passed, an early start must be made to constructing shelters made of more permanent material.

However, it must be acknowledged that there are certain constraints involved in such shelter construction programmes[10].

- Any shelter building or rehabilitation programme takes time.

- Such programmes are costly (although they may produce savings in other sectors).

- As there is a vast range of options for building shelters, and a wide range of criteria have to be taken into account, such programmes are complex to manage. This is a specialized job and requires expertise.

This can often become a highly political issue with local authorities obstructing the building of (semi-)permanent housing when they want to prevent refugees settling for a long period of time.

Longer-term housing should be similar to that with which refugees are already familiar, but should also reflect local conditions[2]. The use of local material is preferable, but its availability may be problematic (e.g. degradation of the environment through deforestation).

In countries such as Afghanistan or the countries of Eastern Europe, where very low temperatures may be experienced in winter, shelter provision is essential for protection against the cold. Although a few solutions have been proposed (e.g. winter tents and the provision of heaters), this is a particularly difficult problem to deal with in an emergency situation.

Once time allows, traditional housing may be built, if the materials are available, and there are sufficient financial resources.

Principal recommendations regarding shelter and site planning

- Site planning and improvement should take place as early as possible in order to minimize overcrowding and make it possible to organize efficient relief services.

- A site should be selected with a view to security, access to water, the provision of adequate space, environmental health risks, and the local population.

- Site planning must ensure the most rational organization of the available space in regard to shelters and the necessary facilities and installations. Where refugees have already settled on a site before any planning could be envisaged, it is not usually advisable to institute radical changes, but improvements and reorganization should be carried out.

- Small sites are preferred. The cultural and social patterns should be taken into account.

- The provision of material for temporary shelters is a high priority when refugees first arrive. These should preferably be single-family shelters, constructed out of local material (when available) by the refugees themselves.

Key references

1. Médecins Sans Frontières. *Public health engineering in emergency situations*. Paris: Médecins Sans Frontières, 1994.

2. UNHCR. *Handbook for Emergencies*. Geneva: UNHCR, 1982.

Other references

3. Toole, M J, Waldman, R J. Prevention of excess mortality in refugees and displaced populations in developing countries. *JAMA*, 1990, 263(24): 3296-302.

4. Simmonds, S, Vaughan, P, William Gunn, S. *Refugee community health care*. Oxford: Oxford University Press, 1983.

5. Oxfam. *Plastic sheeting*. Oxford: Oxfam, 1989.

6. Médecins Sans Frontières. *Prise en charge d'une épidémie de choléra en camp de réfugié*. Paris, Médecins Sans Frontières, 1995.

7. Harell-Bond, B, Leopold, M. *Counting the refugees: The myth of accountability*. [Symposium] London: Refugee Studies Programme, 1993.

8. Van Damme, W. Do refugees belong in camps? Experiences from Goma and Guinea. *The Lancet*, 1995, 346(8971): 360-2.

9. Kent Harding D. *Camp planning*. [draft]. Geneva: UNHCR, 1987.

10. Govaerts, P. *Report on UNHCR shelter workshop, February 1993*. [Internal report]. Brussels: Médecins Sans Frontières, 1993.

6. Health care in the emergency phase

Introduction

The health status of refugee and displaced populations arriving in a camp may still be relatively good (or may already have deteriorated considerably). This will depend on the reasons behind their flight, whether it was precipitated by sudden, dramatic events, a more chronic situation or a famine, and on the duration and hardships of the flight itself. No matter what their condition on arrival, new refugee camps usually provide a very unhealthy environment; indeed, the typical overcrowding, poor water supply and sanitation, and lack of food are the three main underlying factors of high morbidity. In addition, the lack of immunity to new diseases and the psycho-social stress of displacement make refugees more vulnerable to health problems. These factors alone, or in addition to an existing poor health status, are responsible for the excess mortality so often encountered in the emergency phase of refugee situations[16]. They will therefore have to be controlled by a number of public health measures that are described in other chapters. Major interventions, such as the provision of water, food and shelter, make a major contribution towards decreasing excess mortality, but they cannot be implemented very quickly and do not have an immediate impact[1]. It is therefore very important to rapidly provide basic health care as an early measure in any refugee emergency, with the major focus on curative services. Health care can be implemented quickly, and takes effect immediately provided it is well organized and targets priority diseases.

Objectives

The objectives are to help reduce excess mortality and morbidity in the refugee population by ensuring appropriate medical care for all refugees and responding to epidemics.

Health care system

There is no single model for setting up health services in a refugee settlement: this will depend on the specific context, disease patterns, possible outbreaks, the resources available and existing health facilities. However, the model selected should be based on the knowledge that 50% to 95% of the mortality in refugee situations is caused by only four communicable diseases: diarrhoeal diseases, acute respiratory infections, measles and malaria, with malnutrition often acting as an aggravating factor[16]. These killer diseases are easily diagnosed and cured. Early diagnosis and treatment through accessible health facilities, combined with active case finding, are thus the key to successful health care services.

A health care system in refugee emergencies should fulfil the following criteria:

- provide curative treatment for the most common communicable killer diseases;
- reduce suffering from other debilitating diseases;
- have the capacity to carry out active case finding;
- be able to cope with a high demand for curative care;
- provide easy access to different levels of care, including referral services;
- deal with the majority of illnesses at a basic level of care;
- contribute to surveillance activities (by routine data collection);
- combine both curative and preventive services;
- be flexible enough to adapt to any changes in the situation (e.g. outbreaks of disease).

Refugee settings are also characterized by the high number of patients using health services, especially in the early stages[4]: this generally results from the high morbidity, high population density, high demand for health care and easy access to health services. As a result, the health services of the host country, even when reinforced, may not easily cope with a large refugee influx; and this problem may be aggravated by tensions between refugee and resident populations, administrative obstacles and the distance to existing services, which may simply not be adequate for responding to the emergency needs of refugees. For all these reasons, new facilities have to be set up in a high proportion of refugee emergencies.

LEVELS OF HEALTH CARE

When refugee health services have to be set up, a four-tier health care model may fulfil the above criteria. This has proven successful, and contributes significantly to reducing excess mortality under various conditions (See Table 6.1.).

1. Referral Hospital

A small proportion of patients will require the specialized services of a referral hospital (e.g. surgery or major obstetric emergencies)[4]. If possible, these services are provided in an existing hospital in the vicinity of the settlement, and require arrangements for access and transport to be worked out. When access to a local hospital is not possible, or in the case of large camps, field hospitals will have to be erected on the refugee site itself.

2. Central Health Facility (health centre)

This level should be able to deal with most of the morbidity (all common priority diseases), with one central facility for every 10,000 to 30,000 refugees - offering services 24 hours a day, possibly providing basic hospitalization (in-patient service).

3. Peripheral Health Facilities (health post or health clinic)

Decentralized health services, easily accessible to the whole population and providing a very basic level of care should be established on the basis of 1 health post for every 3,000 to 5,000 refugees. This level deals with only a few killer diseases, e.g. diarrhoea and malaria, and refers serious cases to the health centre. It also provides treatment for a few, non-life-threatening diseases (e.g. scabies, conjunctivitis).

4. Home-visitors

An outreach programme is necessary for conducting active case finding and to ensure the link between the fixed health facilities and the population. This is performed by a network of home-visitors based in the population; training and a good supervision system are the keys for the success of this programme. There should be 1 home-visitor for every 500 to 1,000 refugees, and 1 supervisor for 10 home-visitors. Their main tasks initially are active case finding and surveillance.

Table 6.1
Levels of health care in refugee situations (in the emergency phase)

Level	N° structures	Activities	Staff per facility
Referral Hospital	Depending on the situation	– surgery – major obstetrical emergencies – referral laboratory	Variable – 1 nurse for 20-30 beds, 8-hour shifts
Central Health Facilities (health centre)	1/10-30,000 refu.	– triage – OPD* (first level and referral) – dressing and injections – oral rehydration therapy (ORT) – emergency service (24h) – uncomplicated deliveries, minimum reproductive health activities – minor surgery – pharmacy – health surveillance – generally basic hospitalization – referral to hospital – possibly: laboratory, transfusions, on-going measles immunization	Minimum of 5 medical staff: – 1 doctor – 1 HW* for 50 consultations / day – 1 HW for 20-30 beds, 8-hour shifts – 1 for ORT, 1-2 pharmacy, – 1-2 for dressing /injection / sterilization Non-medical staff: – 1-2 registrars, – 1-3 guards 8-hour shifts, – cleaners etc.
Peripheral Health Facilities (health post or clinic)	1/3 - 5,000 ref.	– OPD (first level) – ORT – dressing – referral of patients to higher level – data collection	Total: 2-5 workers – minimum of 1 qualified HW*, based on 1 person for 50 consultations /day – non-qualified for ORT, dressing, registering, etc.
Outreach activities (home-visitors)	Meeting place (other activities conducted from home)	– data collection – home visits and active screening – referral of patients to facilities – health education, information, etc.	– 1 HV* for 500-1,000 ref. – 1 supervisor for 10 HVs – 1 senior supervisor

* **OPD:** *Out Patient Department*
* **HW:** *Health Worker*
* **HV:** *Home-Visitor*
* **Qualified health workers:** *these include nurses, health assistants, medical assistants, midwives, etc.*

Implementation of health care services

PLANNING THE HEALTH CARE SYSTEM

Planning for an appropriate refugee health system must be based on relevant information collected during the initial assessment. The main information required covers:
– existing health facilities and their accessibility (including whether they accept refugees and whether fees are requested),
– population figures (current and anticipated),
– disease patterns and potential outbreaks to be anticipated in the area,
– specific health problems within the refugee population,
– available resources, especially human resources,
– national health policies of the host country and an organization chart.

A plan must then be made for setting up a health care system within the context of the particular situation and this will vary according to whether or not the health facilities of the host country can cope with refugee health needs, or whether new facilities must be set up on the refugee site. Planning should cover the number of facilities required, whether there is a need for a field hospital on the refugee site, which services should be organized in priority, which package of activities should be provided at each level, etc.

Whichever option is selected, it is essential that the Ministry of Health (MOH) and local health authorities are involved in the planning from the beginning and their authorization must be requested. Other aspects of cooperation with the MOH are described below under *Relations with the national health care system.*

When a parallel health system has to be set up

When the host country's health facilities cannot cope with refugee health problems, even when reinforced, new facilities will have to be set up to focus on the specific health needs of the refugees.

Ideally, the four levels of health care should all be set up at the same time, but as it is generally not feasible to do this at the beginning of a large refugee emergency, it is more likely to be achieved in stages. There are some situations where it is not possible to set up all 4 levels, e.g. where there are security problems and insufficient staff. In any case, conditions may change rapidly so a certain flexibility should be maintained. It is also possible to combine different levels of health care and shift tasks from one level to another; for instance, in small refugee populations (fewer than 10,000 refugees), one single facility and a few home visitors will be able to cater for most health needs.

- Services are usually set up in stages
    1. The first stage would normally be the establishment of a central health facility (health centre). The home-visitor network and a referral system to a hospital (nearby or on-site) should be organized as quickly as possible.

2. As health care should not be focused on the central level, a second stage is required to decentralize services by opening peripheral facilities, providing that the necessary human resources, drugs and equipment are available. Decentralization helps to ensure that the whole population is covered and frees the central facility to concentrate on more severe cases.

3. The different activities within each level of care are also developed in stages; for instance, a central facility may start with an out-patient department (OPD) and a small in-patient service, with other services (e.g. deliveries) added progressively.

Implementing these stages is largely dependent on the human resources available; when there are not enough available qualified staff, other staff will have to be trained and the implementation of some services will have to be delayed until this is done.

Under certain circumstances, priorities may differ.

- When an epidemic occurs, all efforts will focus on controlling this and setting up other services will be temporarily suspended. However, the establishment of a home-visitor programme will be crucial to trace cases. In addition, a special treatment unit generally needs to be built (e.g. cholera unit).

- When there is an influx of wounded refugees, particularly when local hospitals cannot cope, in-patient and surgical units will be given priority.

When host health facilities may be used

The reinforcement and expansion of existing health facilities, when feasible, is the best option. This has many advantages: e.g. strengthening local health services will also benefit the host population, even-handed treatment of both refugee and local populations may help avoid resentment against refugees, and resources will not be wasted owing to the duplication of services. It also encourages local authorities to tackle the refugee problem, which is invaluable in the long-term (in protracted refugee situations)[20]. However, this arrangement occurs less frequently, probably because of the obstacles to implementing it. The existing health system may have problems in coping with a large influx of patients or in dealing with acute health problems (e.g. during an epidemic). There may be ethnic or political tensions between refugees and locals. There is a risk of disruption to existing cost-recovery programmes (when free care is ensured for refugees) and a need for increased resources to target a larger population (refugees and residents).

If existing health care facilities are to be used, the following conditions should be in place:
- no current acute health problem requiring large amounts of resources and specific expertise (e.g. large-scale epidemics, influx of wounded people or a bad nutritional status);
- sufficient existing local facilities in the area where refugees settle;
- the size of the refugee population must not be so great as to significantly outweigh that of the local population; it is therefore generally not indicated for large refugee camps;

- no conflict between refugees and the local population (e.g. ethnic, political, etc.);
- a formal agreement should be drawn up between the MOH of the host country, UNHCR and the implementing agency.

Refugee use of local health facilities has been very successfully implemented in some open situations (particularly where refugees were already integrated into local village populations) or in small refugee camps. In Guinea, for example, where about 500,000 refugees from Liberia and Sierra Leone settled in villages (1989-93), the MOH decided to offer all refugees free access to existing health facilities and supplementary health posts were created in areas with particularly high refugee concentrations[20].

Discussions should be held with the local MOH to solve certain complex issues such as fees, additional resources that might be required, national and refugee health policies, etc. See section *Relations with the national health care system* below.

The four levels of health care

1. REFERRAL HOSPITAL

A referral hospital differs from the basic in-patient service that is generally available in the central facility, in the higher level of services it can provide (see below *Central health facilities*): major surgery, management of major obstetrical emergencies, more diagnostic posssibilities (e.g. laboratory and X-ray department), etc. Qualified doctors (particularly specialists) must be present. There are two alternative ways in which this level of health care can be assured.

A/ The best option is to reinforce a local hospital. This would be in preference to setting up a referral hospital on the refugee site, which is not advised for several reasons [1]: the number of patients requiring this level of care is limited providing that other levels of care are available to all refugees; it requires a high input in material and human resources, it can divert attention from other priorities and once established, it is extremely difficult to close.

However, it is imperative that refugee use of a nearby hospital should be well organized.

- The hospital should be reinforced by providing material and/or financial support (e.g. donations of drugs), possibly financial compensations for health staff when a higher workload and regular presence is demanded, and an expansion in capacity (e.g. tents) may be required, as well as additional health staff [1].

- Referral protocols must be established to avoid refugees referring themselves to the hospital; transport to the hospital must be organized and a feedback system to the refugee health services should be agreed upon.

When these issues are not dealt with, problems frequently arise: the referral hospital may be overwhelmed by the number of refugees (presenting spontaneously), the number of staff and the drug supply may not be sufficient to cope, and the result may be a low quality of care with the risk of a high hospital mortality rate.

The resident population must also be taken into account when reinforcing hospital services as there is a risk that these may focus solely on refugees. Ideally, refugees should not receive higher levels of care than the local population. All arrangements must be negotiated with the hospital administration and should result in a written 'terms of agreement'.

B/ A referral hospital may be established on the refugee site if needs clearly cannot be met by an existing local hospital[1,4]. This could happen in the following cases:

– when there is no local hospital accessible to the refugee population because of the difficulty of access, security problems, ethnic tensions, administrative obstacles etc.;

– when the refugee population is very large (for instance above 100,000) and existing services, even when expanded, would be unable to cope with it;

– when there is a significant number of cases requiring surgery, particularly if a very large number of war-wounded arrive and the local hospital does not have the capacity to respond adequately.

In the above situations, it would be preferable to upgrade the in-patient service of a central facility by at least increasing the number of beds and providing surgical services. This needs very good standards of hygiene and sterilization to be in place, an adequate post-operative follow-up, and a capability for carrying out transfusions (including related HIV testing). Additional qualified health staff will also be required, including a highly skilled nurse for overall nursing supervision.

2. CENTRAL HEALTH FACILITIES

Activities

• A good triage system is necessary due to the high number of patients presenting in the health facilities. It allows identification of the most urgent cases, and helps prevent OPD services from being overloaded. This means that patient flow has to be well organized with health screening on entry: urgent cases and those referred by peripheral facilities must be given priority; other patients should be directed to the appropriate service (for ORT, dressings, etc.).

• The out-patient department (OPD) should treat referred cases in priority, but may also provide 'first level' consultations. Separate consultations for women sometimes have to be organized in order to guarantee their access to health care. See *Socio-cultural Aspects* in Part I and *Reproductive health* below.

• An in-patient service, or at least a day-care observation area, is required for the management of severe cases, uncomplicated deliveries, etc.[1] A local hospital located close to the refugee site may sometimes provide these services.

- An emergency service is required for urgent cases arriving at night and during weekends.
- Good nursing care is essential to these activities and must be supervised by an experienced nurse; this should include an adequate sterilization system (for injection material, dressings, etc.).
- Data collection is important for health surveillance.
- A well-organized system must be set up for transferring cases to a referral hospital when patients require a higher level of care (e.g. major surgery).

Organization

There should be at least one central facility for each main population concentration, with a maximum of 30,000 refugees per health centre[1,4]. There is no consensus as to the standard capacity of the in-patient ward based on the size of the refugee population, because bed requirements will be largely influenced by the context of each situation. However, certain factors will help in estimating this: whether or not there is a possibility of referring cases to a local hospital, morbidity patterns (and the occurrence of outbreaks) and available resources. Although an existing building may be used, tents (a minimum of four) are very practical in the emergency phase and allow flexibility in the setup.

Location is important: preferably in a secure place beside the refugee site or in a central location, accessible by road, with sufficient free space surrounding to allow for possible extension. Discussion on the need to set up separate facilities (e.g. in case of a cholera or shigellosis outbreak) is developed in 7. Control of Communicable Diseases and Epidemics.

Staff must include a sufficient number of qualified health workers, and a medical doctor to be in charge of supervision, regular referral consultations and in-patients. Whether or not this person will be required to maintain a full-time presence depends on the qualifications of the staff. The number of staff depends mainly on the patient load, whether or not there are peripheral facilities, and the services provided. The number of staff required to run an OPD should not be underestimated; experience shows that a health worker should not be expected to carry out more than 50 consultations per day.

3. PERIPHERAL HEALTH SERVICES (HEALTH POST OR CLINIC)

The decentralization of health services is necessary in order to meet the heavy use of health services and to ensure accessibility to everyone. When the refugee population exceeds 10,000, the opening of peripheral health services providing a basic level of health care[4] is recommended.

Activities

Activities at this level may vary, depending mainly on the staff available, the possibilities for training them and the major health problems to be dealt with.

- The main service which should be provided is a first line out-patient department (OPD). Standard treatment protocols must be used, based on a limited list of essential drugs. Antibiotics are not always present, and injections at this level are mostly discouraged.

- An ORT unit should be set up in the health post, and rehydration should be continuously supervised.
- Data collection must also be carried out at this level.
- Patient referrals to higher levels should be carefully supervised as there is a danger that peripheral facilities may hold on to severe cases for too long or that staff may underestimate the severity of cases. Strict referral criteria and protocols are thus imperative.

Organization

The number of facilities required - usually varying from 1 per 3,000 refugees to 1 per 5,000 - depends on the situation (i.e. population density). A simple construction consisting of one or two rooms is sufficient and should be located centrally within the area it serves.

A qualified medical staff member is usually required, particularly if antibiotics are to be used. If there are no qualified staff available, either activities should be limited to the treatment of very simple diseases, or serious training should take place. In any case, staff should be trained in the use of essential drugs and therapeutic protocols.

4. OUTREACH ACTIVITIES OR HOME-VISITING

The organization of adequate health services is generally not enough in itself to secure health care for everyone. It has been observed that many patients, even when suffering from serious diseases, do not come to health facilities even when these are very close and treatment is free. This may be due to several factors: a lack of awareness of health services, fear, lack of acceptability, etc. Active case finding via home visits by members of their own community is therefore essential for finding these sick people and encouraging them to come for treatment, and this is one of the major roles of home-visitors (HVs).

The selection and training of home-visitors and the non-medical duties they perform are described in *9. Human Resources and Training*; the medical aspects are dealt with more fully in this chapter. Home-visitors should not be confused with community health workers (CHW), who are a component of long-term primary health care programmes, although some of their tasks may be similar.

Activities

- Screening or active case finding is carried out in regular visits to shelters and in mobilizing the community to check for sick persons (and any malnourished), and is associated with the organization of a referral system and the organization of transport to health services. This is also a key task when outbreaks occur, along with informing the community about health measures and available services.
- Another important task performed by HVs is the collection of data on mortality and population numbers (see *8. Public Health Surveillance*).

- They may be given specific jobs to do, such as following up on treatment compliance (e.g. shigellosis) or tracing defaulters from a specific programme. If culturally acceptable, they may also participate in condom distribution.
- It is not usually recommended that HVs perform curative care activities, unless they have been given a thorough and specific training.

Organization

The number of home-visitors (initially 1 for every 500-1,000 refugees) may be increased, depending on how the situation evolves (outbreaks), and considering any expansion in the range of programmes[1]. HVs should be responsible for home visits and other tasks in the area or section in which they live.

Training should be rapidly organized on case detection and other topics. A supervision system must be ensured; 1 supervisor for every 10 HVs and 1 overall programme supervisor. Meetings should take place regularly, at first daily, then weekly.

HVs should maintain very close contacts with the staff of the health facilities and should be linked to the peripheral facility of their area, to which they refer patients; frequent meetings should be held among them to discuss and share information on the health problems in their areas.

Special issues

REPRODUCTION HEALTH

(See also *Reproductive Health Care in the Post-emergency Phase* in Part III)

During the emergency phase, resources should not be diverted from dealing with the major killers. However, there are some aspects of reproductive health which must also be dealt with at this stage. The UNHCR, together with other agencies, has defined a 'Minimum Initial Service Package' (MISP) to be implemented on site as soon as possible. These minimum services comprise[21]:

- prevention and management of the consequences of sexual and gender-based violence. This includes the provision of emergency post-coital contraception to those women who request it;
- respect for universal precautions against HIV/AIDS (see following topic);
- guaranteeing the availability of free condoms to anyone who requests them;
- simple deliveries and organization of a referral system to deal with obstetric complications;
- planning for provision of comprehensive reproductive health services.

New Emergency Health Kits are available to cover 10,000 people for 3 months, but additional items must be procured to implement all MISP activities.

AIDS AND SEXUALLY TRANSMITTED DISEASES (STDs)
(See also *HIV, AIDS and STD* in Part III)

Although it has not been reported that refugee populations have a higher HIV prevalence, population displacements may occur in areas where there is a high sero-prevalence. Whatever the AIDS situation, special attention should always be paid to this problem. It is essential that the universal precautions against HIV/AIDS are respected by health workers right from the beginning of any emergency in order to avoid accidental AIDS transmission. The following should be ensured[21,22]:

- disinfection and proper sterilization of medical and surgical material, or utilization of single use material;
- restriction of the number of injections;
- protection of health staff: use of gloves, protective clothing, adequate information;
- guarantee of blood transfusion safety and rationalization of blood transfusion indications[18];
- safe handling of sharps;
- proper disposal of waste materials.

Condoms should be made available to those who request them, and staff should make sure that their availability is known. The treatment of AIDS patients is symptomatic.

In the post-emergency phase, other activities targeting AIDS and STDs may receive more attention, see *HIV, AIDS and STD* in Part III.

CHILD HEALTH CARE

As in stable populations in developing countries, death rates in refugee populations are highest in children under 5 years [17]. Child health care in the emergency phase is focused on activities that are the most effective in reducing excess mortality: measles immunization, paediatric curative care, and nutritional activities. Other child health activities, such as Expanded Programme of Immunization (EPI), are not commonly provided during the emergency phase, because they can only prevent a minor proportion of the overall mortality and morbidity at that stage; they will be introduced once the emergency is under control, providing that the population remains stable (see *Child Health Care in the Post-emergency Phase* in Part III)[17].

LABORATORY
(See *7. Control of Communicable Diseases and Epidemics*)

It is not a priority to set up a laboratory in the emergency phase since most diseases will be diagnosed clinically. However, laboratory services may be required under certain circumstances: when drug-resistant malaria is a major problem, in case of certain disease outbreaks (e.g. shigellosis) or when blood transfusions are performed. Once the emergency is under control, a simple laboratory with basic equipment may be set up in health facilities to help to improve the diagnoses and quality of care. Strict indications for laboratory testing should be established.

SURGERY

Surgery is usually not a priority in refugee populations, but the management of surgical emergencies (e.g. war wounded, emergency laparotomy) must be organized rapidly. Preference is given to reinforcing a local hospital, which may require the provision of drugs, surgical material, additional beds, and possibly a surgical team (surgeon and anaesthetist). Transport must be organized between the refugee site and the hospital. Surgery may play a key role when an armed conflict is causing a large number of traumatic injuries[19]; if there is an overwhelming need for surgery, it may be necessary to rapidly deploy a surgical unit to the refugee site. However, this should only be a temporary measure[1]. A high level of hygiene is required: adequate water supply, a sterilization system and strict attention to asepsis. Good nursing is also essential, particularly for post-operative care. Indications for surgery should be clearly defined and limited to casualties and surgical emergencies; for instance, in Burundi (1994), there were a large number of wounded among the Rwandan refugees fleeing the civil war, and special surgical teams were sent in.

TREATMENT OF TUBERCULOSIS CASES

Such programmes should not be undertaken in the emergency phase. This topic is dealt with in the *Tuberculosis Programme* in Part III.

MENTAL HEALTH
(See also *Psycho-social and Mental Health* in Part III)

Specific programmes to address mental health issues may be required. These programmes usually have to be prepared in the emergency phase but will only be effectively developed in the post-emergency phase. It should be kept in mind that a proportion of the patients seen in OPD health services may be psychologically traumatized refugees presenting psycho-somatic complaints.

Specific aspects of health care organization

Health care programmes should be coordinated with and involve all the partners: the local health authorities, the refugee community and all agencies involved in refugee assistance.

Agreement should be reached on the common use of some standardized systems in order to improve and then maintain the coherence in the services offered by all parties involved:

– clinical and therapeutic protocols,
– essential drugs and drug supply,
– patient flow and referral system,
– data collection,
– health coordination and relations with the national health care system.

CLINICAL AND THERAPEUTIC PROTOCOLS

Standard medical protocols are essential in refugee health care, especially if refugee, national and expatriate staff have different prescription habits. They are also very useful for training staff and crucial for promoting a common approach when different organizations are involved in curative care. Standardization procedures need to be dealt with at coordination level, and protocols should be available for every health care level in accordance with essential drug lists (see below).

In principle, the national treatment protocols should be the guide. However, in practice, they may be lacking, or are not suited to the type of health problems and medical supplies typical of refugee emergencies, and need to be adapted. Therefore, international agencies such as WHO[11], CDC[17], MSF[6,9] or Oxfam[2] have developed guidelines that are adapted to the priority health needs of refugee and displaced populations, and handy to use at the start of a programme. Whatever standard tools are used, they should be adapted as soon as possible to the particular refugee situation, under the supervision of the health coordination body (see *10. Coordination*). A small number of clinical and therapeutic guidelines adapted to specific refugee programmes in particular countries have been developed by some agencies (e.g. UNBRO[8], Oxfam[7] and ARC).

In addition to clinical guidelines, diagnostic flow charts might be useful. WHO has designed flow charts for some major health problems such as diarrhoeal diseases and respiratory infections[11,6]. These are mostly used for staff training, to assist in the management of specific problems (e.g. dysentery and malaria), and to identify patients for referral in order to ensure that cases are treated at the appropriate level.

ESSENTIAL DRUGS AND DRUG SUPPLY

An essential drugs policy is vital for any effective health care system, ensuring a supply of safe, effective and affordable drugs to meet priority health needs, and encouraging a rational and appropriate approach to the use of drugs. It is particularly necessary to have standardized protocols for drugs when dealing with refugee situations because of the large number of health workers and organizations involved, and the varied circumstances in which refugees are to be found[10]. A list of essential drugs should be decided for every level of health care, taking into account staff qualifications, the type of services provided, local disease patterns and treatment protocols. UNHCR, together with other NGOs, has developed standard lists of essential drugs and supplies, although these will have to be adapted to each individual situation[10].

A safe and effective drug supply system must be ensured from the start of any medical interventions. Emergency health kits have been developed on the basis of standard treatment protocols in emergencies. The best known is the 'New emergency health kit', which was conceived in collaboration with WHO, UNHCR, UNICEF, MSF and other agencies, and has been adopted by many organizations and national authorities. The contents of each kit are intended to meet the needs of 10,000 people for 3 months, based on an average attendance of 4 new cases per person per year[9] (see *8. Public Health Surveillance*). The kit is designed for use at two levels (peripheral and central facilities)[9].

It is very easy to use kits in the first stages of refugee programmes because they facilitate a swift and effective response to an emergency situation. However, additional drugs may be required in the light of specific morbidity patterns and drug sensitivity (e.g. chloroquine-resistant malaria and multi-resistant shigellosis) and these should be ordered as early as possible. Drug shortages may be frequent because of the high drug consumption in refugee programmes due to frequent high attendance rates (higher than the average expected 4 new cases per person per year) and bad prescription habits. Requirements must be assessed rapidly and further supplies ordered on the basis of projected consumption and morbidity patterns, and taking into account the high drug consumption and the necessity of holding a reserve stock[9].

The donation of drugs (e.g. by a government) is a frequent source of problems due to the inappropriate drugs received and expiry dates that have almost lapsed. When these donations cannot be avoided, WHO regulations for donations should be followed[24].

In large-scale emergencies, the management of drugs and medical material is generally a full-time job at the start of the programme, and a senior staff member should be in charge of the organization and management of central stock, setting up a delivery system to supply health facilities, etc. Once the acute phase of the emergency is passed, drug consumption and the rational use of medical items should be monitored; this will also facilitate further ordering. Guidelines on organization of medical store, drug management and drug use are available in reference documents[9,10].

REFERRAL SYSTEM

The referral system (see Figure 6.2) between services must be well organized, avoiding bottlenecks as well as delays in the management of severe cases.

There are certain principles that should be observed:
– every refugee should have easy access to a basic level of health care;
– priority must be given to severe cases so that they can be dealt with quickly;
– referral criteria and protocols should be established at every level of care;
– transport should be organized for referral to facilities outside the refugee site.

Referrals may take place in the same facility (e.g. referral consultation), from one level of care to another (e.g. from health post to health centre) or from a health facility to another programme (e.g. to a feeding centre) or conversely. Referrals normally require formal agreements between all the programmes concerned, and standardized procedures. This is particularly crucial when referring to services outside the refugee site.

The referral system must be particularly efficient during outbreaks, when suspect cases detected by home-visitors or the peripheral facility must be promptly referred to the relevant treatment unit.

Figure 6.2
Referral of patients between health facilities on the refugee site:
chart showing camp services and the referral flow of patients.

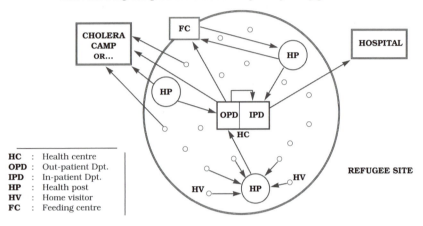

HC :	Health centre
OPD :	Out-patient Dpt.
IPD :	In-patient Dpt.
HP :	Health post
HV :	Home visitor
FC :	Feeding centre

DATA COLLECTION
(See *8. Public Health Surveillance*)

The collection of health data must be organized as soon as health services are established, with reporting on a daily or weekly and later a monthly basis. Four types of data should be collected:

- **Vital statistics**: these mainly concern population figures and the number of deaths in the settlement and are collected by home-visitors.

- **Routine data on morbidity**: these are limited to the most common diseases and those which are potentially epidemic and are based on strict case definitions. This data allows early warning of epidemics and an estimate of morbidity patterns.

- **Routine data on medical activities** (monitoring the different activities): only a limited amount of data will be useful during the emergency phase, principally concerning the number of consultations, admissions, exits and deaths in the in-patient service.

  When the total number of consultations in the refugee settlement are known, it becomes possible to make a monthly calculation of the 'attendance rate' (number of new cases in OPD per person per year extrapolated from monthly data to arrive at annual attendance rate). This is a measure of how much the medical services are used by the population. The attendance rate is particularly high in refugee populations: it varies around 0.5-1 NC/person/year in stable populations, while an average of 4 NC/person/year is expected in refugee populations[14].

When the attendance rate is low (say under 2 NC/person/year), the reasons for this must be assessed, and may include poor access to health care or the insufficient capacity of the existing facilities. It may for instance indicate a need to decentralize or expand health services. When access for specific groups is poor (e.g. ethnic minority or women), it may be necessary to make changes in the health staff or provide separate services for these groups.

Where the attendance rate is too high (say above 5 NC/person/year) - and rates as high as 10 NC/person/year were observed in Goma in 1994 - this may be due to an error in estimating the denominator e.g. the non-refugee population may be using the same facilities, or an over-utilization of services. The supply of free drugs to patients definitely plays a role in very high attendance rates.

The hospital mortality rate (percentage of the number of deaths over the number of exits) is useful for monitoring the quality of care.

- **Data provided through studies** carried out within a health facility may cover aspects of morbidity (e.g. plasmodium index among patients), drug-sensitivity for some treatment or health behaviour (e.g. treatment compliance), but is not often required in the emergency phase.

A health worker should be made responsible for the collection of routine data in each facility. The medical coordinator is responsible for the overall supervision, analysis, interpretation and reporting of data.

HEALTH COORDINATION
(See also 10. Coordination)

The integrated organization of health programmes is based on coordination between the partners involved. Good coordination is required not only between the different medical programmes, but also with other programmes affecting refugee health (water and sanitation, food distributions, etc.). Coordination is particularly essential when a large number of agencies are working on the same site, in order to avoid a situation where some programmes overlap while other needs are not met.

Health coordination must be carried out in line with certain principles:

- Health sector coordination teams should be established at central level (national or regional) and at field level (on site). They must involve the Ministry of Health (MOH). If a UNHCR medical coordinator is present, this person may play a key role.
- Health coordination at the central level may be under the leadership of the MOH or UNHCR; at the field level, it is the role of either the local health authorities or a health agency.
- The individual responsibilities of each of the partners involved should be clarified and the division of tasks formalized (e.g. written terms of agreement).
- Regular meetings among partners at both levels should be organized early on in order to define common health strategies, adapt health programmes, divide tasks according to changing needs, share information, discuss any

specific health problems (e.g. a current outbreak) and work on guidelines and standard policies for assistance programmes.

- The reporting system should be decided by the health coordination team, which must agree upon the information required and the standard forms to be used; the regular collection of reports and their dissemination should be centralized by one of the partners.
- The use of standardized guidelines and policies by all partners concerned is imperative in any coordinated medical assistance.

Relations with the national health care system

As stated above, refugee health services and staff fall under the responsibility of the host health authorities and their authorization is required before starting up any relief activities. Coordination is thefore very important. A formal agreement is required, outlining the responsibilities on each side. This aspect is too often overlooked when relief organizations rush in to deal with an emergency.

Health authorities, at the national and/or local level, may assist medical NGOs by providing local health staff, medical guidelines and information on local morbidity patterns, such as potential epidemic diseases. Refugee assistance programmes should be in line with the national health policies of the host country whenever possible. However, some policies may not be applicable during the emergency or may have to be adapted; for example, there are different strategies and target age groups for measles immunization in refugee emergencies.

- When new facilities have to be set up

  An agreement should be reached with the national health authorities on the services to be provided, medical protocols, health staff, and referral to local services. Negotiations on issues such as refugee health policies may sometimes be arduous, particularly when these policies clearly differ from the national ones.

  Certain complex issues require special attention and clear agreement:

  - **Health staff** (see *9. Human Resources and Training*): Diplomas hold by refugee health staff trained in their country of origin may not be recognized by the host MOH; the same may sometimes be true for expatriate medical staff. Salaries may pose a difficult question as the salaries paid by foreign agencies are often higher than those of the MOH. Although this may be justified by the hardships involved and a higher workload, a drain on qualified health staff transferring to work in refugee camps may endanger the national health system. It may be useful to hire both refugee and national staff to run health facilities as they may complement each other in regard to knowledge of health problems and language. However, cultural and ethnic differences between refugees and national staff must also be taken into consideration as these may affect accessibility to health services for some refugee groups.

– **Level of health services**: It frequently occurs that the health services in the camps provide a higher quality of care than the local services. Although major differences in quality should obviously be avoided, this may be difficult to guarantee because the greater availability of drugs in refugee assistance programmes already creates a difference in the quality of care offered from the start. The best strategy is to reinforce the local services, e.g. through supplies of drugs and equipment. Refugee health services that are of a higher quality and free of charge may also attract the local population to attend; they cannot be refused, particularly not the urgent cases. Nonetheless, this influx may overwhelm refugee facilities and create competition with the local services; when these are based on a system of cost recovery, this system may even be endangered.

– **Disease outbreak**: If there is an outbreak of disease, this will generally not be confined to the refugee population: indeed, there is a high risk that the resident population will be affected as well. It is imperative in such a case to notify the health authorities and agree upon common strategies. The relief agencies working on a refugee site cannot overlook the local resident population at risk, and additional back-up must sometimes be provided to local services.

• When the existing health facilities are to be used

When the refugee population are to use existing health facilities, certain issues must be discussed and agreed upon.

– **Fees**: Refugees should generally have free access to health care, but cost recovery systems have been introduced in many countries, and health care financing of the existing system is generally walking on a tightrope. It will therefore be necessary to arrange compensation for facilities offering free access to refugees (either financially or materially, e.g. through donations of drugs). UNHCR is generally involved in this aspect where refugees are concerned; for instance, in Guinea, the MOH decided to offer free care to refugees in local facilities in 1989 and UNHCR covered the fees for refugees at the same rate as Guinean patients would pay[20].

– **Resources**: As attendance in existing facilities increases, these should receive additional resources to help them cope: additional staff, drug supplies, tents to increase capacity, possibly supplementary funding. The adequacy of the existing structures also needs to be assessed.

– **National health policies**: These need to be adapted to the specific refugee health needs, and training of national staff in dealing with refugee emergencies may be needed.

Principal recommendations regarding health care in the emergency phase

- The health authorities must be contacted and involved from the outset of medical programmes.

- Whenever possible, the existing facilities of the host country should be used. However, in most camp situations, new services have to be set up. Health services should focus on basic curative care.

- Ideally, four levels of health care should be envisaged:
    - a referral hospital,
    - a central facility,
    - peripheral facilities and
    - outreach activities.

  As soon as a central facility is up and running, some services should be decentralized in order to improve accessibility to health care and avoid the central facility becoming swamped. Whether or not a hospital will be required in the camp and what its capacity should be depends on the local situation.

- Some basic tools are essential for organizing effective health care: treatment protocols, lists of essential drugs for each level, a clear referral system for patients, good coordination, including relations with the national health authorities, and a system of data collection to ensure health surveillance from the start and early warning of epidemics.

- Health services have to be flexible: they must be adapted to the evolving situation and changing needs. If an outbreak occurs, the need for curative care may be very high and additional capacity will be required.

✎ References

1. UNHCR. *Handbook for emergencies*. Geneva: UNHCR, 1982.

2. Mears, C, Chowdhury, S. *Health care for refugees and displaced people*. Oxford: Oxfam Practical Health Guide No. 9, 1994.

3. UNICEF. *Assisting in emergencies : A resource handbook for UNICEF field staff*. New York: UNICEF, 1986.

4. Simmonds, S, Vaughan, P, William Gun, S. *Refugee community health care*. Oxford: Oxford University Press, 1983.

5. Castilla, J. *Refugee camp programmes for Somalis in Kenya*. [Evaluation Mission]. Brussels: AEDES, 1993.

6. Médecins Sans Frontières. *Clinical guidelines, diagnostic and treatment manual*. Paris: Hatier, 1993.

7. Oxfam Refugee Health Unit, Somali Ministry of Health. *Guidelines for health care in refugee camps*. Oxford: Oxfam, 1983.

8. United Nations Border Relief Operations. *Medical guidelines for the Thai Kampuchean border*. August 1988.

9. Médecins Sans Frontières. *Essential drugs. Practical guidelines*. Paris: Hatier, 1993.

10. UNHCR. *Essential drugs policy*. Geneva: UNHCR, 1989.

11. WHO. *The New Emergency Health Kit*. Geneva: WHO, 1990.

12. Johns, W. *Establishing a refugee camp laboratory*. Save the Children Fundation, 1987.

13. CDC. Guidelines for collecting, processing, storing and shipping diagnostic specimens in refugee health care environments. *MMWR*, 1992, 41(Annex A).

14. AEDES. *Système d'information sanitaire*. Brussels: AEDES, 1994.

15. Moren, A, Rigal, J, Biberson, P. Populations réfugiées. Programme de santé publique et urgence de l'intervention. MSF-F, Epicentre. *Rev Prat*, 1992, 172: 767-76.

16. Toole, M J, Waldman, R J. Prevention of excess mortality in refugees and displaced populations in developing countries. *JAMA*, 1990, 263(24): 3296-302.

17. CDC. Famine-affected, refugee, and displaced populations: Recommendations for public health issues. *MMWR*, 1992, 41(RR-13): 1-76.

18. Médecins Sans Frontières. MSF and AIDS. *Medical News*, 1994, 3(5): 5-10.

19. Allegra, D T, Nieburg, P I. *Emergency refugee health care - A chronicle of experience in the Khmer assistance operation 1979-1980*. CDC, Atlanta, GA, 1984: 1-191.

20. Van Damme, W. Do refugees belong in camps? Experiences from Goma and Guinea. *The Lancet*, 1995, 346(8971): 360-2.

21. *Reproductive health in refugee situations. An inter-agency field manual*. Geneva: UNHCR, 1995.

22. Global Programme on AIDS. *Preventing HIV transmission in health facilities*. Geneva: WHO, 1995. GPA/TCD/HCS/95.16.

23.   Médecins Sans Frontières. *Guide of kits and emergency items*. Paris: Médecins Sans Frontières, 1996.

24.   WHO, UNHCR, UNICEF, ICRC, IFRCRCS, MSF, CAHWCC, OXFAM. *Guidelines for drug donations*. Geneva: WHO, 1996. WHO/DAP/96.2.

7. Control of communicable diseases and epidemics

Introduction

The primary causes of morbidity and mortality among refugees and displaced populations are measles, diarrhoeal diseases, acute respiratory infections, malnutrition and, in areas where it is endemic, malaria. Studies indicate that these diseases account for 51% to 95% of all reported deaths in refugee populations[1]. Most of these health problems are communicable diseases (the only exception being malnutrition). Other communicable diseases, such as meningococcal meningitis, hepatitis, typhoid fever, typhus, relapsing fever, etc, have also been responsible for outbreaks in refugee camps[2,8]. Outbreaks or epidemics may occur in refugee populations at any time: in the emergency, post-emergency or chronic phase.

There are 3 major sources of communicable disease in a refugee population:

- Refugees may bring infection with them from their home environment (e.g. malaria or trypanosomiasis) or from the areas they travelled through before arriving.

- The disease may be present in the new environment and the local population; refugees who have not acquired immunity (e.g. against malaria or cholera) are therefore at greatest risk.

- Disease may surface in the camp itself as a result of overcrowding, poor sanitary conditions, etc.

A poorly planned refugee settlement is one of the most pathogenic environments, due to the typical overcrowding, poor water supply and sanitation, and inadequate shelter, which are the main risk factors for communicable diseases. In addition, the poor nutritional status of many refugee populations and their lack of acquired immunity from some diseases, combined with disruptions to the immunization services, all contribute to increasing their vulnerability. Psycho-social factors, such as stress, family disruption and change of environment, which destroy many of the refugees' coping mechanisms, also make them more vulnerable to illness.

The communicable diseases that are most common among non-displaced populations tend therefore to be more easily spread and more severe among refugee populations, presenting higher incidence and mortality rates. Furthermore, camp conditions facilitate the spread of other diseases, with the risk of epidemics increasing dramatically (meningitis, cholera, dysentery, etc.)[3].

Most of the risk factors in refugee settings can be eliminated or their impact reduced, i.e. a major proportion of epidemics and the high mortality related to communicable diseases will be averted through preventive measures and appropriate case management[2,3].

The general measures which should be taken in order to control communicable diseases are indicated in the introductory chapter to Part II, *The Ten Top Priorities*.

Objectives

The main objective of disease control is to reduce the excess overall mortality among a refugee population. To achieve this goal, interventions must aim at reducing the morbidity caused by the killer diseases and lowering their related mortality (case fatality). This includes measures intended to prevent or stop epidemics.

GENERAL MEASURES FOR COMMUNICABLE DISEASE CONTROL

- General preventive measures aimed at reducing the number of cases are the most effective for the control of communicable diseases[5]. These measures are not specific to any given disease and consist mainly in improving the environment and the living conditions of refugees: decreasing overcrowding by a proper organization of the site, providing shelters, ensuring water supplies, excreta disposal, food supply, vector control, etc. In addition, mass immunization against measles is extremely effective and must always be given the highest priority. These topics are all dealt with in other chapters.

- Outreach activities should be undertaken by home-visitors conducting early case finding and active screening to cover the whole population. Suspected cases should be rapidly referred to the health facilities.

- In addition, control of the 4 biggest killer communicable diseases (measles, diarrhoeal diseases, acute respiratory infections and malaria) requires the implementation of a basic health system: health facilities must be rapidly set up to ensure the early and adequate treatment of the main diseases. This is essential for reducing mortality and preventing the further spread of disease.

- Epidemic control implies a need for a good surveillance system (see *8. Public Health Surveillance*). If data suggest the occurrence of an outbreak, there must be an early and appropriate response; its effectiveness will be enhanced if contingency plans have been drawn up in advance.

General measures are described below and measures specific to each disease are developed in the relevant sections of this chapter.

EPIDEMIC PREPAREDNESS

General contingency plans should be prepared in any refugee emergency in order to enable health teams to react as quickly as possible if an epidemic is declared.

Planning should cover a range of measures[2]:

- Information should be obtained on potentially epidemic diseases that may occur in the refugee site area or could be brought in by refugees. This can usually be provided either by the Ministry of Health (MOH) in the host country and the country of origin, or from international agencies.

- A surveillance system must be ready to detect new epidemic diseases as soon as they appear and standard case definitions established, although these may have to be adapted once an epidemic is declared. It is important to train health staff in the use of case definitions in order to ensure early detection of epidemic diseases.

- Standard protocols for epidemic diseases must be made available for use in prevention, diagnosis and treatment procedures. These may be requested from the host country MOH or from international agencies (e.g. WHO or CDC). Case definitions and standard protocols must be drawn up but, whenever possible, should be adapted to the local conditions: whether or not a laboratory is available, the level of qualification of health workers, local characteristics of the causative agent (drug resistance and serotype), acquired immunity of the refugee population, etc. These protocols can be worked out by health teams with the help of experts, and should be agreed upon in health coordination meetings.

- A laboratory must be identified, whether locally or in another country, for providing confirmation of cases. Sample material for the most common tests (stools and serum) should be available on site, and a few 'rapid tests' may also be stored locally. A reference laboratory should also be identified, at regional or international level. This may, for example, be required for antibiotic sensitivity testing of *Shigella*, or for viral haemorrhagic fever. See below under *Laboratory*.

- Sources of relevant vaccines should be identified in case a mass campaign is required to control an epidemic (e.g. measles or meningitis). A stock of measles vaccine must be available, as immunization remains a priority throughout.

- Reserves of material and medical supplies should be prepared and stored in an easily accssible place, exclusively reserved for use in the event of an epidemic. These reserves will usually include oral rehydration salts, intravenous fluids, immunization material, tents, plastic sheeting, etc. A cholera kit should be held in reserve in most situations.

- Possible treatment sites must be identified. Since cholera is a risk in most situations, an appropriate site within the settlement should be identified and prepared for a cholera unit to be set up if required; it may even be built in anticipation (see section *Control of diarrhoeal diseases* later in this chapter).

- The accessibility of health services must also be ensured: health facilities should be accessible to all sections of the settlement, and outreach activities carried out by home-visitors should ensure that the whole population is reached.

- The availability of human resources and their level of skills must be assessed and upgraded if inadequate. Training needs should be determined. Responsibility should be worked out in advance for the specific tasks that have to be distributed among the different members of the health teams which will be involved in controlling an outbreak (surveillance activities, curative care, immunization, etc.). In situations where there is a high risk of certain epidemics (cholera, dysentery or meningitis), training courses may be organized in anticipation of an epidemic. Several guidelines on outbreak control, covering many of the diseases likely to be met with, are available and may be used for training (references for these are indicated at the end of each section dealing with a specific disease).

Interventions in epidemics of communicable diseases

INVESTIGATING THE EPIDEMIC[4,5,6]

When an epidemic is suspected, the following steps should be undertaken immediately by the team in the field, without waiting for external support. Although epidemiologists may be required in certain outbreaks, their arrival may be delayed and their work will in any case rely on the quality of information collected initially by field teams.

- **Confirmation of the existence of an epidemic**: reports and rumours of outbreaks are frequent among refugee populations and should always be followed up.

  An epidemic is defined as an excessive number of cases of a given disease in relation to prior experience according to place, time and population[9]. This implies comparison of the incidence of the disease with a previous incidence at a similar time of year and in the same population, which is usually not possible in regard to refugee populations. Hence, it can be difficult to decide whether there is an epidemic or not, and criteria for epidemic thresholds should be established for the diseases for which this is possible. For instance, for a few specific diseases, one case reported in a refugee camp is sufficient for an epidemic to be declared (e.g. cholera); for other diseases such as meningitis, two consecutive doublings of the weekly incidence may be required. However, many diseases do not have a defined threshold for declaring an epidemic. Any suspected or confirmed epidemic must be reported immediately to health coordinators and local health authorities.

- **Confirmation of the diagnosis**: the causative agent must be identified by assessing suspected cases. Diagnosis should be confirmed either on a clinical basis by senior staff (e.g. for measles), or by laboratory tests, in which case specimens need to be taken (e.g. serum, faeces or cerebrospinal fluid) and sent to a reference laboratory for further tests (see below *Laboratory*).

- **The case definition**: this is an essential tool for epidemic investigation which should be rapidly established or adapted. Cases can be classified as suspected, probable or confirmed on the base of diagnostic criteria.

- **Case registration**: in addition to the basic information collected through a routine surveillance system, information on every case should be registered on a separate form. This should include at least age, location, date of onset and outcome; for some diseases, additional data on immunization status, water source, symptoms, treatment and duration of the disease may be collected.

- **Sorting data**: data should be sorted as follows:
  - time: an epidemic curve should be drawn showing the distribution of cases over time; for instance, this makes it possible to know if the peak of the epidemic has been reached, and helps to foresee how the epidemic will evolve;
  - place: it may be useful in outbreaks of certain diseases to map cases geographically with date of onset and observe where and how the disease spreads;
  - person: weekly attack rates should be calculated, as well as the distribution of cases by age, sex, and other variables.

- **High risk groups**: these can be suspected by comparing the attack rates in different groups, especially in regard to age and sex. Confirmation of a risk difference may require further study. The identification of these high risk groups helps to target them better through preventive and curative measures; for instance, high risk groups in shigellosis epidemics should always receive antibiotic treatment.

- **Studies**: in some epidemics, routine data does not give sufficient information about the source of the epidemic, risk factors, local characteristics of the causative agent (resistance, serotype, etc.), mode of transmission, etc. Methods such as case control studies, retrospective epidemiological surveys, or environmental assessments may have to be employed to identify transmission modes, risk factors in regard to severity, etc., but these often require the help of epidemiologists.

OUTBREAK CONTROL[5,7]

There are twin objectives to epidemic controls: to lower the number of cases (by preventive measures) until the epidemic is stopped and to reduce the mortality among cases (early detection of cases and treatment). The implementation of these control measures should not wait until the epidemic is fully investigated. Control measures vary widely depending on the disease and are dealt with in the relevant sections of this chapter.

Control strategies fall into 3 major categories of activity:

1. Attack the source, i.e. reduce the sources of infection to prevent the disease spreading to other members of the community. Depending on the disease, this may involve the prompt diagnosis and treatment of cases

(e.g. cholera), isolation of cases (e.g. viral haemorrhagic fevers) and controlling animal reservoirs (e.g. plague).

2. Protect susceptible groups in order to reduce the risk of infection: immunization (e.g. meningitis and measles), better nutrition and, in some situations, chemoprophylaxis for high risk groups (e.g. malaria prophylaxis may be suggested for pregnant women in outbreaks).

3. Interrupt transmission in order to minimize the spread of the disease by improvements in environmental and personal hygiene (for all faeco-orally transmitted diseases), health education, vector control (e.g. yellow fever and dengue), and disinfection and sterilization (e.g. hepatitis B).

A special issue: the laboratory in refugee situations

IN THE EMERGENCY PHASE

Setting up a clinical laboratory is not a priority in the emergency phase of assistance to refugees or displaced persons. The most commonly reported diseases in this period and the main causes of death can be identified clinically, and their treatment will be presumptive or symptomatic.

On the other hand, as soon as an infectious agent is suspected of being the possible cause of a major outbreak, every means must be employed to ensure a precise identification (see above, page 148, under *Investigating the epidemic*). This essentially means having sample material available for testing and a reference laboratory network (e.g. Institut Pasteur) to turn to for confirmation, whenever necessary[10]. Simple sampling techniques exist for blood or stool testing on filter paper, for example, for the identification of cholera *vibrio* or unexplained fevers. Testing and sampling kits must be available in the field whenever there is a risk of an outbreak[10]. Moreover, in cases where meningococcal meningitis is suspected or there is a risk of epidemic, it is wiser to have a kit for rapid diagnosis using cerebrospinal fluid (rapid test)[10,11].

In any hospital facility performing transfusions, it is essential not only to have serum tests for determining blood types, but also equipment for rapid HIV screening[10,12]. Rapid screening tests for viral antigens of hepatitis B (HBS) may also be considered, depending on the material and human resource capabilities of the hospital. Screening for syphilis is a more difficult issue, as simple tests like the VDRL lead to multiple cross-reactions from other antigens, and it is rarely possible to perform more complex tests such as RPR in emergency situations.

Only material required for performing the above-mentioned techniques would normally be considered essential emergency equipment. Besides, it is advisable to identify a reliable laboratory nearby (e.g. in a neighbouring hospital) for necessary tests that cannot be performed in the refugee setting. This also implies that health workers should know how to collect and send the samples.

However, there may be exceptions to this very limited programme:

- A medical team may need to carry out an assessment of the drug resistance of certain malaria plasmodium strains. This may have to be done during the emergency phase because of the grave consequences of treatment failures (see section *Malaria control* below)[13]. Such an evaluation needs specialist advice and equipment.

- *Shigella dysenteriae* type A (Sd1) and other agents responsible for dysentery outbreaks require specific and rapid investigation. Identifying the bacteria requires culture as it dies rapidly outside the body. The major problem with such epidemics is that antibiotic resistance develops rapidly. Monitoring this resistance by regular antibiotic sensitivity testing is of prime importance for the control of an epidemic of this type. If there is no reference laboratory able to test, culture and carry out sensitivity tests, equipment will have to be supplied to set up a laboratory and staff will have to be specially trained (see section *Control of diarrheoal diseases* below)[14].

AFTER THE EMERGENCY PHASE

Once the emergency phase is past, a laboratory performing basic complementary tests may be necessary as a diagnostic aid[10,15]. Its use and limitations should be carefully assessed, including indications on which health staff are permitted to request testing or refer specimens. A basic laboratory is not expensive, but local staff will usually require extra training or refresher courses on laboratory techniques.

The main tests requested are usually malaria smears and stool examinations (for intestinal parasites). As each test requires a certain amount of time for preparation and microscopic observation, there is an obvious danger of decreasing their reliability by overloading laboratory staff. It is therefore wise to impose strict limits on laboratory testing and the referral of specimens[10].

Microscopic diagnosis of tuberculosis should only be planned if all other measures for managing the disease have already been implemented (see *Tuberculosis Programme* in Part III).

Some epidemics of certain tropical parasitoses, which are public health priorities among the displaced people in some regions, require screening, and complicated and cumbersome treatment: for instance African trypanosomiasis and visceral leishmaniasis (see *Human african trypanosomiasis* and *Leishmaniasis* in appendix 4). The laboratory has a primary role to play here in regard to screening tests and decisions about therapy, and the equipment and expertise required are beyond the scope of a basic clinical laboratory.

Control of the main communicable diseases

Control of the most common communicable diseases - diarrhoeal diseases (including dysentery and cholera), acute respiratory diseases, measles and malaria - is dealt with in sub-sections of this chapter.

The control of rarer or less severe diseases, which experience has proven to be potentially epidemic or endemic in a refugee context, is treated in Annex 3. The diseases covered are meningococcal meningitis, hepatitis, haemorrhagic fevers, including yellow fever and dengue, typhus, relapsing fever, typhoid fever, influenza, leishmaniasis, plague, trypanosomiasis, Japanese encephalitis, schistosomiasis, poliomyelitis, whooping cough, tetanus, scabies, conjunctivitis and Guinea worm. The control of sexually transmitted diseases, including AIDS, and tuberculosis is dealt with by individual chapters in Part III (see *HIV, AIDS and STD,* and *Tuberculosis Programme*).

Principal recommendations regarding the control of communicable diseases and epidemics

- The 4 major communicable diseases responsible for most mortality (diarrhoeal diseases, respiratory infections, measles and malaria) must be brought under control.

- Preventive measures are the most effective, and health facilities are essential for the early management of cases.

- Health teams must be ready to react to epidemics by preparing contingency plans in regard to material and staff requirements, protocols, health facilities, etc.

- Every outbreak requires a response specific to the disease.

✎ References

1. Moren, A, Rigal, J, Biberson, Ph. Populations réfugiées. Programme de santé publique et urgence de l'intervention. MSF-F, Epicentre. *Rev Prat*, 1992, 172: 767-76.

2. CDC. Famine-affected, refugee, and displaced populations: Recommendations for public health issues. *MMWR*, 1992, 41(RR-13): 1-76.

3. Toole, M J, Waldman, R J. Prevention of excess mortality in refugees and displaced populations in developing countries. *JAMA*, 1990, 263(24): 3296-302.

4. Hausman, B. *Guidelines for epidemics: General procedures*. Amsterdam: Médecins Sans Frontières, 1994.

5. Simmonds, S, Vaughan, P, William Gun, S. *Refugee community health care*. Oxford: Oxford University Press, 1983.

6. Dabis, F, Drucker, J, Moren, A. *Épidémiologie d'intervention*. Paris: Arnette, 1992.

7. UNHCR. *Operational guidelines for health and nutrition programmes in refugee settings*. Geneva: UNHCR, 1987.

8. CDC. *Guidelines for collecting, processing, storing, and shipping diagnostic specimens in refugee health-care environments.* Atlanta: US Department of Health and Human Services - Public Health Services CDC, 1992.

9. Morton, R F, Hebel, J R. *Epidemiology and biostatistics.* Baltimore: University Park Press, 1990.

10. Lacroix, C. *Guide du laboratoire médical.* Paris: Médecins Sans Frontières, 1994.

11. Médecins Sans Frontières. *Conduite à tenir en cas d'épidémie de méningite à méningocoque.* Paris: Médecins Sans Frontières, 1993.

12. Médecins Sans Frontières. *La pratique transfusionnelle en milieu isolé.* Paris: Médecins Sans Frontières, 1997.

13. WHO. *Antimalarial drug policies. Data requirements, treatment of uncomplicared malaria and management of malaria in pregnancy.* Geneva: WHO, 1994.

14. WHO. *Guidelines for the control of epidemics due to Shigella dysenteriae type 1.* Genève: WHO, 1995. WHO/CDR/95.4.

15. WHO. *Manual of basic techniques for a health laboratory.* Geneva: WHO, 1980.

16. Médecins Sans Frontières. *Laboratory diagnosis.* Amsterdam: Médecins Sans Frontières, 1995.

A - Control of diarrhoeal diseases

Introduction

Diarrhoeal diseases represent a major public health problem in developing countries. Each year, at least 4 million children under 5 years of age die from diarrhoea, 80% of them under 2 years old. *Rotavirus, Colibacillus* and *Shigella* are the most commonly identified infectious agents[10].

An inadequate water supply (both in quantity and quality), poor sanitation, overcrowding and malnutrition are the main factors implicated in the occurrence, spread and severity of diarrhoeal diseases. Malnutrition and diarrhoeal diseases are particularly closely linked; malnutrition increases the severity and duration of diarrhoea, and diarrhoea may cause malnutrition[12].

Among refugee and displaced populations, diarrhoeal diseases are a major cause of morbidity and count as one of the main killer diseases; in the refugee camps of Somalia (1980), Ethiopia (1982), Malawi (1988) and Goma (Zaire, 1994), 28-85% of deaths were attributable to diarrhoeal diseases[3,7]. However, most deaths from diarrhoea can be easily prevented by oral rehydration therapy (ORT).

SURVEILLANCE

Surveillance of diarrhoeal diseases is included in the routine surveillance system and as far as possible should be in line with the host country's national programme for the control of diarrhoeal diseases (CDD).

Cases of bloody and non-bloody diarrhoea should be recorded separately and it should be indicated whether they fall into the under-five or over-five age group. Deaths from bloody and non-bloody diarrhoea should be recorded separately in the mortality surveillance whenever possible, depending on the ability of staff to determine cause of death by interviewing families (verbal autopsy, see *8. Public Health Surveillance*). This information enables the detection of dysentery or cholera epidemics.

Medical staff should be alerted when one of the following observations are made:

– adult deaths (or deaths over 5 years) due to diarrhoea,

– an increase in the number of adult cases with diarrhoea and dehydration,

– a significant increase of cases of bloody diarrhoea (dysentery cases),

– a rise in the case fatality rate.

These observations should be followed up by a rapid laboratory confirmation of cholera or shigellosis cases. Procedures for taking specimen and laboratory tests to be performed are available in guidelines[15,16].

PREVENTION

Preventive measures consist of improving the standards of water and sanitation (see 3. *Water and Sanitation*) and ensuring adequate general nutrition. They involve:

- an adequate and accessible supply of clean water;

- an adequate disposal system for human excreta (latrines or defecation field);

- improved personal hygiene by providing soap in sufficient quantities and through health education with regard to environmental, food and personal hygiene;

- a regular and adequate food ration for everyone, and the promotion of breast feeding;

- control of food safety through health education for those selling food in a market and for the general population, although this is often not practical.

CASE MANAGEMENT

Apart from the case management specific to each diarrhoeal disease, dehydration and malnutrition should be prevented or treated.

- Early rehydration is the most important treatment for preventing death and requires the organization of oral rehydration therapy (ORT) units. An ORT unit must be set up in every health facility (hospital, health centre and health post) and feeding centre, as diarrhoeal diseases always represent a major problem in refugee populations. In practice, at the start of an intervention, a lack of trained staff may make it impossible to open a sufficient number of ORT units; but at least one ORT corner should rapidly be set up in the central health facility, followed by others once staff have been trained. It is important to decentralize ORT units so that the population has easy access to them and the highest possible coverage of diarrhoeal cases can be ensured.

  Further decentralization might be considered in situations such as epidemics: small ORT units scattered around the camp supported by trained staff (e.g. community health workers) may supplement existing health facilities[7]. These units should detect serious cases (dysentery and severe dehydration) and refer them to health facilities, ensure rehydration throughout the day of other cases and may be coupled with active case-finding by home-visitors. However, this strategy is only feasible when the staff are sufficiently well trained to identify severe cases and refer them immediately, and when close supervision is ensured. These conditions are often not present, at least not in the first stages of an emergency.

  Unfortunately, the organization of rehydration centres is frequently a weak point in refugee relief programmes: ORT centres are not seen as a priority when there is no outbreak of diarrhoea: their set-up is generally delayed (until a month after beginning an emergency programme in many cases) and their numbers insufficient[9]. In addition, they are often limited to distributing oral rehydration salts (ORS) packs and the information provided to patients is not sufficient to ensure the continuity of rehydration and the quality of the solution once they are back home.

A major and common problem is that most people, whether mothers of dehydrated children or health staff, do not believe in oral rehydration. Patient compliance with oral rehydration treatment is therefore difficult to achieve and additional efforts will be required to improve it through targeted health education by medical staff and home-visitors. A clear explanation of how to prepare the solution at home is essential.

• Feeding and breast-feeding must be continued and are particularly important in view of the strong relationship between malnutrition and diarrhoeal diseases (see above).

EPIDEMICS OF SEVERE DIARRHOEAL DISEASES

These have become increasingly common among displaced and refugee populations over the last few years. The responsible pathogens are most likely to be the same agents that cause diarrhoea in non-refugee populations in developing countries. Epidemics due to *Shigella dysenteriae* type 1, *Vibrio cholerae*, and *Escherichia coli* 0157 are the ones most frequently encountered and are dealt with in this chapter[5].

Shigellosis

Shigella is the most frequent cause of dysentery (see other causes below). *Shigella dysenteriae* from serogroup type 1 (or Sd1) differs from the other *Shigella* serogroups in 3 ways[1]:

1. It is the only cause of large-scale and prolonged dysentery epidemics.

2. Antimicrobial resistance occurs more frequently.

3. It is the most virulent organism, causing more severe, prolonged and frequently fatal illness, with high case fatality rates[1].

Infection with Sd1 is most common in overcrowded areas with poor sanitation and water supplies. Refugee populations are thus at especially high risk[1].

A major characteristic of shigellosis is that it is highly contagious. The infectious dose is very low as compared, for example, with cholera: the ingestion of as few as 10 to 100 organisms can cause the disease (while the cholera infectious dose is counted in millions).

A major concern about *Shigella* is its extraordinary ability to develop strains multi-resistant to antibiotics. Sd1 has shown resistance to a wide range of antimicrobials such as ampicillin, cotrimoxazole and more recently nalidixic acid. Recent studies have shown that resistance patterns can vary considerably over time and within defined areas[3]. But a major obstacle to monitoring and quantifying antibiotic resistance is the fragility of the micro-organism (culture failures are frequent). The consequences of multi-resistance are increasing difficulties in case-management and the high cost of treatment (because of newer drugs required). While the mechanisms involved in the development of resistance are not fully identified, it is clear that health staff and patients are both partly responsible: health staff by large, uncontrolled or incorrect use of the drugs - resulting in over or under-prescription - and the patient by poor treatment compliance. Rapid and simple tests for diagnosis are still in the experimental stage.

EPIDEMIC DESCRIPTION

Dysentery epidemics due to Sd1 occur mostly in highly endemic areas, but it is likely that most developing countries are at risk[1,2]. Epidemics have been reported throughout the world, including countries in Latin America, Asia and Africa.

Some epidemic characteristics differ between stable situations and refugee settings:

- In stable populations, overall attack rates vary by around 5%. All age groups are concerned (while endemic shigellosis affects a higher proportion of children). Around half of the infections are symptomatic, and around 10% of them are severe enough to require hospitalization. Case fatality rates (CFR) range from 10%-20% with inadequate treatment and from 2%-5% with appropriate treatment (hospital data)[2]. Seasonal variations are observed, though not in the same manner in all countries (a higher incidence can occur in both rainy or dry seasons).

- Among refugee populations, there have been large-scale outbreaks of shigellosis, especially in Africa (Rwanda[4], Tanzania[6], Zaire[14]), causing high mortality rates. The overall attack rates have reached levels above 30%[1], with weekly incidence rates ranging from 2%-10% (Rwanda, 1994[13]). In most reported outbreaks, children under five were the most affected, with attack rates twice those observed among the over-fives[6]. It has been observed that the overall attack rate in camps seems to be related to population density. The disease does not appear to be more serious in refugee settings - except when there is a high level of malnutrition. On the contrary, CFRs can be even lower than in open situations because good treatment compliance is easier to ensure: CFR based on hospital data was 1% in Goma (Zaire, 1994) where treatment was 5 days of ciprofloxacine[13]. However, a major proportion of shigellosis deaths in large refugee settlements occur at home[6].

OUTBREAK CONTROL

Outbreak investigation

- In the absence of a clear epidemic threshold, an epidemic should be suspected if one of the following is observed in the routine data collection:
  - an unusual or sudden rise of new cases in weekly reports,
  - an increase in the proportion of dysentery within diarrhoeal cases,
  - an increased number of deaths from bloody diarrhoea.

Stool specimens should be collected from dysentery cases and sent for analysis in the early stages of an outbreak in order to identify the causative agent and determine the antibiotic resistance patterns (initially and for monitoring). The preparation of specimens is complex and culture failures are frequent (28% of positive stool samples among clinical shigellosis cases in Rwanda, 1994)[13]. Strict procedures must be followed (see below) and detailed information is available in reference documents[1,11,15,16]. Once *Shigella* has been confirmed as the causative agent of the epidemic, cases should be diagnosed clinically[1].

However, antibiotic resistance must be monitored periodically: tests should be carried out on specimens (on at least 20 specimens with Sd1) every one or two months, or if a new resistance is suspected on clinical grounds.

- The case definition should be standardized immediately, using the recommended case definition for dysentery[1]:

> **Case definition for dysentery[1]:**
> any case of diarrhoea with visible blood in the stools.

In theory, medical staff should check for the presence of blood in the fresh stools of suspect cases, or at least when there is doubt[1]. However, it may be difficult to convince staff to respect this recommendation[3,6].

- For surveillance and reporting purposes, the number of deaths from bloody diarrhoea must be recorded in routine mortality data and staff should be trained in verbal autopsy if required. For each case, the registered data should include the date of onset, origin, age, treatment and outcome (including eventual treatment failure).

CFRs based on hospital data must be monitored to assess the efficacy of the treatment.

> **Principles to be followed when taking stool samples in a *Shigella* epidemic[1]**
>
> - Selection of cases for bacteriological sampling should respect these criteria:
>   - onset of illness less than 4 days before sampling,
>   - current bloody diarrhoea,
>   - no antibiotic treatment received,
>   - patient consent.
> - A sufficient number of samples must be tested: 20 samples minimum per site.
> - An appropriate laboratory is selected, located as close as possible to the settlement.
> - A specific transport medium must be used, and the specimen should be kept refrigerated.

Preventive measures

Person-to-person transmission plays an important role and the promotion of personal hygiene is therefore the best preventive measure. Moreover, there is a risk of transmission by water and food as large numbers of Sd1 are excreted in stools, and as *S. flexneri* and *S. sonnei* can survive for up to six months in water and some foodstuffs (little is known about Sd1 survival in the environment).

Preventive measures are those described for all diarrhoeal diseases, but some deserve particular attention given *Shigella* characteristics:

– sufficient quantities of water should be available;

– soap should be available: several studies have shown the important impact of soap distribution, e.g. in Bangladesh it reduced the secondary infection rate from 32.4% among controls to 10.1% among the targeted population[2];

– the use and maintenance of latrines should be promoted;

– attention should be paid to food preparation and consumption;

– adequate food rations should be ensured.

Some potential vaccines are on trial.

Case management

- **High-risk patients**, i.e. those most at risk of dying from dysentery, must be identified and receive appropriate attention. According to WHO, high risk patients are [1]:

  – children under 5 years,

  – adults above 50 years,

  – any case which is dehydrated, has had convulsions, or is seriously ill when first seen,

  – older children or adults who are obviously malnourished.

  Ideally, all severe dysentery cases should be hospitalized and receive effective antibiotic treatment under strict medical supervision. If sufficient space is available in in-patient facilities, other high-risk patients can also be hospitalized. Otherwise, they are treated by the out-patient department with careful follow up.

- **Therapy with an effective antibiotic** is the mainstay of treatment for Sd1. This therapy lessens the risk of serious complications and death, and should ideally be given to all dysentery patients. However, there are major obstacles to the feasibility and effectiveness of such a strategy: the very high number of cases in epidemics which makes it unrealistic, the rapid variation in Sd1 resistance to antibiotics during an epidemic, poor patient compliance with the current 5-day treatment course, and the high cost of effective drugs which limits their availability[1,2].

In practice, the use of antibiotics will depend on the availability of effective antimicrobials[1]:

– If an effective antibiotic is available for all cases, it should be given to every patient, under the direct observation of health staff.

– When the supply of an effective antibiotic is insufficient to treat all cases, for instance when it is too expensive (see below), antibiotics should be reserved for patients who have to be hospitalized, i.e. those at higher risk of dying (high-risk patients and patients whose clinical state worsens without antimicrobial therapy); other cases receive only supportive therapy (rehydration and nutrition).

The selection of an effective antibiotic is a complicated problem because the variations in resistance patterns make it impossible to make clear recommendations (and it must be kept in mind that *in vitro* susceptibility does not always mean efficacy *in vivo*). Information should be gathered on recent susceptibility testing of Sd1 strains from a nearby area or from the current outbreak. Nalidixic acid has been the drug of choice in most areas, but resistance to it is increasing rapidly (close to 100% resistance in the main areas of Central Africa in 1994)[13]. Sd1 currently remains sensitive to recent quinolones (e.g. ciprofloxacine), but their use might be a complex issue because they are very expensive and contraindicated for pregnant women; their use in children is still debated because of a lack of data on their side-effects (WHO trials are currently under way)[1]. However, they remain the only alternative when resistance to nalidixic acid is high.

In practice, the selection of an antibiotic should take the following into account:

– when information on resistance is not available, nalidixic acid can be used until the results of susceptibility testing are obtained;

– when resistance to nalidixic acid is above 50%, quinolones should be used. As this treatment is very expensive, only severely ill patients should receive antibiotics, and under medical supervision (ideally as in-patients).

The problem of treatment compliance is mainly related to the treatment duration[1,2]. An assessment of the compliance with a 5-day course of nalidixic acid in Rwandan refugee camps in 1993, revealed a rate of 72% at day two and 45% at day five, in spite of several measures taken to improve it[4].

Measures to improve treatment compliance may include:

– ensuring accessibility to treatment by the provision of a sufficient number of peripheral facilities;

– instructing medical staff in how to educate patients on the need to complete treatment;

– instruction/supervision of home-visitors on the active follow-up of cases under treatment [3,4];

– possibly offering incentives to complete the treatment (e.g. food rations).

Other possible measures must be explored and tested locally, accompanied by a regular monitoring of compliance rates. The development of a single-dose treatment would clearly constitute a major advance in the area.

- **Adequate nutrition** is essential for a good prognosis. If possible, hospitalized patients should receive frequent small meals; if resources are sufficient, ambulatory cases should be given a supplementary dry food ration[1,4]. Severe cases in convalescence should be admitted into feeding programmes (see below).

- **The rehydration of patients** is not as important in shigellosis as in acute watery diarrhoea, since complications and mortality are not primarily caused by dehydration[1]. However, dehydration should be looked for in all cases and rehydration initiated early, because it is associated with a greater severity of the illness[1].

Organization of treatment services

In the case of large epidemics in refugee settings, the organization of services to treat shigellosis cases usually involves two operational aspects to deal with the high load of patients: the verticalization and the decentralization of services, usually in association.

- The vertical organization of services, consisting in the setting up of dysentery services separate from other health services, is usually advisable during large outbreaks. This offers several advantages: it allows better case handling (as compared to what could be provided in the existing, over-stretched services), it restricts the transmission to other patients given the high contagiousness of shigellosis, and it facilitates the standardization of protocols and allows a better monitoring of antibiotic resistance.

Separate services organized for the management of dysentery cases include:

- a shigellosis treatment unit providing in-patient care. It is often the only feasible solution to caring for the 10-25% of total dysentery cases that need hospitalization (according to WHO hospitalization criteria). This unit may be a new structure or a special ward in the general in-patient facility, but must at least have a separate entrance and sanitation facilities. The isolation of patients is not required, providing adequate nursing barriers are present;

- a separate consultation facility (with separate entrance and waiting room) for the treatment of ambulatory cases. This should improve patient compliance through closer follow up;

- a separate drug-dispensary area may also be useful as it makes it easier to cope with a high number of patients (especially when treatment is given daily), to provide comprehensive information on the necessity of completing the course of treatment, and to monitor treatment compliance;

- a special feeding unit may be included to ensure their nutritional recovery;

– Home-visitors are asked to perform specific tasks: the active case-finding of dysentery cases, referral to treatment centres, and follow-up of patient compliance. Home-visitors must quickly be trained in these tasks and should be linked to the treatment centre for their area.

If the number of cases is low and existing health structures can cope with the additional caseload, verticalization is not particularly recommended.

• The decentralization of treatment centres, i.e. the setting up of peripheral centres where treatment is provided, has the major advantage of improving accessibility to patients (services are closer to hand), thus reducing the waiting time as compared to that in overcrowded central facilities. Decentralization is particularly justified when attack rates are high (they may go as high as 30%), thus affecting a very large portion of the population. The usual procedures are listed as follows:

– Ambulatory cases are treated in peripheral centres where they can receive rehydration and antibiotic therapy[4]. There are two options: special temporary facilities are opened to operate only during the outbreak, or the normal curative health services are expanded by opening additional facilities which may remain afterwards (see *6. Health Care in the Emergency Phase*).

– Patients requiring hospitalization are usually referred to a central in-patient unit; the decentralization of such units is not advised.

However, such decentralization can only function properly if adequate and continued supervision is ensured. There is always a high risk when treatment is provided to serious cases by under-skilled staff without intensive supervision, and severe cases are not referred in time to appropriate units, or that antibiotic treatment is provided to patients other than those with shigellosis.

Cholera and shigellosis outbreaks have occurred simultaneously in refugee or displaced camps (Malawi 1992, Angola 1992, Zaire 1994). In these cases, the question arises whether to separate shigellosis cases from cholera cases. There is no clear advantage in separating them as the disinfection measures are similar in either case. However, given how highly contagious shigellosis is, it might be advisable to set up two different units in the same compound to prevent cross-contamination.

E. *coli* 0157:H7

E. coli 0157:H7 is another cause of dysentery, and has produced localized outbreaks of dysentery in Europe and North America. Such outbreaks have not often been documented in refugee settings: *E. coli* 0157:H7 has been proven to be the cause of an outbreak among Mozambican refugees in Swaziland in 1993, and was probably the causative agent of another outbreak in the Lisungwi refugee camp (Malawi) in 1992[14]. However, it is probable that such epidemics have occurred and been misclassified as dysentery due to *Shigella*. Since dysentery due to *E. coli* does not respond to antibiotic treatment, it is important to rule out *E. coli* in case of a suspected shigellosis outbreak.

OTHER CAUSES OF DYSENTERY

Other causes of endemic dysentery are *Campylobacter jejuni*, *Salmonella* and *Entamoeba histolytica*.

E. histolytica does not cause epidemic disease. But since healthy carriers of *E. Histolytica* cysts are frequent in developing countries, it has been identified in several Sd1 outbreaks and was initially thought to be the cause of them. Finding cysts of *E. histolytica* in bloody stools during an epidemic does not indicate that it is the cause of the epidemic.

✎ Key references on shigellosis

1. WHO. *Guidelines for the control of epidemics due to Shigella dysenteriae type 1*. Genève: WHO, 1995. WHO/CDR/95.4.

2. Cobra, C, Sack, D A. *Strategic response to epidemic dysentery in Africa*. Baltimore: School of Public Health, Johns Hopkins University, 1994.

Other references

3. Murray, J, Espey, D. *Sentinel disease surveillance and antibiotic resistance patterns of Shigella dysentery type 1 in Burundi, 12/11/93 - 01/22/94*. Mission Report, February 1994. Atlanta: IHPO/CDC, 1994.

4. Paquet, C, Leborgne, P, Lebague, Sasse, A, Varaine, F. Une épidémie de dysenterie à *Shigella dysenteriae* type 1 dans un camp de réfugiés au Rwanda. *Cahier Santé*, 1995, 5(3): 181-4.

5. Toole, M J, Waldman, R J. Refugees and displaced persons: War, hunger and public health. *JAMA*, 1993, 270(5): 600-5.

6. Paquet, C, Sasse, A, Varaine F, Leborgne P. Epidémies de dysentérie et déplacement de population en Afrique de l'Est. *Medical News*, 1994, 3(2): 51-2.

7. CDC. Famine-affected, refugee, and displaced populations: Recommendations for public health issues. *MMWR*, 1992, 41(RR-13): 1-76.

8. CDC. Public health consequences of acute displacement of Iraqui citizens, March-May 1991. *MMWR*, 1991, 40(26): 443-7.

9. Brown, V. *Evaluation des interventions en urgence de Médecins Sans Frontières. Impact des évaluations Epicentre*. Paris: Epicentre, 1992.

10. Médecins Sans Frontières. *Laboratory diagnosis*. Amsterdam: Médecins Sans Frontières, 1995.

11. Lacroix, C. *Protocole pour la culture de shigelle*. [doc. interne]. Paris: Médecins Sans Frontières, 1993.

12. Tomkins, O, Watson, F. *Malnutrition and infection. A review*. ACC/SCN State of the art series. Nutrition Policy Discussion Paper No.5. London: UN Center of Human Nutrition, 1989.

13. Paquet, C. *Caractéristiques de l'épidémie de dysenterie dans les populations déplacées d'Afrique Centrale en 1994*. Paris: Journées Scientifiques 1994-1995, Epicentre, Médecins Sans Frontières, 1994.

14. Paquet, C, Perea, W, Grimont, F. Aetiology of haemorrhagic colitis epidemic in Africa. *The Lancet*, 1993, 342: 175.

15. Lacroix, C. *Guide du laboratoire médical*. Paris: Médecins Sans Frontières, 1994.

Cholera

The seventh pandemic of *Vibrio cholerae* O:1 biotype *El Tor* began in Indonesia in 1961, and in 1993, 78 countries reported 376,845 cases with a global case-fatality rate of 1.8%[1]. Another cholera serogroup, *Vibrio cholerae* O:139 was identified in 1992 in India. This vibrio might represent the beginning of a new cholera pandemic particularly since it is not affected by previous immunity to O:1.1. In Asia and the former states of the USSR, *V. cholerae* O:139 also represents a new danger for the next few years.

Cholera transmission usually takes place via the faecal-oral route; infection is acquired after ingestion of a high number of vibrios present in water or food. Where there are large population concentrations, with poor hygiene conditions, direct transmission from person to person may be suspected. Cholera infection does not lead to severe diarrhoea in every individual: among infected persons, 75% of them will have no symptoms, 20% will have mild or moderate diarrhoea, and only 5% a severe clinical infection (or clinical cholera)[9].

In refugee camps, overcrowding, poor sanitation and inadequate water supplies combined with the disorganization of services have considerably increased the risk of cholera epidemics[1].

In Malawi (1988), a first epidemic arose among Mozambican refugees, and many further outbreaks occurred in the following years, some outbreaks lasting more than 3 months[8]. In 1994, a major cholera outbreak (V.O:1) hit the newly arrived Rwandan refugees in Goma (Zaire), lasting only a few weeks after the influx, but it is estimated that there were between 58,000 and 80,000 cases in the first weeks (around 1,000 cholera-related deaths per day) out of an estimated population of 500,000 to 800,000 refugees[14].

Although cholera is a major killer, it should be remembered that acute diarrhoea - due to other causes than cholera - kills far more than cholera in refugee settings.

EPIDEMIC DESCRIPTION

Two serogroups, *Vibrio cholerae* O:1 and *Vibrio cholerae* O:139, are responsible for cholera outbreaks. *Vibrio cholerae* O:1 occurs as two biotypes - classical and *El Tor*. Each biotype also occurs as two serotypes - *Ogawa* and *Inaba*. These two serotypes may coexist in the same epidemic. The transmission modes and clinical effects are similar for all these serogroups, biotypes and serotypes; the recommendations for dealing with outbreaks are thus the same.

According to WHO, a cholera outbreak should be suspected when[4]:
- a patient older than 5 years develops severe dehydration or dies from acute watery diarrhoea, or
- there is a sudden increase in the daily number of patients with acute watery diarrhoea, especially patients who pass the 'rice water' stools typical of cholera.

In refugee or displaced settlements, any adult death by dehydration is thus highly suspect.

An outbreak is declared as soon as there is a single bacteriologically-confirmed case.

In open situations, the attack rate mostly varies from 1-2%, while in refugee camps, around 5% of the population may be expected to develop clinical cholera. The rate has been even higher in some epidemics; for instance, in the cholera epidemic in Goma (Zaire, 1994), the attack rate was 8% and it is assumed that all refugees were infected (compare above: 5% of all those infected develop a clinical cholera)[3,14].

Attack rates vary in line with the population's previous immunity, sanitary conditions, the level of overcrowding, the accuracy of records and the case definition used[5].

Cholera is a disease that can rapidly kill if left untreated: up to 50% of patients may die in the absence of treatment. The case fatality rate (CFR) depends on the case definition used, the handling of cases and the quality of records. The CFR is usually higher in the first 2 weeks of the outbreak[19]. A low CFR can be achieved by a combination of factors: adequate preparedness, rapid action, good public awareness, good collaboration among international agencies and with the local authorities, few security problems and no major staff problems[6]. In any cholera epidemic, the objective should be to achieve a CFR below 2%[5].

Epidemics in refugee camps generally last from 3 weeks to more than 3 months[17].

OUTBREAK PREPAREDNESS

In most refugee or displaced populations, cholera is a significant health risk, and a particularly high one when populations come from, pass through or settle in a cholera-affected area[17]. In such higher-risk situations, plans for responding to an eventual cholera outbreak should be prepared well before the emergence of the first cases, ideally as soon as refugees begin to gather (or prior to arrival when possible).

Planning should make it possible to limit the extent of an outbreak and reduce both the CFR and the cost of the response.

Preparedness plans contain several elements:

1. The early detection of the first patients with cholera is of prime importance and a routine surveillance system should be prepared to detect them.
   - The number of diarrhoeal cases and deaths due to diarrhoea, occurring in both adults and children, should be recorded daily.
   - A cholera case definition for suspected cases should be established, based on clinical criteria. In most countries where cholera is endemic, the national programme has determined a case definition which can be applied. In other situations, e.g. where cholera is not endemic, a standard case definition can be used but should be adapted once the epidemic is confirmed (see case definitions under *Outbreak investigation* below)[4,5].

2. Clear protocols should be prepared on how to deal with suspected cases of cholera. A reference laboratory should be identified, and material for collecting stool specimens be available[4]. The confirmation of suspected cases is described below under *Outbreak investigation*.

3. Cholera treatment units should be prepared before the outbreak. This requires the identification and preparation of sites, arrangements for stocks of material and drugs, and organization of the patient flow[3,4]. Cholera treatment kits have been developed by several agencies; MSF kits provide for the treatment of 625 cholera patients per kit, based on 500 patients receiving intravenous treatment. Such kits (at least one) should be pre-positioned in the area so as to be rapidly available when required.

It is questionable as to whether there is a necessity to have fully-prepared cholera units before cases occur. However, a site for a cholera unit should at least be identified and prepared (e.g. cleaned and fenced). When there is increased risk of an outbreak, e.g. when there is an outbreak in a neighbouring area, all the required material (logistical equipment and drugs) should be available immediately (see under *Requirements for cholera units* below). As soon as an outbreak is declared, the decision to open cholera units should be taken without delay. A referral system (from health facilities to cholera units) should be planned in advance.

4. Measures in regard to the water supply and sanitation should be reinforced and the standard objectives (e.g. water supply of 20 litres per person per day) should be reached as soon as possible. Water chlorination products should be on hand. Cemeteries should be planned.

5. Home-visitors and health workers should receive extra training in the detection of suspected cholera cases, rehydration techniques and prevention of disease. Additional staff should be identified: skilled and unskilled people will be needed to work in the cholera units and to reinforce other aspects of outbreak control, e.g. water and sanitation measures (see the requirements listed in Table 7.1, page 169). Individual job descriptions should already be prepared in advance[6].

6. Cholera vaccines exist but their effectiveness is not yet proven; parenteral vaccine against cholera has not been recommended since 1971[4]. New oral vaccines have been developed against the *V. cholerae* O:1 (but provide no protection against O:139) and are currently being tested. They provide a better short-term protection than the parenteral one; they protect against death and severe illness[11,13,14]. The most promising vaccine so far, the WC/BS vaccine, has to be administered in two doses, with a seven-day interval between doses; protection starts after a further week. These new vaccines may appear attractive for use in refugee crises, but their use is not yet recommended in refugee emergencies[14,19].

7. Although it is important that health education should be provided to the refugee population, its success largely depends on their previous level of knowledge. If the population is not aware of diarrhoeal diseases, more personnel will have to be trained to supervise defecation fields and latrines, chlorinate and protect water, etc.

OUTBREAK CONTROL

Outbreak investigation

As soon as cholera cases are suspected, they must be confirmed by laboratory investigation as soon as possible[4]. Specimens (e.g. around 10) should be sent to an international reference laboratory to identify the vibrio and test its antibiotic sensitivity. Several methods of collecting samples may be used, but the preferred one is the use of filter paper in a small plastic container[5]. A rapid test (ELISA) is currently under study, but so far does not present any advantage over the classical test. However, treatment should start and other measures should be implemented immediately, without waiting for laboratory confirmation[7]. Once the vibrio has been identified, further stool testing is no longer necessary.

Once the outbreak has been confirmed, it is important to use a simpler case definition to allow a larger-scale and earlier detection of cholera cases; for instance, WHO case definitions differ according to whether cholera is already present or not[4].

> **WHO case definition for suspected cholera[4]:**
> A case of cholera should be suspected when :
> – in an area where the disease is not known to be present, a patient aged 5 years or more develops severe dehydration or dies from acute watery diarrhoea;
> – in an area where there is an outbreak of cholera, any patient aged 5 years or more develops acute watery diarrhoea, with or without vomiting.

> **MSF case definition for presumed cholera[5]:**
> any patient developing a rapid onset of severe watery diarrhoea (usually with vomiting), resulting in severe dehydration.

Each case definition presents disadvantages: the second WHO case definition leads to the inclusion of diarrhoeal cases which are not due to cholera, while a too restrictive (or too specific) definition would lead to underestimating the number of cholera cases.

Active case finding

As the onset of cholera disease is very abrupt, cases should be detected and treated as early as possible. Trained home-visitors and health workers should actively screen the population to detect suspected cases. Any dehydrated patient should be immediately admitted into the cholera unit to receive treatment; mild cases may be treated in existing health facilities (by oral rehydration), providing that the detection and referral of severe cases is properly organized. In some situations, where resources and capacity allow, all suspected cases are referred to the cholera unit, at least for observation. In open situations, more resources are required in order to ensure quick identification and transportation to the cholera unit.

Case management

Patients must be quickly rehydrated with oral rehydration salts (ORS) or Ringer's lactate, depending on the level of dehydration and conscious level. Recommendations on the proportion of patients that need intravenous treatment vary with the guidelines: the WHO states that 80%-90% of cholera patients can usually be adequately treated with ORS solution alone, and that 20% of the patients can be rehydrated by intravenous treatment[4]. However, experience has shown that this proportion is too low for refugee settings and that it can reach 75%, probably because the proportion of severe dehydration is higher[5]. It is therefore advised to base the perfusion requirements on an estimated 75% of patients requiring intravenous treatment[5,15]. Careful supervision of rehydration is necessary to ensure that patients are rehydrated quickly enough, but also to prevent excess fluid being administrated (especially among children)[7,18].

Short-course antibiotic therapy can reduce the duration of excretion of the vibrio in stools and the volume of stools, and is still recommended by WHO for severely dehydrated patients[4]. Doxycycline is the preferred antibiotic because only a single dose is needed, and it does not put extraburden on the disease management[4,5]. Nevertheless, *Vibrio El Tor* is increasingly resistant to all common antibiotics, and *V. cholerae* O:139 is also becoming resistant to some antibiotics[2]. Sensitivity testing - when available - should be undertaken. In outbreaks where the vibrio is sensitive to doxycycline, a single dose of doxycycline will be given to severe cases[4]. When it is not sensitive to doxycycline, the use of antibiotics is usually not recommended in practice, because the benefits do not outweigh the extraload it puts on the health services. Antibiotics will never be given outside the rehydration unit, and in any situation priority should always be given to rehydration[1,5].

Cholera treatment unit

The decision to open such a unit should be taken early (e.g. when 5 new cases are being admitted daily)[5]. As contacts between patients and the community have to be restricted, the cholera unit should be located apart from the other health care facilities, but not too distant from the population so as to ensure easy access. Movements into and out of the unit are controlled; only the staff involved in the management of the unit and one family member (the same person for the duration of the treatment) should be admitted.

Regular disinfection is important. Fresh chlorine solutions and washing facilities must be available and it is essential to assure the safe disposal of excreta and vomit.

Cholera treatment unit requirements

The estimated number of daily patient admissions should be calculated on the basis of the expected attack rate (around 5% in camp situations), the size of the population, the expected duration of the outbreak (which should be estimated at 1 month to ensure optimal bed capacity), the average length of hospitalization (3 days) and the stage reached in the outbreak (there will be more patients at the beginning).

For instance, in a camp population of 50,000 people:

– 2,500 cases can be expected during the course of the outbreak (attack rate of 5%);

– around 1,875 cases may require intravenous treatment (75% of cases).

Staff requirements are based on the principle that 3 teams of 3 people each are required for every 20 beds (a team composed of 1 qualified health worker and 2 cleaners) to provide around-the-clock coverage.

Table 7.1
Resources required for cholera treatment units[5,6]

	Resources required	**Remarks**
Bed capacity	Around 50 beds for a population of 10,000, i.e. 30-40 beds for IV treatment 10-20 beds for oral rehydration	Based on an attack rate of 5%, duration of 1 month, 3 days of stay and 75% cases with IV treatment
Human resources	1 health worker for IV treatment/ 20 beds/8 hours 2 unskilled workers for other tasks/ 20 beds/8 hours 1 medical supervisor per 60 beds 1 coordinator per cholera unit	3 shifts of 8 hours to cover 24 hours staff previously trained and clear job descriptions
Drugs	ORS: 10 litres per patient Ringer's lactate: 8 litres per patient requiring intravenous treatment	WHO recommends to plan for 6 litres of Ringer's lactate per patient, and 20% of patients under intravenous treatment (IV).
Sanitation	Drinking water (50 litres/patient) Latrines: 1/25 patients, 2 for the staff Laundry facilities, showers, foot bath, waste pit, etc. Place to wash corpses and a morgue Incinerator for used medical material	Chlorine solutions to be prepared (in specific concentrations depending on the utilization)

In open situations, the attack rate is usually around 1% and the estimate of requirements can be adapted accordingly. However, it is important to assess the treatment habits of the local health staff in the area; they may tend to over- or under-use infusions, and therefore require greater supervision to ensure correct treatment.

Control of the transmission

- Good control of excreta and water treatment (chlorination) are the most effective measures for limiting the spread of cholera. These should ensure a safe and sufficient water supply, adequate water storage on site and at household level, soap distribution, and provision of latrines or at least defecation fields. See also *3. Water and Sanitation*. Other measures dealing with waste and education on personnel hygiene are also important[8,16].

- Corpses present a high risk of infection and great care must be taken in handling them. It is vital to ensure corpse disinfection with a chlorine solution, control of their transportation, and the prevention of physical contacts between the family and the corpses. It is debatable as to whether or not there is benefit to be gained by chlorine disinfection of patients' homes; it should not be considered a priority in refugee settings as resources would be better employed in encouraging personal hygiene[5].

Spraying the whole site with insecticide is hardly feasible but the priority for controlling flies should be given to waste disposal areas.

- Prophylaxis with antibiotics (e.g. doxycycline 200 mg/week) can be given to staff and patient helpers to calm any anxiety about becoming infected. However, it does not replace hygiene measures, and it is generally not effective since the vibrio is multi-resistant[4].

Experience shows that some control measures are ineffective:

- Mass chemoprophylaxis has never succeeded in limiting the spread of cholera. It diverts attention and resources from effective measures and contributes to the emergence of antibiotic resistance[4].
- Selective chemoprophylaxis is not recommended in refugee camps; it has been shown that focusing on other activities (i.e. water supply, sanitation and prompt treatment) results in a more effective use of resources[7].
- Travel restrictions do not prevent the spread of cholera. They require large-scale control systems and are ineffective[4].
- The use of new oral vaccines to control cholera outbreaks is not so far indicated. Indeed, this might even have negative consequences as other aspects of cholera control could be overlooked as a result[17].

Information and coordination

Local authorities, refugee leaders and all health staff should be informed as soon as an outbreak is declared. They will help to inform the population about the services available, hygiene measures to be taken, etc. It is also essential that there is good coordination among all the operating partners involved in the intervention, in order to control the epidemic effectively.

EPIDEMIOLOGICAL FOLLOW-UP

Cholera cases and deaths should be recorded daily, and indicated on a daily curve. The same case definition is used to record cases from the beginning to the end of the outbreak. Since a simple case definition is used, other causes of dehydration will probably also be included. Deaths are recorded in the treatment unit, and throughout the site by home-visitors. For every case and death, data should be collected on the patient's age, sex, and if possible, the section of the camp where s/he lived. The attack rates and case fatality rates are calculated every week (globally and by age group). It may also be useful to indicate the attack rate for each section of the camp on a map.

Case-control studies to assess the source of an outbreak can only be carried out in the early days. Later, the increasing number of healthy carriers (75% of those infected) makes the data difficult to interpret.

The use of water analysis in a cholera outbreak is questionable. The number of faecal coliforms is still the main indicator for faecally contaminated water, or residual chlorine when water has been treated with chlorine. ELISA tests (rapid laboratory test) can be carried out on water samples but only give qualitative results. In any case, priority is given to providing sufficient quantities of treated water during an epidemic.

AFTER THE OUTBREAK

At the end of the outbreak, some stool samples may be analysed to confirm the disappearance of the vibrio (at this stage, it is useless to analyse all characteristics of the vibrio). The seasonal recurrence of cholera may be expected. In the long term, improvements to water supplies, sanitation and personal hygiene are the best means of preventing cholera[4].

Cholera outbreaks take place in areas with poor sanitary conditions. Other diarrhoeal diseases, such as shigellosis, can be associated with or follow a cholera epidemic; therefore the surveillance system cannot be relaxed (see section *Shigellosis*).

➦ *References*

1. Cholera in 1993, Part I. *Wkly Epidemiol Rec*, 1994, 69(28): 205-12.

2. Cholera in 1993, Part II. *Wkly Epidemiol Rec*, 1994, 69(29): 213-20.

3. Médecins Sans Frontières. *Cholera outbreak: Goma, Zaïre, July-August 1994. A preliminary overview, 14 August 1994*. [Internal report]. Paris: MSF, 1994.

4. WHO. *Guidelines for cholera control*. Geneva: WHO, 1993.

5. Médecins Sans Frontières. *Prise en charge d'une épidémie de choléra en camp de réfugiés*. Paris: Médecins Sans Frontières, 1995.

6. Médecins Sans Frontières. *Emergency assistance for the cholera epidemic of Kismayo and surrounding areas. Final operation report*. Brussels: Médecins Sans Frontières, 1995.

7. CDC. Famine-affected, refugee, and displaced populations: Recommendations for public health issues. *MMWR*, 1992, 41(RR-13): 1-76.

8. Bitar, D, Moren, A. *Epidemiological surveillance of cholera among Mozambican refugees in Malawi, 1988-1991*. Journées Scientifiques 1991-92. Paris: Epicentre, Médecins Sans Frontières, 1992.

9. CDC. Update: Cholera - Western Hemisphere, and recommendations for treatment of cholera. *MMWR*, 1991, 40(32): 562-5.

10. Boelaert, M, Suetens, C, et al. Cholera treatment in Goma. *The Lancet*, 1995, 345: 1567.

11. Sanchez, J L, Vasquez, B, Begue, R E, et al. Protective efficacity of oral whole-cell/Recombinant-B-subunit cholera vaccine in Peruvian military recruits. *The Lancet*, 1994, 344: 1273-5.

12. Steffen, R. New cholera vaccines-for whom ? *The Lancet*, 1994, 344: 1273-6.

13. Suharyono et al. Safety and immunogenicity of single-dose live oral cholera vaccine CVD 103-HgR in 5-9-year-old Indonesian children. *The Lancet*, 1992, 340: 689-694.

14. The Goma Epidemiological Group. Public health impact of Rwandan refugee crisis: What happened in Goma, Zaire, in July, 1994? *The Lancet*, 1995, 345: 339-44.

15. Médecins Sans Frontières. *Guide of kits and emergency items. Decision-maker guide*. 3rd edition. Paris: Médecins Sans Frontières, 1996.

16. Hatch, D L, Waldman, R J, Lungu, G W, Piri, C. Epidemic cholera during refugee resettlement in Malawi. *Int J Epidemiol*, 1994, 23(6): 1292-9.

17. WHO. *The potential role of new cholera vaccines and control of cholera outbreaks during acute emergencies. Report of a meeting*, 13-14 February 1995, Geneva. Geneva: WHO, 1995. CDR/GPV/95.1.

18. Siddique, A K, Salam, A, Islam, M S, et al. Why treatment centres failed to prevent cholera deaths among Rwandan refugees in Goma, Zaire. *The Lancet*, 1995, 345(8946): 359-61.

19. Pierce, N F, Robinson, D, Rigal, J, Dualeh, M. Cholera treatment. *The Lancet*, 1994, 344: 1022.

B - Measles control

Introduction

Measles ranks as one of the leading causes of childhood mortality, and is still endemic in most developing countries despite the major efforts of the Expanded Programme on Immunization (EPI) in regard to measles immunization.

Measles is a very contagious disease, and can be associated with high mortality, severe complications, and an increased vulnerability to other infections over the following weeks or months, causing malnutrition and delayed mortality. In developing countries, children under 5 years represent the highest proportion of cases, and up to 25% of cases are children under 9 months. Mortality is especially high in the youngest age group and among the malnourished[7].

Outbreaks of measles are common among refugee and displaced populations, especially in camps situations, and refugees have been recognized as one of the highest risk groups for measles outbreaks by the WHO[17]. Furthermore, measles has often been the leading cause of mortality among children in these populations. Overcrowding seems to play a major role, increasing the risk of infection at an early age and the severity of the disease in all age groups[10]. Case fatality rates, ranging from 2% to 21% in stable populations, can reach very high values in refugee settings (33% in Sudan)[1].

However, the high mortality rate due to measles can be prevented by immunization and early case management. Mass immunization is one of the first actions that should be initiated in a refugee situation (see *2. Measles Immunization*). As this strategy is now widely recognized, fewer measles outbreaks have been reported among refugees since 1990. Nonetheless, severe outbreaks have occurred recently in refugee camps (Zimbabwe, Somalia and Nepal) where mass vaccination was not promptly implemented[11].

Table 7.2
Measles morbidity and mortality rates in refugee situations

Among children under five	Attack rate	Case fatality rate (%)
Sudan (Wad Kowli), 1985[3]	97/1,000/month	33
Malawi, 1988-89[5]	9/1,000 (overall)	17
Nepal, 1991[15]	0.9-1.7/1,000/month	unavailable

Prevention

Measles immunization should be given the highest priority in the early phase of refugee programmes, whether or not there are cases of measles and whether or not refugees have been immunized in the home country. This topic is described in chapter *2. Measles Immunization.* It is performed through a mass immunization campaign targeting the age group between 6 months and 12-15 years, and should usually be coupled to mass prophylaxis of vitamin A[1,13]. Fixed immunization points should then be rapidly organized in health facilities to reach children who have not been immunized (e.g. new arrivals) and to administer a second dose to those receiving a first dose before the age of 9 months.

In open situations, where the refugees are living in the local community, the target age groups of the local population should also be vaccinated.

Case management

- Active case finding, using a standard case definition (see below) should be conducted by home-visitors and health workers during outbreaks, and all suspected cases should be referred to a health facility. The screening system (triage) in health facilities should be reinforced to ensure that measles cases are dealt with promptly.

- The strict isolation of measles cases is most probably not effective, since cases are mainly contagious before they present to health facilities[1]. However, it is advisable to separate measles cases from other patients in hospitals and therapeutic feeding centres (e.g. in tents) in order to limit transmission to others. The malnourished should not be withdrawn from feeding programmes when presenting with measles infection, as they are particularly in need of nutritional supplements[2].

- Measles-related mortality is mostly due to complications such as pneumonia, gastro-enteritis, severe malnutrition and meningoencephalitis. Appropriate treatment should deal with these complications, and is described in guidelines [1,2,16]. It consists mainly in oral rehydration therapy for diarrhoea, antibiotics for secondary infections and diazepam to control convulsions. In all measles cases, the following is indicated: treatment of fever, increased fluid intake, encouragement of good oral hygiene and prophylaxis against conjunctivitis (eye ointment).

- It is known that measles aggravates vitamin A deficiency, and several studies have shown that the administration of high doses of vitamin A markedly reduces the risk of measles-associated morbidity and mortality in hospitalized children[18]. High doses of vitamin A (at least 2 doses) should be given to measles cases, even in areas where vitamin A deficiency is not a significant health problem[13,16,19].

- Continued feeding should be ensured: mothers should be educated to continue feeding and breast-feeding, and children should be enrolled in supplementary feeding programmes. The nutritional status of all cases should be closely monitored[1].

Surveillance

The existing surveillance system (see *8. Public Health Surveillance*) should ensure the early detection and registration of measles cases, whether or not all children are believed to have been immunized. The system is based on routine data provided by out-patient facilities, hospitals and death registrations, and complemented by data collected through periodical surveys (e.g. immunization coverage surveys)[2].

A standard case definition must be used for the diagnosis of measles cases, for instance the one recommended by the EPI.

Case definition for measles[4,13]:

– a generalized rash lasting 3 or more days AND;

– fever AND;

– one of the following: cough, runny nose or red eyes

Health workers at every level should be trained to recognize the clinical symptoms of measles. Every clinically-suspected case should be reported immediately and investigated by the medical officer in charge. It is also imperative to screen all new arrivals to a camp in order to detect measles cases (and ensure systematic immunization).

For each measles case, data should be collected on age, sex, immunization status, determination of possible exposure (e.g. contact with other measles case), and outcome of the illness.

Immunization coverage should be assessed by using routine data and conducting immunization coverage surveys if required, according to EPI protocol for coverage survey[14]. Even if immunization coverage is high, efforts should still be made to identify and target pockets of low coverage[5] (see *2. Measles Immunization*).

Outbreak control

OUTBREAK INVESTIGATION

Even among immunized populations, outbreaks of measles are to be expected[1,4,13]. There is no standard threshold for determining a measles outbreak, and - in principle - a specific threshold should be developed on the basis of local epidemiology and immunization programmes. However, in refugee settings, the reporting of even a single case should trigger immediate investigation and a rapid response[1,13]. A suspected case may be considered as a 'confirmed measles case' if it meets the standard clinical case definition (see above)[13].

The analysis of the collected data (see above) should include at least construction of an epidemic curve, graphing of the age distribution of cases and estimation of the vaccine efficacy. This is important to determine the immunization strategies.

The age distribution of cases will be used to review the upper age limit for vaccination; older children and adults may also need to be vaccinated if these age groups are affected[6,13].

Field vaccine efficacy should be assessed when vaccine failures are suspected. A first estimate of vaccine efficacy may be obtained from routine data, using the method described in WHO/EPI documents[8]. Other studies (cohort study or case-control study), using sample surveys, can provide more accurate information but require specialists and are generally not conducted in the emergency phase (see also *2. Measles Immunization*). Measles vaccine efficacy is around 85% at 9 months of age, and 50% at 6 months. If the calculated vaccine efficacy is below 80% during an outbreak, the immunization and cold chain practices should be assessed[13].

- The age at which cases have been immunized should be checked, as well as the administration of a second dose at 9 months to those immunized before that age.

- If the vaccine efficacy appears to be low across all age groups, the cold chain should be reviewed to ensure that it has been properly functioning.

IMMUNIZATION ACTIVITIES

The main control measure is to accelerate the immunization as measles transmission is not rapid enough to infect all susceptible individuals before they can be vaccinated; there is also some evidence that measles vaccine may reduce the severity of the disease if administered within 3 days of exposure to the measles virus[1,12].

Based on the analysis of data, the strategies for immunization may need to be adapted.

- The target age group previously discussed (see *Prevention*) may be extended to cover adolescents and adults if these groups are also affected[6].

- During a mass campaign conducted in refugee settings, it is recommended to vaccinate all individuals within this age group, whether or not they can present a record of previous immunization (non-selective vaccination)[15]. This is especially important if the vaccine efficacy is revealed to be low. A second vaccine dose has no adverse effect, but it provides an even better protection.

- Only in situations where the initial mass campaign has been correctly conducted, ensuring a good coverage level, satisfactory vaccine efficacy, and the distribution of vaccination cards, it can be envisaged to limit immunization to those with no record of measles vaccination (selective immunization; see also *2. Measles Immunization*).

INFORMATION AND EDUCATION

The refugee community, the local health authorities, and the health staff must be informed of the current epidemic.

Home-visitors and community health workers must undertake health education activities. The main objectives should be to encourage mothers to bring their children for immunization, to inform them that some children may still develop measles after immunization, to persuade them to take sick children for treatment and to educate them on home care (continued feeding, hydration, etc.)[13].

Principal recommendations regarding measles control

- In a refugee situation, a measles immunization campaign is an absolute priority and takes place whether or not there are cases of measles. It targets children between 6 months and 15 years. A high vaccine coverage must be maintained through an on-going immunization of new arrivals and in health facilities. This coverage must be assessed regularly.

- Any suspected case of measles should be immediately assessed; health workers must be trained to detect measles early on. Measles cases require symptomatic care, administration of high doses of vitamin A, and treatment for complications. Feeding must be continued.

- In case of a measles outbreak, investigating the outbreak is important, and allows reassessment of immunization strategies. More effort must be concentrated on immunization. Appropriate education of the refugee communities and the health staff is also essential.

▧ *Key references*

1. Toole, M, Steketee, R W, Waldman, R J, Nieburg, P. Measles prevention and control in emergency settings. *Bull WHO*, 1989, 67(4): 381-8.

2. Médecins Sans Frontières. *Conduite à tenir en cas d'épidémie de rougeole*. Paris: Médecins Sans Frontières, 1996.

Other references

3. Shears, P, Berry, A M, et al. Epidemiological assessment of the health and nutrition of Ethiopian refugees in emergency camps in Sudan, 1985. *Brit Med Jour*, 1987, 295:314-7.

4. Cutts, F. *Measles control in the 1990s: Principles for the next decade*. Geneva: WHO, 1990. WHO/EPI/GEN/90.2.

5. Porter, J D, Gastellu Etchegorry, M, et al. Measles outbreaks in the Mozambican refugee camps in Malawi: The continued need for an effective vaccine. *Int J Epidemiol*, 1990, 19(4): 1072-7.

6. CDC. Famine-affected, refugee, and displaced populations: Recommendations for public health issues. *MMWR*, 1992, 41(RR-13): 1-76.

7. WHO. *Measles control in the 1990s: Plan of action for global measles control.* Geneva: WHO, 1992. WHO/EPI/GEN/92.3.

8. WHO. *Directives pour l'étude et la surveillance des flambées épidémiques des maladies cibles du programme.* Geneva: WHO, 1984. WHO/EPI/GEN/84.7.

9. Médecins Sans Frontières. *Clinical guidelines, diagnostic and treatment manual.* Paris: Hatier, 1993.

10. Aaby, P, et al. Overcrowding and intensive exposure as determinants of measles mortality. *Am J Epidemiol*, 1984, 120(1): 49-60.

11. Toole, M J, Waldman, R J, et al. Refugee and displaced persons. War, hunger and public health. *JAMA* , 1993, 270(5): 600-5.

12. WHO. *Efficacy of measles immunization shortly after exposure in preventing disease transmission.* Geneva: WHO, 1989, EPI/RD/PROTOCOL/89.1.

13. WHO. *Measles outbreak response.* A background document prepared for the Global Advisory Group Meeting. Washington D C: EPI/WHO, 1993.

14. WHO. *Training mid-level managers: The EPI Coverage Survey.* Geneva: WHO, 1991. WHO/EPI/MLM/91.10.

15. Marfin, A A, Moore, J, Collins, C, et al. Infectious disease surveillance during emergency relief to Bhutanese refugees in Nepal. *JAMA*, 1994, 272(5): 377-81.

16. WHO. *Case management of measles - a policy document* [draft]. Geneva: WHO/EPI, 1993.

17. Clements, C J, Strassbourg, M, Cutts, F T, Torel, C. The Epidemiology of measles. *World Health Stat Q*, 1992, 45: 285-91.

18. WHO. *Clinical research on treatment of measles: report of a meeting. Banjul, Gambia, November 1993.* Geneva: WHO, 1995. WHO/EPI/GEN/95.07.

19. Sommer, A. *La carence en vitamine A et ses consequences: Guide pratique du dépistage et de la lutte.* Geneva: WHO, 1995.

C - Control of Acute Respiratory Infections (ARIs)

Introduction

Acute Respiratory Infections (ARIs) are a major cause of both morbidity and mortality throughout the world, but particularly so in developing countries, where 25% to 30% of deaths among children under 5 years are caused by ARIs; 90% of them are attributable to pneumonia alone[1,3,4]. Furthermore, it must be remembered that respiratory complications from measles, whooping cough and diphtheria (all preventable by immunization) are also ARIs and together account for 15% to 25% of all ARI deaths[3].

ARIs can be categorized as mild, moderate or severe: the great majority of ARIs are mild and recover spontaneously, while a small percentage evolve into pneumonia, which is fatal in 10% to 20% of untreated cases. ARIs can also be divided into upper (e.g. common cold, otitis media and pharyngitis) and lower respiratory tract infections (e.g. bronchitis, bronchiolitis and pneumonia). Most upper ARIs are mild or moderate, almost all ARI deaths are due to lower ARIs, mainly pneumonia (e.g. bronchitis is relatively common and rarely fatal)[6].

ARIs also represent a heavy burden for health services, since under-fives generally suffer between 4 and 8 episodes of ARIs per year. Between 30% and 50% of paediatric consultations and between 30% and 40% of paediatric admissions are attributable to ARIs. Furthermore, ARIs are the conditions that are most frequently associated with the unnecessary use of antibiotics (i.e. antibiotic administration for mild cases of ARIs) and other drugs in out-patient services[1].

The risk factors for the spread of pneumonia are low birth weight, malnutrition, poor breast-feeding practices, specific nutritional deficiencies (e.g. vitamin A), chilling in infants, indoor air pollution (e.g. smoke from cooking fuels and tobacco), urban air pollution and overcrowding. The first two factors are the most important: children with low birth weight and those suffering from malnutrition are at an especially high risk of death from ARIs. The causative agents of ARIs may be viral or bacterial (mainly *Streptococcus pneumoniae* and *Haemophilus influenza*).

WHO interventions in regard to ARI control are focused on the reduction of mortality: the main strategy for achieving this is correct case management, i.e. the early and adequate diagnosis and management of cases. This requires an accessible health system, training for health staff and establishment of simple treatment protocols[6]. The most effective preventive measure is the immunization of children (measles, diphtheria and pertussis).

ARIs are among the leading causes of death among refugee populations as well[2]. Refugees are probably at higher risk from ARIs because of the significant presence of risk factors in refugee settings: malnutrition, vitamin A deficiency, chilling in infants (due to poor shelter), overcrowding, indoor pollution (e.g. bad ventilation in shelters)[1,3,5]. Although it is difficult to know if there is a higher ARI incidence in refugee populations, it may be assumed that infections will be more severe, leading to higher case fatality rates.

Surveillance

Morbidity data is based on the clinical case definition commonly used for ARIs in emergency surveillance, which is based on symptoms and has a low specificity.

> **Example of a case definition for moderate to severe ARIs[11]:**
> any case of fever with cough and rapid breathing
> (50 or more breaths per minute)

Differentiation may be made between upper and lower respiratory infections, but health staff require good training to diagnose this properly; this might not be a priority during the emergency phase. On the other hand, mortality data on cause of death, if available, will be more useful for measuring the importance of ARIs in the population although they may be difficult to obtain, e.g. by verbal autopsy (see *8. Public Health Surveillance*).

Prevention

Non-specific measures can be taken to reduce the risk factors for the development of pneumonia: improving the nutritional status of children; administering supplements of vitamin A; reducing overcrowding and limiting chilling in young infants by the provision of proper shelters and the distribution of blankets (see *5. Shelter and Site Planning*)[4,7].

Immunization against measles, diphtheria and whooping cough (only in the post-emergency phase as far as the two latter diseases are concerned; see *Child Health Care in the Post-emergency Phase* in Part III) is the most important preventive measure recognized so far[4]. New vaccines have recently been developed against *Haemophilus influenza* B and *Streptococcus pneumoniae* and are currently undergoing population-based trials[1]. They represent hope for the future in the fight against the high mortality rates resulting from pneumonia[3].

Case management

The importance of ARI case management lies in the early recognition and adequate treatment of pneumonia, as correct case management is the cornerstone for the prevention of deaths from pneumonia. Therefore, health staff should proceed with a careful assessment of all children presenting with cough, and/or difficult breathing, by analysing history and clinical signs. This assessment should also include checking for signs of malnutrition, as this is an important risk factor for mortality (see below *Specific management*). It is therefore important to train health staff with little prior knowledge on how to identify pneumonia[3,4]. Guidelines for diagnosing pneumonia are given in several reference sources[6,8].

- The management of pneumonia consists of antibiotic treatment (at home or in a health facility) and supportive measures. In most cases, antibiotics can be orally administered but severe pneumonia requires intravenous antibiotics[4,8]. Where oral therapy is concerned, the national policies of the host country will help to decide the type of antibiotic: cotrimoxazole remains the drug of choice for the present because it is easy to administer and is cost-effective in the ambulatory treatment of pneumonia[9,10]; possible alternatives are amoxycillin and chloramphenicol. Ensuring compliance with the antibiotic treatment (frequently over a 5-day period) is a common problem. For intravenous treatment, ampicillin or chloramphenicol are used[11].

  Supportive measures, such as the administration of oral fluids for the prevention of dehydration, antipyretics to reduce high fever, and protection from chills and draughts are essential. Furthermore, it is of paramount importance to continue feeding the child.

- Management of other types of ARI ('coughs and colds') only need supportive treatment as they are generally caused by viruses. However, they are frequently mistreated with antibiotics.

- Management of ARIs in severely malnourished children warrants special attention: they should be referred to a hospital both for assessment (rapid breathing and chest indrawing are less sensitive as predictors of pneumonia in severely malnourished children) and for treatment[9]. Indeed, recent evidence suggests that severely malnourished children with cough or difficult breathing should receive presumptive antibiotic treatment when admitted either for ARIs or for nutritional rehabilitation[9].

  Management of most ARI cases can thus be carried out at the health post level (supportive measures and oral antibiotics), but cases of pneumonia or ARIs in severely malnourished children must be treated in an environment where intravenous antibiotics can be administered (health centre with an adequate level of in-patient care, therapeutic feeding centre or hospital).

  It is therefore imperative to properly train health staff in the clinical criteria of pneumonia, and in the need to refer such cases rapidly; flow charts have been developed for this[8].

Principal recommendations regarding to the control of acute respiratory infections

- A majority of deaths from acute respiratory infections are due to neumonia. The main strategy for reducing ARI mortality is the early diagnosis and adequate management of cases, especially of pneumonia cases. Pneumonia treatment consists of antibiotic administration and supportive measures.

- Malnutrition is an important risk factor for ARI mortality; the management of ARIs in severely malnourished children warrants thus special attention.

- The most effective preventive measure is the immunization of children, which protect them against measles, diphtheria and pertussis.

➤ References

1. WHO. *Programme for control of acute respiratory infections. Sixth programme report 1992-1993.* Geneva: WHO, 1994. WHO/ARI/94.33.

2. CDC. Famine-affected, refugee, and displaced populations: Recommendations for public health issues. *MMWR*, 1992, 41(RR-13): 1-76.

3. WHO. *Acute respiratory infections.* Geneva: WHO, 1990. WHO/ARI/90.17.

4. Paquet, C. Control of acute infant respiratory infections in developing countries. *Medical News*, 1992,1(2): 3-8.

5. Babille, M, De Colombani, P, Guerra, R, et al. Post-emergency epidemiological surveillance in Iraqi-Kurdish refugee camps in Iran. *Disasters*, 1994,18(1): 58-75.

6. WHO. *Acute respiratory infections in children: Case management in small hospitals in developing countries.* Geneva: WHO, 1990. WHO/ARI/90.5.C.

7. Mears, C, Chowdhury, S. *Health care for refugees and displaced people.* Oxford: Oxfam, 1994.

8. Médecins Sans Frontières. *Clinical guidelines, diagnostic and treatment manual.* Paris: Hatier, 1993.

9. WHO Division of Diarrhoeal and Acute Respiratory Disease Control. *Interim Report 1994.* Geneva: WHO/CDR, 1994.

10. Sidal, M, Oguz, O, et al. Trial of co-trimoxazole versus procaine penicillin G and benzathin penicillin + procaine penicillin G in the treatment of childhood pneumonia. *J Trop Pediatr*, 1994, 40(5): 301-4.

11. Marfin, A A, Collins, C, Moore, J. Infectious disease surveillance during emergency relief to Bhutanese refugees in Nepal. *JAMA*, 1994, 272(5): 377-81.

D - Malaria control

Introduction

Although the degree of malaria transmission varies greatly from one part of the world to another, more than 80% of cases are observed in tropical Africa[4]. The most frequently occurring species of plasmodium are *Plasmodium falciparum* and *Plasmodium vivax*. *P. falciparum* is the predominant species in tropical Africa (where more than 90% of cases are due to *P. falciparum*), Eastern Asia, the Pacific region and in the Amazon area. This strain causes severe malaria and high mortality[4,9]. *P. vivax* is found mainly in North Africa, Central and South America and south-east Asia[18].

The majority of malaria deaths occurs in Africa, and among non-immune individuals in areas where appropriate treatment is not available[4].

The drug resistance of *Plasmodium falciparum* is increasing; resistance to chloroquine has spread to most countries: in 1993, among the countries where *P. falciparum* is endemic, only those of Central America have not recorded resistance of *P. falciparum* to chloroquine[4]. Resistance to other drugs such as mefloquine has also developed in some areas. Chloroquine-resistant *P. vivax* has been reported as well. This rapid evolution is making malaria treatment increasingly complex.

Over recent years, there has been an increasing number of malaria epidemics in endemic areas. This is due to many factors, including wars and disasters, which play an obvious role by provoking the displacements of population which may be non-immune, and the collapse of public health services. The severity of epidemics is aggravated by the spread of *P. falciparum* to *P. vivax* affected areas in Asia, and also the increasing drug resistance[9].

Malaria is frequently a leading cause of morbidity, and an important cause of death among adult refugees in some areas (Sudan[5,13], Malawi[1], Mozambique[6] and Thailand[8]). It is already a major health problem in many countries hosting refugee populations.

Malaria incidence can also be particularly high among refugees who have settled in an area of higher endemicity than their region of origin, and outbreaks may result[1]. For instance, in Pakistan in 1981, the prevalence of malaria infection (parasitic rate) among Afghan refugees was almost double that in the local population since the refugees came from an area of lower transmission and thus had lower levels of immunity than the local people[3]. It is suggested that this low immunity also increases the risk of drug-resistance.

On the other hand, the migration of infected people from highly endemic areas to refugee sites in areas where there is a low transmission level will not particularly increase the risk of malaria epidemics, since these are more dependent on the presence of vectors than on other factors.

Table 7.3
Malaria morbidity and mortality in refugee or displaced populations

	Incidence rate (per 1000 per month)	Proportional mortality (%)
Thailand (1987-89)[8]	600	24
Sudan (1985)[13]	70-112	5
Rwanda (1994)[14]	120-240	10-30

Malaria is a health problem that is permanently evolving and several measures for malaria control are either under discussion or currently being tested. It is therefore difficult to set clear recommendations for dealing with the disease, but the different strategies and factors to be taken into account in decision-making are discussed below.

Prevention

Preventive measures in a refugee setting include individual protection (e.g. mosquito-net) and community protection (e.g. insecticide spraying). Prevention is becoming more important, although not always easily implemented, since malaria treatment is hindered by the spread of drug resistance. In order to implement these measures, it is necessary to gather information on the epidemiology of transmission. For example, information on previous exposure among refugees is useful for estimating immunity levels and instigating appropriate action.

CHEMOPROPHYLAXIS

1. Mass chemoprophylaxis is not so far recommended[9]. It is extremely difficult to implement and monitor on a very large scale, and it can accelerate the development of drug resistance and decrease naturally acquired immunity.

2. Chemoprophylaxis of high risk groups is only recommended by WHO in exceptional circumstances as it is difficult to implement: since resistant *P. falciparum* is spreading to most areas, there are problems in regard to the toxicity and cost of alternatives to chloroquine, and the level of compliance is usually poor[9]. Complex decisions have to made as to whether to start chemoprophylaxis and which drug to use; they should be based on factors described below.

   • Chemoprophylaxis of pregnant women is a subject of debate globally, and current recommendations are not clear. The benefits are a decrease in illness episodes, anaemia and placental parasitaemia, and a positive effect on birth weight (although the impact on perinatal outcome is not yet clear)[20]. It is most effective when started early in pregnancy and among primigravidae, particularly in preventing anaemia[21]. Among the obstacles above mentioned, the financial side is of particular concern in areas of chloroquine-resistant malaria due to the high cost of alternative drugs and the large number of pregnant women (normally 5% of a population).

Depending on the malaria situation, the following recommendations can be given:

– in areas where chloroquine resistance is absent or low, chemoprophylaxis may be used: WHO recommends starting early in pregnancy with a treatment of chloroquine, followed by weekly chemoprophylaxis[21];

– where chloroquine resistance is high, chemoprophylaxis should generally not be used, particularly if *P. falciparum* is only sensitive to toxic and expensive drugs; but other strategies must be adopted to protect pregnant women, such as early detection and treatment of cases [20]. Other types of chemoprophylaxis are currently being tested: for instance, some studies are testing the use of a single treatment dose of sulfadoxine-pyrimethamine (Fansidar) in the second and third trimester[7]. The advantages are better compliance and lower costs.

Decision-makers in refugee situations should contact the Ministry of Health (MOH) for information on national policy and seek advice from medical experts (e.g. in agency headquarters) when choosing the most appropriate strategy for the situation.

• Chemoprophylaxis of severely malnourished children must also be considered. Where malaria is endemic and chloroquine resistance is not a major problem, chloroquine prophylaxis can be given, and is easy to implement for groups attending feeding programmes; prophylaxis using other antimalarial drugs is not presently recommended. Presumptive malaria treatment should be given automatically on admission, whichever drug is chosen, and may be repeated periodically.

VECTOR CONTROL

Vector control may currently be one of the main tools of malaria control. However, its efficacy varies, depending on transmission levels, endemic levels, vector and human behaviour patterns[9]. Among vector characteristics, the most determinant are biting habits (indoor or outdoor) and resistance to insecticide [9]. Where malaria transmission is low, unstable or seasonal, vector control can considerably reduce incidence and prevalence, while in areas of intensive and stable transmission, it has not generally produced a long-term effect on prevalence. In refugee populations, vector control measures should be considered, but the strategic decisions should be left to sanitation specialists[9].

• When selecting a refugee settlement area, special care should be taken - wherever possible - to avoid proximity to vector breeding sites, such as ponds, small streams or swamps. However, this choice is rarely dependent on the relief organizations (see *5. Shelters and Site Planning*). Efforts should therefore be made to reduce vector sources by eliminating breeding sites. This can be achieved either by getting rid of unnecessary collections of water where possible or making those that remain unsuitable for vectors by the use of larvicides [19].

- Periodic spraying of shelters with residual insecticide reduces transmission and is recommended in refugee camps, particularly among populations with low immunity[9]. It can be implemented in the early phases of a refugee settlement, with the involvement of the host country's national malaria services. For instance, in refugee camps in Pakistan (1990), spraying tents had been shown to significantly reduce the transmission of *P. falciparum*[14]. The residual effect may last up to 6 months, depending on several factors, including the absorption quality of building material[19]. The selection of a residual insecticide is based on vector resistance, toxicity, cost and national regulations, and the relevant information is available in guidelines[24]. Health facilities should also be treated to provide individual protection to patients.

- Mosquito nets (bed nets) impregnated with residual insecticide provide good individual protection by acting as a barrier, killing mosquitoes on contact, or repelling and driving them out of shelters. Mass distributions of impregnated nets can have a significant impact on malaria transmission by reducing the mosquito population and creating a shield effect, thus even benefiting people who do not themselves use nets[11,17]. Its effect on reducing malaria prevalence and incidence levels has been the subject of several studies[10,16]. As the residual effect of pyrethrinoids lasts from 6 to 9 months, mosquito nets should be impregnated twice a year.

  Although distributions of insecticide-impregnated mosquito nets to refugees are generally recommended, the decision ultimately depends on several factors: transmission levels, mosquito biting habits, the immune status of the population, financial constraints and, in particular, the sleeping habits of the population[11]. A main obstacle is the cost, although this should be compared to the cost of malaria treatment which may be very high in multi-drug-resistant areas; a mefloquine treatment costs around US$10 (IDA, 1996) while an impregnated bed-net costs around US$8 (S-E Asia, 1993)[17].

  Buildings can also be protected by placing mosquito screens over all possible entrances.

Case management

Since malaria prevention can be difficult to implement within the constraints of many refugee emergencies, particular attention should be given to the prompt and effective management of malaria illness. There is no standard treatment for malaria because of its growing resistance to certain drugs and the different immunity levels in refugee populations. Whenever possible, treatment schedules should be in line with the national malaria programme of the host country, but adapted in line with epidemiological patterns among refugees. Several guidelines are available from WHO and health agencies[2,18,22,23].

1. DECIDING WHOM TO TREAT

- In general, there are 3 main options in regard to the diagnosis and treatment of uncomplicated malaria:
  - treat all cases of fever (presumptive malaria treatment);
  - treat all clinical cases according to a clinical case definition (e.g. fever excluding other infections);
  - treat only cases confirmed by blood smear (this requires a definition for a threshold of parasite density).

The first two strategies have the advantage of reducing malaria mortality, especially among children. They are indicated in highly endemic areas and for non-immune populations, where clinical signs are more valid for the diagnosis of malaria (high positive predictive value of clinical criteria)[5,7,8]. In these situations, clinical criteria and diagnostic protocols for malaria can be improved by comparing the blood smears of cases with clinical signs, with those of a control group (which makes it possible to estimate the positive predictive value)[7].

However, in other situations, the clinical diagnosis is not specific (positive predictive value around 50%)[5,8], and these two strategies entail the unnecessary treatment of non-malaria cases and subsequent potential toxicity, drug over-consumption and an increased risk of drug resistance[9,2]. Treatment limited to laboratory-confirmed cases will help to avoid these problems, but this requires equipment and skilled staff, and tends to overload existing laboratory capacities[9].

- In refugee situations, the ideal strategy in principle is to treat cases with confirmed *parasitaemia*, but this is only rarely possible in practice. Therefore, if a laboratory is not available or is overloaded, or in highly endemic areas and among non-immune populations, treatment will be administered to clinically-presented cases. However, laboratory confirmation is essential in situations where drug resistance is a problem, especially if a species other than *P. falciparum* (e.g. *P. vivax*) is present and requires a different treatment scheme[9].

Every refugee programme must select and standardize the strategy most appropriate to the local situation. This will certainly be better defined in the post-emergency phase, when epidemiological trends can be further assessed.

2. SELECTING A THERAPY

The choice of a treatment protocol is based on several parameters[2]: the plasmodium species, the sensitivity of the parasite to anti-malaria drugs, the severity of the malaria attack and membership of specific high-risk group (e.g. children, pregnant or non-immune). In the case of chloroquine resistance, the choice of an alternative drug (first or second line) should be consistent with national malaria policies. It is sometimes necessary to select several first line drugs[9]. For instance, in the Rwandan refugee camps in Northern Kivu (Zaire, 1994), CDC recommended sulfadoxine-pyrimethamine (Fansidar) as the first-line therapy for high risk groups and chloroquine for others[7].

A treatment strategy must be defined in every situation, with appropriate therapy according to the following indications[9]:

- first-line treatment,
- severe or complicated malaria,
- high-risk groups,
- therapeutic failures.

Table 7.4
Main drugs used in the treatment of malaria

Drug	Indications	Contraindications
Chloroquine	P. malariae and ovale P. falciparum and vivax if sensitive malaria prophylaxis	
Sulfadoxine-pyrimethamine	chloroquine-resistant P. falciparum (if sensitive)	pregnancy, but debated
Mefloquine	chloroquine-resistant P. falciparum (if sensitive)	pregnancy, children under 15kg (numerous side effects)
Quinine	cerebral malaria resistant P. falciparum	
Primaquine	P. falciparum (gametocide) P. vivax to reduce relapses	G 6PD deficiency
Artemisine	multi-resistant malaria (so far limited to Southeast Asia)	

The following general recommendations are listed below (see guidelines[2,18]):

- For P. vivax, ovale and malariae, and for falciparum in areas with low, or no chloroquine resistance, uncomplicated malaria is treated by an oral regimen of chloroquine.

- For P. falciparum where chloroquine resistance is high, an alternative first-line drug will be used. In areas where drug resistance is quickly spreading to other drugs (e.g. Southeast Asia), first-line drugs must be continuously adapted to drug sensitivity.

- Treatment failure should be suspected if a patient remains symptomatic after 3 days of treatment (correctly taken) and the blood smear is still positive. Alternative therapy should be instituted immediately with a drug selected on the basis of local resistance (e.g. quinine, mefloquine, artemisine, etc.)[1,2].

- Severe malaria requires hospitalization and parenteral treatment with quinine (or parenteral chloroquine before referral to hospital or artemisine derivatives). Appropriate therapy should be instigated to treat and prevent seizures or other complications (anaemia, hypoglycaemia, etc.).

- Supportive therapy includes the control of fever, hydration and treatment of anaemia with folic acid (not iron, unless the malaria is associated with iron deficiency).

Surveillance

There is no standard case definition for malaria; it must be determined according to local factors: endemicity level, population immunity, health staff skills, etc. Ideally, MALARIA ILLNESS (malaria signs and symptoms) should be differentiated from MALARIA INFECTION (presence of parasites in the blood smear), but this is rarely possible in emergency settings[1].

Example of a case definition for malaria[9]:

a case of fever excluding other infections,
preferably confirmed by laboratory.

Note that a threshold of parasite density should ideally be defined locally in populations presenting acquired immunity.

The information collected depends on the availability of a laboratory. Wherever possible, a blood smear test should be carried out for all suspected cases (although this may not often be feasible). However, in hyperendemic areas, the relationship between parasitaemia and clinical status is low, and a clinical case definition is generally preferable higher positive predictive value (see above)[5,8].

- **In the emergency phase**, a blood smear examination is indicated at least in the following cases[2,9]:
  – the diagnosis and follow-up of severe cases,
  – identification of species, especially in areas of drug resistance,
  – assessment of treatment failure.
  It should also be used to regularly evaluate the clinical diagnosis (see above).

- **In the post-emergency phase**, a laboratory should be set up in all refugee settings where malaria is a significant problem.

Routinely collected data may provide a fair picture of the malaria situation among refugees, although they are biased because the refugees attending health services are not representative of the overall population.

Routine data for malaria surveillance should include the following[9]:

– number of malaria cases, making it possible to get an approximation of incidence rates;

– age distribution of cases: this helps to determine whether the population is newly exposed (high prevalence in all age groups), previously exposed (prevalence high in children and low in adults) or subject to a low transmission (low prevalence in all age groups)[19];

– number of severe or complicated cases: this is usually represented by the number of malaria cases requiring hospitalization[9];

– number of malaria deaths: this makes it possible to calculate the case fatality rate;

– treatment failures: the response to drug treatment is an essential variable. When drug resistance is suspected in a population, a simple and systematic assessment can be made by checking (using experienced staff) the blood smears of cases on day one and day three of treatment[9]. If this test indicates the presence of drug resistance, further in-depth studies can be conducted by specialists (see below);

– laboratory data: makes it possible to determine the species involved.

However, studies may have to be carried out where malaria is a major problem[19]. They may take place in the emergency phase if a new drug resistance is suspected, or if an epidemic occurs, but are more often indicated in the post-emergency phase. Although expensive and requiring specialists, the following studies may have to be conducted[9]:

- Drug sensitivity studies may be required when a new drug resistance is suspected[27].

- Parasitological surveys can be used to assess the prevalence of malaria infection on the basis of a random sample. This can be useful to determine the prevalence of the various plasmodium species (e.g. in south-east Asia) and to develop specific recommendations for prophylaxis and treatment[26].

- Morbidity surveys can help to assess the incidence of malaria disease on the basis of blood smears from patients.

- Laboratory quality control surveys may also be carried out[25].

OUTBREAK CONTROL

Malaria outbreaks are reported with increasing frequency and may be influenced by many factors (entomological, parasitological, immunological, meteorological, etc.). In refugee populations, the main risk factors are population displacement in general, but especially the migration of populations with a low acquired malaria immunity to hyperendemic areas, the increase in vector-human contacts resulting from overcrowding, the specific type of parasite species, and the increase in drug resistance[9]. Malaria epidemics can be sporadic (after a displacement), periodic or seasonal.

Outbreak investigation

No clear definitions or thresholds for epidemics have been determined. An epidemic should be suspected when there is a local increase in malaria morbidity and/or mortality. In the occurrence of an outbreak due to a febrile illness and causing deaths, blood smears (even post-mortem) will confirm or exclude a malaria epidemic[9].

Special measures in outbreak control

There are only a few specific actions which can be implemented when an outbreak is suspected: health services providing prompt diagnosis and the treatment of cases should be reinforced; treatment can be administered to all fever cases and may sometimes be dispensed by home-visitors after appropriate training; home-visitors should at least undertake active case finding and prompt referral. Shelter spraying and other vector control measures may be considered after prior evaluation by specialists and discussions with the MOH[9].

▄ *References*

1. CDC. Famine-affected, refugee, and displaced populations: Recommendations for public health issues. *MMWR*, 1992, 41(RR-13): 1-76.

2. Nosten, F. *Paludisme*. Paris: Médecins Sans Frontières, 1992.

3. Suleman, M. Malaria in Afghan refugees in Pakistan. *Trans R Soc Trop Med Hyg*, 1988, 82: 44-7.

4. World malaria situation in 1991. *Wkly Epidemiolog Rec*, 1993, 68(34): 245-52.

5. Mercer, A. Mortality and morbidity in refugee camps in Eastern Sudan: 1985-1990. *Disasters*, 1990, 16(1): 28-42.

6. Toole, M J, Waldman, R J. Prevention of excess mortality in refugees and displaced populations in developing countries. *JAMA*, 1990, 263(24): 3296-302.

7. CDC. *Malaria assessment. Rwandan refugee programme in the North Kivu region, Zaire*. [Internal report]. Atlanta, CDC, 1994.

8. Decludt, B, Pecoul, B, Biberson, Ph, et al. Malaria surveillance among the displaced Karen population in Thailand. April 1984 to February 1989. Mae Sot, Thailand. *Southeast Asian J Trop Med Public Health*, 1991, 22(4): 504-8.

9. WHO. *Comité OMS d'experts du paludisme*. Dix-neuvième rapport. Geneva: WHO, 1989. WHO/CTD/92.1.

10. Beach, R F, et al. Effectiveness of permethrin-impregnated bed nets and curtains for malaria control in a holoendemic area in Western Kenya. *Am J Trop Med Hyg*, 1993, 49(3), 290-300.

11. Bermejo, A, Veeken, H, et al. Insecticide-impregnated bed nets for malaria control: A review of the field trials. *Bull WHO*, 1992, 70(3): 293-296.

12. Moren, A, Bitar, D, Navarre, I, Gastellu-Etchegorry, M, Brodel, A, Lungu, G, et al. Epidemiological surveillance among Mozambican refugees in Malawi, 1987-89. *Disasters*, 1991, 15(4): 363-72.

13. Shears, C, Berry, A M, et al. Epidemiological assessment of the health and nutrition of Ethiopian refugees in emergency camps in Sudan, 1985. *Br Med J*, 1987, 295: 314-7.

14. Bouma, M J, Parvez, S D, Sondorp, E. Treatment of tents with permethrin for the control of vector-borne diseases. *Medical News*; 1992, 1(4): 5-8.

15. Médecins Sans Frontières, Mission Rwanda. *Situation épidémiologique des camps de réfugiés, au 1 mars 1993*. [Internal report]. Kigali: Médecins Sans Frontières, 1993.

16. Karch, S, Garin, B, Asidi, N, et al. Moustiquaires imprégnées contre le paludisme au Zaïre. *Ann Soc Belge Med Trop*, 1993, 73(1): 37-53.

17. Jacquier, G. Mosquito net impregnation technique, Maela. *Medical News*, 1993, 2(3): 22-4.

18. Médecins Sans Frontières. *Clinical guidelines, diagnostic and treatment manual*. Paris: Hatier, 1993.

19. Simmonds, S, Vaughan, P, William Gunn, S. *Refugee community health care*. Oxford: Oxford University Press, 1983.

20. Garner, P, Brabin, B. A review of randomized controlled trials of routine antimalarial drug prophylaxis during pregnancy in endemic malarious areas. *WHO Bull*, 1994, 72(1): 89-99.

21. Brabin, B J. *The risks and severity of malaria in pregnant women*. Geneva: TDR, WHO. Applied Field Research in Malaria Report, 1991.

22. WHO. *Management of severe and complicated malaria. A practical handbook*. Geneva: WHO, 1991.

23. WHO. *Antimalarial drug policies. Data requirements, treatment of uncomplicared malaria and management of malaria in pregnancy*. Geneva: WHO, 1994.

24. Médecins Sans Frontières. *Public health engineering in emergency situations*. Paris: Médecins Sans Frontières, 1994.

25. Lacroix, C. Quality control for microscopic malaria screening. *Medical News*, 1993, 2(6): 22-6.

26. Hurwitz, E S. *Malaria among newly arrived refugees in Thailand, 1979-1980*. In: Allegra, D T, Nieburg, P & Grabe, M. Emergency refugee health care - A chronicle of the Khmer refugee assistance operation 1979-1980. Atlanta: CDC, 1980: 43-7.

8. Public health surveillance

Introduction

Surveillance is defined as a routine activity involving the regular collection and analysis of quantitative data (see below). It is an essential component of any public health programme[3].

> **A definition of public health surveillance**
>
> The ongoing, systematic collection, analysis and interpretation of health data essential to the planning, implementation, and evaluation of public health practice, closely integrated with the timely dissemination of these data to those who need to know. The final link in the surveillance chain is the application of these data to prevention and control. A surveillance system includes a functional capacity for data collection, analysis and dissemination linked to public health programmes[19].

The objective of surveillance is to provide information on a regular basis for use in decision-making: in other words, surveillance is information for action. In practice, it makes it possible to determine health priorities, plan and guide public health programmes and provide warning of rare and unexpected health problems (particularly an outbreak of a communicable disease). In the context of refugee and displaced populations, there are three further reasons why surveillance is imperative:

– the extreme vulnerability of refugees to the risk of epidemics, malnutrition and, more generally, any acute health problems (see 7. *Control of Communicable Diseases and Epidemics*);

– the sudden changes that can occur during the emergency phase, both in the population itself (size and composition) and in health conditions;

– the need to have quantitative data on which to base information on the refugee situation for communicating to partners (UN agencies, the host country's ministry of health - MOH, NGOs, etc.), and possibly to the media and/or donors.

These specific aspects of refugee situations highlight the need for implementing an appropriate surveillance system as an extension of the initial assessment right from the start of an intervention. Surveillance therefore constitutes one of the top ten priorities for refugee programmes and should be an integral part of all relief activities. Unfortunately, it is a priority that is all too easily neglected during the emergency phase as resources and staff are diverted to sectors perceived to have greater needs, for instance, hospitals and feeding programmes[21].

Some methods of data collection are not included in the surveillance although they may be undertaken on an ad hoc basis in response to signals from the surveillance system; they include cross-sectional surveys, outbreak investigations and some qualitative methods, and are discussed below under *Other health information-gathering methods.*

Objectives

The data supplied regularly by the surveillance system should direct intervention in the following ways:

– by providing early warning of epidemics (and allowing a rapid response),
– by determining the main health problems among the refugee population and following their trends over time,
– by assisting the planning of interventions and ensuring resources are properly targeted,
– by acting as a guide for programme implementation,
– by evaluating the coverage and effectiveness of programmes,
– by providing information on the refugee situation (for eventual witnessing - 'témoignage'), or on current activities,
– by constituting a data bank (optional) that might be useful for training or operational research.

Principles

Implementation of a surveillance system should be guided by the following principles:

– during the emergency phase, data collection should only cover the principal health problems, i.e. those which produce the highest mortality and morbidity[9,21];
– data collection should be limited to public health matters which both can and will be acted upon, i.e. problems that can be effectively prevented or treated[9];
– the system should be as simple as possible;
– the frequency with which data is transmitted and analysed should be adapted to the situation, i.e. weekly in the emergency phase and monthly thereafter;
– responsibility for organizing and supervising the surveillance system should be clearly assigned to an individual and/or an agency, and close coordination between all partners (UN agencies, NGOs and the host country's MOH) is essential[9];
– data analysis should take place at field level, where it will be translated into action;
– the surveillance system should be flexible in order to respond to new health problems or changes in programme activities.

Data coverage and sources

In general, 5 categories of data are gathered. These cover[11]:

- demography,
- mortality,
- morbidity,
- basic needs,
- programme activities.

1. DEMOGRAPHY

This category of information essentially covers the size and composition of the refugee population and is required in order to plan interventions and to constitute the denominator for calculating mortality, morbidity and other rates. The demographic indicators most frequently required in refugee settings are the total population, the number of children under 5 years of age, and new arrivals and departures. A first estimate of the population size is generally obtained during the initial assessment (see *1. Initial Assessment*), but must be regularly updated during the surveillance.

Information	Sources	Indices	References
Population	– host country authorities – UNHCR and other agencies – community leaders – home-visitors (periodic census) – (repeated rapid household sample surveys)	– total number of refugees – number of under-fives – number of new arrivals and departures	17% of total

Sources of demographic data

One of the main tasks of home-visitors (HVs) is to collect data in those sections of the refugee site for which they are responsible. They should report new arrivals and departures, and undertake a regular census in their area (e.g. every month)[9]. Population data can also be obtained from the updated records of operational partners, such as UNHCR, the agency in charge of food distribution, refugee leaders, etc. However, the population figures given by one source may differ from those provided by another and these different figures should be compared in order to estimate the most likely figure. Whatever estimate is arrived at, it is important that all the operational partners agree on the same figures and sources to be used as the basis for planning and evaluating programmes.

2. MORTALITY

The Crude Mortality Rate (CMR - see definition in Table 8.2) is the most useful indicator in the emergency phase as it alone measures the gravity of the situation and follows its evolution. Calculating mortality rates per 10,000 population per day enables each situation to be compared against reference values (see below). The expected CMR in a developing country is in the order of 25 deaths/per 1,000 population/per year, i.e. 0.68/10,000/day; but in emergencies it can rise above 1/10,000/day[4,11].

Recording the cause of death is often difficult when death takes place outside health facilities. The information which refugee representatives or home-visitors obtain from the community in family interviews is generally not very reliable. Data should therefore be limited to very common diseases such as diarrhoea and acute respiratory infection, or to any specific disease that may be causing an outbreak.

Information	Sources	Indices	References[4,11]
Deaths	– cemetery: 'grave watchers' – hospital – community: home-visitors, leaders, representatives of camp sections, etc.	– crude mortality rate – under 5 specific mortality rate	< 1/10,000/day < 2-4/10,000/day
Causes of death	– hospital – community: home-visitors (verbal autopsy)	– proportional mortality (%)* – cause-specific mortality rate	

* also called cause-specific mortality proportion

Sources of mortality data

When cemeteries or burial sites are clearly identified, they represent the best source of information on the number of deaths occurring in the community; this system requires the permanent presence of previously trained staff ('grave watchers'), assigned to provide 24-hour coverage and report on the number of daily burials; they should be closely supervised[11]. In some situations, data provided by religious facilities might be an alternative to cemetery surveillance.

Medical records in health facilities provide reliable information (especially on cause of death) but this source of information is not sufficiently representative, given that many deaths occur within the home setting. Therefore, information from the community itself is needed, usually provided by home-visitors and refugee leaders. The free distribution of religious/burial material (e.g. incense, shroud, etc.) could be used to encourage families of the deceased to report deaths. Attention should be paid to the frequent over - and particularly under - reporting of deaths in the community, depending mainly on the method of registration used. The reported mortality is likely to increase when the method of data collection changes from passive to active reporting, and this should not be misinterpreted as a real increase in mortality.

Identification of the most likely cause of death in the community can be performed by home-visitors or staff specifically trained in the 'verbal autopsy' method. This is a technique that involves a structured interview with the family of the deceased, asking questions intended to identify symptoms associated with the most frequent causes of death. However, this technique is not easy and requires previous staff training. It is described in more detail in other reference works[21].

3. MORBIDITY

Diseases are selected for surveillance because of their significance for public health issues. Two categories of disease should be covered:

– the common diseases, responsible for an important proportion of mortality, such as common diarrhoea, malnutrition, acute respiratory infections and malaria; and

– the potentially epidemic diseases, such as measles, meningitis and cholera, which can all be associated with a high mortality, and for which control measures exist.

Information	Sources	Indices	References[4,11]
Common diseases	Out-patient department (OPD)	incidence rate (/1,000/ week) (proportional morbidity)	see chapters on specific diseases
Epidemic diseases	OPD and in-patient special treatment unit possibly home-visitors	number of cases/week incidence rate (/1,000/ week) attack rate	see chapters on specific diseases for some diseases: 0 cases

Sources of morbidity data

Health care facilities are the main source of morbidity data. Even though all cases of a given pathology do not pass through the health system, the objective of disease surveillance is trend assessment and not exhaustive registration.

Home-visitors (HVs) can sometimes participate in disease surveillance, but this should be limited to special situations, when more exhaustive and detailed data are needed on a specific problem for a given period of time (i.e. epidemic).

A case definition should be worked out for every disease selected. These definitions must be simple and clear, adapted to the level of staff qualifications and to the available diagnostic means (most diagnoses will be based on clinical signs). They should be sensitive enough to enable an epidemiological alert. Health workers should be trained to use these case definitions for recording data. Table 8.1 presents examples of clinical case definitions for the surveillance of morbidity in developing countries.

Table 8.1
Examples of clinical case definitions for use in public health surveillance in refugee settings

Illness	Definition
Measles (EPI definition)	generalized rash lasting > 3 days AND temperature > 38°C AND one of the following: cough, runny nose, red eyes
Dysentery (WHO)	3 or more liquid stools per day and presence of visible blood in stools
Common Diarrhoea	3 or more liquid watery stools per day
Acute Respiratory Infection (moderate to severe)[21]	fever, cough and rapid breathing (> 50 or more per min.)
Malaria	temperature > 38.5°C and absence of other infection
Malnutrition	weight for height index < -2 Z-Scores or kwashiorkor
Meningitis	sudden onset of fever > 38.9°C and neck stiffness or purpura

4. BASIC NEEDS

This category covers water, sanitation and food supplies as well as shelter and other essential non-food items such as soap, cooking fuel, water containers, etc. It is especially important that health agencies monitor this sector in the emergency phase because, if basic needs are not met, there will be a direct effect on the health status of the population. Therefore, health staff have an important role to play as watchdogs, monitoring overall living conditions[11]. UNHCR, WHO, UNICEF and other international relief organizations have defined standards with which the data gathered can be compared (see below).

Information	Sources	Indices	References
Water quantity	agency in charge of water supply community (HVs)	litres/person/day	15-20 litres/person/day
Food available	agency in charge of distribution community (HVs) food basket monitoring	Kcal/person/day	> 2,100/kcal/person/day
Sanitation	agency in charge observation on site	number refugees/ latrines	< 20 refugees/latrine
Shelters	agency in charge community (HVs)	shelter space per person	> 3,5 m²/person
Other items (blankets, fire-wood, etc.)	agency in charge community (HVs)	items available per household	depending on the item

Sources of basic needs data

The main sources of data, based on distribution records, are the agencies in charge of these different sectors; but these data should be compared with information from the community itself, mostly gathered by home-visitors, and direct observation in the camp (for instance, regularly counting the number of latrines). Data sources and collection methods in regard to food availability are developed in *4. Food and Nutrition.*

5. DATA ON PROGRAMME ACTIVITIES (PROGRAMME INDICATORS)

During the emergency phase the main concern is to gather data on priority programmes such as measles vaccination, water supply, sanitation, basic curative care and feeding programmes. Only simple indicators should be gathered, and in limited numbers. For example, monitoring the out-patient department mainly involves collecting data on the number of new cases attending consultations, and not on injections and dressing, that are of very little use for decision-making. When the situation moves into a post-emergency phase and other health programmes are implemented, such as reproductive health and child health services, the indicators should cover other fields, such as the number of ante-natal consultations, the number of vaccine doses administered within the Expanded Programme on Immunization (EPI), etc.

Information	Sources	Indices	Références
Health activities OPD, in-patient, immunization feeding centres etc.	registers of the programmes concerned (repeated vaccine coverage surveys)	n° consultations/week attendance rate n° admissions/week hospital mortality rate measles vaccine coverage and others	around 4 NC*/ person/ year > 90% of the target pop.
Other public health activities (water supply, latrines etc.)	see below: *Basic Needs*	see below: *Basic needs*	see below *Basic needs*

* NC: NEW CASE

Sources of data

Most data sources and collection methods are described in the relevant chapters (see *2. Measles Immunization, 4. Food and Nutrition, 6. Health Care in the Emergency Phase,* etc.). Information-gathering requires a system of registers for every programme - or tally sheets for immunization. (See below.)

Some general considerations in regard to data collection

It is not vital that data are recorded by age group and gender. However, during the emergency phase, under-fives should be recorded separately as they constitute a group at specific risk; in addition, gender break-down for mortality allows to detect sex-specific mortality differences. Later on, in the post-emergency phase, more detailed data may be gathered to determine other differences according to age and sex, and within other high-risk groups (e.g. pregnant women, the elderly, etc.).

One of the qualities required of a good surveillance system is flexibility, especially in emergency situations: it should therefore always be possible to add an indicator to the system in place (e.g. unexpected epidemic diseases).

In open situations, where refugees or displaced persons are integrated into the local population, it is generally much more difficult to collect data, particularly on demography and number of deaths. Only a very efficient system of home-visitors or community workers, covering the whole displaced population, is able to provide correct and representative data.

Summary of sources and methods

The main information sources in a refugee camp are:
- the health and nutritional facilities, other programme facilities and the cemetery,
- the agencies in charge of programmes,
- the community itself through home-visitors.

- Data is usually gathered on a daily basis. Every medical facility and every programme likely to be a source of public health information should keep a register in which information is recorded on a daily basis. For example, medical staff in charge of consultations at the OPD should keep a register of the age, address (camp sector or home village) and diagnosis of every patient.

  Using the same principle, a register should be established for all programmes, including the cemetery (grave watchers), and staff should be trained in recording information.

- A network of home visitors (HVs) should be set up early on as this facilitates the collection of demographic data (population size, composition and movements) and mortality data, which can be assessed through regular visits to shelters. HVs can also be used to complement information collected routinely when specific problems have been identified (by surveys or focus groups), and for other tasks described in the chapter *9. Human Resources and Training* (active case-finding, health education, etc.).

  This network should be implemented in the very early weeks of intervention, and should comprise one or two HVs for every 1,000 refugees.

Definitions should be established for all data selected (e.g. case definitions for disease). The same definition should be used whatever the source and the method of data collection. For instance, case definitions can be developed for the different causes of death[21].

Analysis and transmission of data

Information is organized and disseminated by means of a weekly report in the emergency phase and a monthly report once the situation has stabilized. These reports should be simple, composed of crude indicators and interpreted within the context of the particular situation.

DATA ANALYSIS

It is important that data analysis be conducted at field level. Essentially this means sorting and analyzing the data gathered in terms of time, place and persons (i.e. who is sick, where and when). Appropriate epidemiological indices have to be calculated for each of the data categories in order to allow comparisons. The crude mortality rate and the under-five mortality rate are the two basic indices for data on mortality (expressed per day); these should be computed and followed over time. The trends in the most frequent pathologies can be followed via incidence rates. Information on the absolute number of cases is useful for the rarer but potentially epidemic diseases (e.g. hepatitis) for which very few cases are needed to signal the beginning of an epidemic. Table 8.2 presents the definitions of these different indices.

Table 8.2
Frequently used indices for describing mortality and morbidity in public health surveillance [20,4]

Health indices	Numerator	Denominator	Expressed per number at risk
MORTALITY			
Crude mortality rate (CMR)	total number of deaths reported over a given period of time	estimated mid-period population	1,000 or 10,000
Under-five specific mortality rate	number of under-five deaths reported over a period of time	estimated mid-period under-five population	1,000 or 10,000
Cause-specific mortality rate	number of deaths attributed to a specific cause over a period of time	estimated mid-period population	1,000 or 10,000
Cause-specific mortality proportion	number of death attributed to a specific cause over a given period of time	total number of deaths from all causes reported over the same period	100 or 1,000
MORBIDITY			
Incidence rate	number of new cases of a specified disease reported over a given period of time	estimated mid-period population at risk	variable: 10^x (1000, 10,000 or 100,000)
Attack rate	number of new cases of a specified disease reported over the duration of the epidemic	total population at risk over the same period	variable : 10^x
Prevalence	number of current cases, new and old, of a specified disease at a given point in time	estimated population at risk at the same point in time	variable : 10^x

The comparison of epidemiological indicators, calculated over a given period (week or month), with normal or reference values, constitutes the first phase of data analysis. With regard to mortality and morbidity, it must be taken into account that the reference values were obtained from large populations for use at national level. When applied to small refugee populations (population denominator less than 10,000), these references might lead to either an under-estimation or an over-estimation of the situation.

This is why surveillance really begins once the trends of these indicators can be followed in time. For example, although the CMRs were similar in Sudan in 1985 and in eastern Ethiopia in 1988, 6 months after refugee camps had opened, time trend analyses show that the situation in Sudan had largely improved over the 6 months, while the situation in Ethiopia had deteriorated. The only way to visualize these trends in time is to produce graphs that are updated on a weekly or monthly basis. The analytical essence of surveillance data is based on the interpretation of these graphs.

Analysis according to PLACE basically means comparing the data taken from several camps, or different locations within one settlement.

Analysis according to PERSON is initially restricted to comparing the under-five group with the general population, which may be important for mortality rates and the incidence of certain diseases.

Analyses of both place and person can also be illustrated in graph form.

DATA INTERPRETATION

The major objective of the analysis is to single out the priorities for current activities. Interpretation of data may rely on reference and norm values or on thresholds that have been set for certain indicators, but again it is the time trend, i.e. the slope of the curve, that counts the most. The main question is whether things are getting better or worse. Trends should be related to the events occurring in the settlement and the programmes being carried out. It should also be taken into account that several indicators interact on each other: for instance, the measles incidence rate, the under-five specific mortality rate and the malnutrition prevalence rate.

Data should always be cautiously interpreted by taking into account the numerous possible surveillance biases. For instance, it should always be kept in mind that disease observed in a health centre represents only what is happening among the people who have access to this health centre, that the decrease observed in a mortality rate may be due to a relaxation of mortality surveillance and that certain sensitive data (e.g. population size) are sometimes manipulated.

Communication

Data that has been collected and analysed must be passed on to decision-makers, the staff involved, and partners. This communication aspect is an essential component of a surveillance system and includes:
- feedback,
- dissemination of information,
- specific communications.

The first two are routine activities to be carried out with the same frequency as transmission and analysis, i.e. weekly and monthly.

Feedback consists of returning processed information to those who supplied the raw data in the first place (medical personnel, community leaders, home-visitors, etc.). The main aim is to maintain motivation for data gathering and to adjust or refine programme activities accordingly. Feedback generally takes place during informal meetings and staff training sessions. Although feedback is an essential component of a surveillance system, it may be difficult to ensure in the first stages of an emergency. However, after the acute phase is passed, more attention should be paid to this because, without feedback, surveillance is doomed to failure.

Information is disseminated to decision-makers and medical officers both inside and outside the refugee settlement. All the individuals and institutions receiving surveillance reports should be listed, and the list must include the host country's MOH. The regular report (weekly or monthly) should combine a summary of the data for the given period, a few graphs showing the main time trends of indicators and commentaries helping to interprete the graphs. During the emergency phase, the series of graphs must necessarily include the mortality rates expressed in deaths/10,000/day from the beginning of the intervention. (See example of surveillance report in appendix 5.)

Special communications could be undertaken for specific problems, such as an epidemic or a disastrous food situation. This often involves drawing up a document that combines surveillance data and survey data. However, priority should always be given to the actual intervention being implemented to bring the problem under control.

Important messages must always be made very clear through a special emphasis on visual communication, i.e. graphic presentation. Note that the graphic presentation of data constitutes the basis for data organization and communication. Graphs should be as simple as possible and carry only a single message. The use of three-dimensional graphs or combinations of bars and lines should be avoided along with any other complicated options. The rule is to use bars to present absolute numbers (population, cases of a disease and admissions to hospital) and to use lines to present rates (incidence and mortality). The title should be self-explanatory and contain all the following information: topic, time, place and group covered (e.g. incidence of measles among under-fives, Mankokwe refugee camp, Malawi, 1987-91).

Implementing a surveillance system

A surveillance system is implemented in two stages.

1. THE EMERGENCY PHASE

During the first days of refugee programmes (ideally, concomitant with the population displacement itself), surveillance is the extension of the initial assessment and relief workers should not wait for medical facilities and programmes to be organized in order to implement it. At this stage, two types of information are required in priority: the number of refugees and the number of deaths. The CMR is computed every day to assess the gravity of the situation and its evolution. After the first few weeks, a limited number of priority indicators are gathered and analysed once a week: population size, mortality, basic needs, principal diseases and main programme activities.

The emergency phase lasts until basic requirements have been met and the major medical problems brought under control, and is characterized by a CMR reduced to 1/10,000/per day or below (by convention).

2. THE POST-EMERGENCY OR CONSOLIDATION PHASE

During this period, most of the indicators are reported monthly rather than weekly. The choice of morbidity indicators can be broadened, although they should remain limited to the diseases for which action is feasible. Programme indicators should follow diversification in programmes (e.g. ante- and post-natal consultations, EPI, family planning and health education) but should be limited to one or two indicators per programme. At this stage, the refugee surveillance system could begin to integrate some characteristics of the national health information system (HIS) of the host country although it must continue to remain sensitive to new health problems; for instance, when certain host country vertical medical programmes are extended to the refugee population (e.g. EPI), specific reporting and surveillance systems must be implemented in line with MOH policy. In the longer term, if the refugee situation enters a chronic phase, refugee surveillance may gradually be integrated into the national HIS.

Organization and responsibilities

Information is usually communicated to 3 different levels (see flow chart):
- field level, i.e. the refugee population, medical facilities, home-visitor network, agencies operating in the field, etc.;
- national level, i.e. the MOH of the host country, officials of UN agencies and representatives of other agencies participating in refugee relief programmes; all settlements in a region or country will be taken into account;
- supra-national level, i.e. the headquarters of agencies and donors.

The medical coordinator on the refugee site is the pivot of the surveillance system. Information sources (registrars, grave watchers, etc.) should be identified and organized by those in charge of specific programmes, while the medical coordinator supervises the collection, revision and correction of data, and finalizes analysis and interpretation. This person should also transmit the information to the other levels and ensure that feedback reaches the relevant people in the field.

One person should be designated within each programme or facility to take responsibility for the daily collection and reporting of data.

Evaluating a surveillance system

An evaluation of the surveillance system can be undertaken at the beginning of the post-emergency phase, when it is clear that the refugee situation is likely to persist and it becomes necessary to redefine objectives, re-assess the situation, and adapt the surveillance system. Methods for evaluating health information systems have been designed by epidemiologists from the Center for Disease Control (CDC), and can be applied to public health surveillance in refugee situations[3]. Evaluation should consider usefulness as the principal quality of a good system: for instance, whether the system signalled outbreaks, or whether the diseases under surveillance are important in terms of public health. In refugee camp situations where there is a better knowledge of denominators, surveillance has immediate objectives and medical personnel are motivated, evaluations can often be conducted more easily than in open situations.

Special issue: other health information-gathering methods

As previously mentioned, some health information methods are not part of surveillance, but must be undertaken regularly in refugee settings.

Cross-sectional surveys measure the frequency of a characteristic (malnutrition, vaccination status, mortality, etc.) in a population based on a sample. If well done, these surveys supply quality information but of a pin-point nature. They are not useful for assessing trends over a period of time, unless they are repeated at regular intervals (e.g. repeated nutritional surveys). Such surveys are indicated at the start of an intervention (see 1. Initial Assessment), when a problem is revealed by the routine surveillance system (e.g. an increase in hospital admissions of malnutrition cases can lead to a nutritional survey in the camp), or in the framework of a programme evaluation (e.g. vaccination coverage survey carried out at the end of a mass immunization campaign).

An outbreak investigation should follow on from an early warning provided by the surveillance system. Analysis of specific surveillance data gives information on the distribution of cases (who is affected, where and when). Further epidemiological studies (case-control or retrospective cohort studies) may identify the source of the disease or risk factors associated with its transmission.

Qualitative methods, such as semi-direct interviews and focus groups, make it possible to obtain information on, for example, the refugees' personal perception of health problems and of the relief programmes implemented. These methods are often required to complement the surveillance system in an attempt to address problems it has identified. For example, a surveillance that picks up an under-representation of children among sick patients seen at an OPD can lead to the organization of focus group discussions with groups composed of a dozen or so mothers dealing with access to health care.

Principal recommendations regarding Public health surveillance

- The surveillance system is essential to direct refugee programmes by providing early warning of epidemics, by determining the main health problems and by acting as guide for programme planning, implementation and evaluation. It should be established early in any refugee intervention, as an extension of the initial assessment.

- Data collection should be simple and limited to those public health problems which both can and will be acted upon. The 5 categories to be covered by data collection are demography, mortality, morbidity, basic needs and programme activities. Only a limited number of simple and standardized indicators should be used. The surveillance system should be flexible, especially in emergency situations.

- In the emergency phase, the crude mortality rate is the most useful indicator as it alone measures the gravity of the situation. Morbidity data should mainly cover the common diseases that are the major causes of death and the potentially epidemic diseases for which control measures exist.

- In the post-emergency phase, other data and indicators will be added, according to changing morbidity profile and new programmes.

- Data should be analysed and transmitted to decision-makers by means of a weekly report in the emergency phase and a monthly report once the situation has stabilized. Data should first be analysed in the field, with feedback provided to field staff and local authorities. The most important application of data is in the interpretation of trends over time (using graphs).

References

1. Benenson, A. *Control of communicable diseases in man.* 15th edition. Washington DC: American Public Health Association, 1990, pp. 280-4.

2. Bitar D. *Surveillance of cholera among Mozambican refugees in Malawi, 1988-1991.* [Internal report]. Paris: Epicentre, 1991.

3. CDC. Guidelines for evaluating surveillance systems. *MMWR*, 1988, 37(S-5).

4. CDC. Famine-affected, refugee, and displaced populations: Recommendations for public health issues. *MMWR*, 1992, 41(RR-13): 1-76.

5. Dabis, F, Drucker, J, Moren, A. *Epidemiologie d'intervention*. Paris: Arnette, 1992.

6. Decludt, B, Pecoul, B, Biberson, P, Lang, R, Imivithaya, S. Malaria surveillance among the displaced Karen population in Thailand, April 1984 to February 1989, Mae Sod, Thailand. *Southeast Asian J Trop Med Public Health*, 1991, 22(4): 504-8.

7. Desenclos, J C, Michel, D, Tholly, F, Magdi, I, Pecoul, B, Desvé, G. Mortality trends among refugees in Honduras, 1984-1987. *Int J Epidemiol*, 1987, 19(2): 367-73.

8. Manoncourt, S, Dopler, B, Enten, F, et al. Public health consequences of the civil war in Somalia. *The Lancet*, 1992, 340:176-7.

9. Moren, A, et al. Epidemiologic surveillance among Mozambican refugees in Malawi, 1987-1989. *Disaster*, 1991, 15(4): 363-72.

10. Moren, A, Stefanaggi, S, Antona, D, Bitar, D, Gastellu-Etchegorry, M, Tchatchioka, M, et al. Practical field epidemiology to investigate a cholera outbreak in a Mozambican refugee camp in Malawi, 1988. *J Trop Med Hyg*, 1991, 94: 1-7.

11. Hakewill, P, Moren, A. Monitoring and evaluation of relief programmes. *Trop Doctor*, 1991, 21, Suppl 1.

12. Pécoul, B, Cohen, O, Michelet, M J. Mozambique: Mortality among displaced persons. *The Lancet* (letter),1991, 338: 650.

13. PHCMAP. *Primary health care management advancement programme. Surveillance of morbidity and mortality*. The Aga Khan University, 1993.

14. Shears, P, Lusty, T. Communicable disease epidemiology following migration: Studies from the African famine. *Int. Migration Rev*, 1987, 21: 783-95.

15. Toole, M J, Waldman, R J. An analysis of mortality trends among refugee populations in Somalia, Sudan, and Thailand. *WHO Bul*, 1988, 66: 237-47.

16. Toole, M J, Waldman, R J. Refugees and displaced persons: War, hunger, and public health. *JAMA*, 1993, 270: 600-5.

17. UNHCR. *Handbook for Emergencies*. Geneva: UNHCR, 1982.

18. Wharton, M, Chorba, T L, Vogt, R L, Morse, D L, Buehler, J W. Case definitions for public health surveillance. *MMWR*, 1990, 39 (RR-13): 23.

19. CDC. CDC *Surveillance update*. Atlanta: CDC, 1988.

20. The EIS Officer's manual of practical epidemiology. *CDC/EPO*, 1988.

21. Marfin, A A, Moore, J, et al. Infectious disease surveillance during emergency relief to Bhutanese refugees in Nepal. *JAMA*, 1994, 272(5).

9. Human resources and training

Introduction

Human resources are one of the most important resources in relief programmes. They include both expatriate and local staff (either refugees or nationals of the host country), working together in close cooperation. A major factor - and principal constraint - in deciding and planning programmes is the difficulty of ensuring a supply of appropriate staff and managing them efficiently.

The specificity of refugee emergencies is such that they require a large number of staff to be recruited rapidly, at least in the initial stages. This does not mean that staff can be recruited at random and en masse however critical the situation may be; hiring hundreds of people for jobs that are only vaguely defined will soon result in chaos. Such an approach would not save time; on the contrary, much more time would be required later on to reorganize the staff. A rational and professional approach is therefore necessary.

The availability of human resources varies widely according to the country and refugee context. For instance, basic medical staff may sometimes be difficult to find because of the remoteness of the refugee settlement and security problems, while in other instances, highly qualified staff may be available locally. When staff do not have the required skills, training will be necessary and specific courses (e.g. for measles immunization) should be started in the first stages of an emergency.

Another specificity of refugee programmes is the essential role played by home-visitors. These are refugees chosen from among the population who ensure the link between their community and the relief services. Home-visitors must be promptly recruited at the beginning of an emergency.

Human resource management is generally a major undertaking, although one that is often underestimated. Responsibility for it should be clearly assigned to a senior staff member at the start of a refugee programme.

Objectives

The major objective is to provide human resources capable of performing the different tasks involved in refugee programmes, and to organize these efficiently. The overall goal is the effective and coordinated implementation of the 10 top priorities (see *Part II, The Ten Top Priorities: Introduction*).

Determining human resource requirements

The number of staff required, and their qualifications, must be properly defined for every refugee intervention. The estimation of staff needs cannot just be a rough guess but must be based on the activities to be carried out, and not the other way round (i.e. deciding on activities according to the resources available). Staff requirements should be defined in a series of steps.

DETERMINING STAFF REQUIREMENTS STEP BY STEP

- Refugee health needs are assessed in the initial assessment and appropriate programmes defined in response to them. These will usually cover the 10 top priorities.

- The target population for each programme should be defined; for instance, measles mass immunization targets children between 6 months and 15 years, i.e. 40% to 50% of the population.

- A list of activities and the tasks to be performed within them should be established for every programme.

- The different categories of personnel required to execute these tasks must be identified.

- A job description should be prepared for each category of staff, describing in detail the tasks to be undertaken, the means available to execute them and the level of competence required (see below). This should take into account the qualifications of available staff: the less qualified the staff, the shorter the list of tasks.

- The number of staff required may then be calculated, based on the estimated work load, which depends on the target population, and the time required to perform every task; for instance, one health worker should not be expected to perform more than 50 consultations per day. Day-shifts, night-shifts and days off should be taken into account.

Thus staff requirements cannot be based on a set of pre-determined standards, and flexibility must always be maintained in order to adapt to fluctuations in the workload and changes in programmes[1]. For instance, additional staff will be necessary if there is a large influx of newcomers or a large-scale outbreak of disease requiring new facilities to be set up (e.g. cholera/shigellosis units). Manpower needs will be particularly high in the first weeks of an emergency when the infrastructure has to be set up (e.g. clinics, latrines, etc.), but should then begin to decrease.

Estimates for staff requirements for each activity are given in Table 9.1. These figures are based both on experience and existing guidelines, and may be used as indicators for staff needs in camp situations where new staff must be recruited. Other suggested staffing figures are available in specific guidelines and UNHCR documents[1]. In open situations, where refugees are scattered among the local population, fewer staff would normally be required because access to and utilization of services is generally lower than in camps, and staff from existing local facilities participate in refugee assistance (particularly the health facilities).

Table 9.1
Minimum staff requirements for different activities in a camp setting
(see relevant chapters)

Activity or service	Staff requirement
Mass immunization campaign[15]	1 vaccination team (20 people, including 2 vaccinators and 1 cold chain technician) to immunize 500-700 people per hour 1 supervisor (e.g. nurse)/1-2 teams
Health services: – Out-Patient Department (OPD) (at central or peripheral level)	1 qualified health worker/50 consultations/day medical doctor for supervision non-qualified staff for registration (1), dressing/sterilization (1-2), oral rehydration (1-2), delivering drugs, etc. 1 watchman / 8-hour shift
– In-Patient Department (IPD) (at central level)	1 medical doctor (minimum) 1 qualified health worker/20 beds/8 hour shift 1 nursing supervisor/IPD (hygiene, sterilization, dressing etc.) 1-2 for pharmacy staff for data collection 1-2 watchmen/8 hour shifts
Home visiting	1 home-visitor/500-1,000 refugees 1 supervisor/10 home-visitors 1 supervisor/programme (e.g. nurse)
Cholera unit[11]: (around 200 beds)	1 health worker/20 patients/8 hour shift 2 non-qualified workers for other tasks (cleaning, oral rehydration, etc.)/20 beds/8 hour shifts 1 medical supervisor for 60 beds 1 logistician 1 coordinator per cholera unit other staff for registration, watchmen, etc.
Nutritional centres[10]: – Wet supplementary feeding centre (250 beneficiaries)	1 general supervisor for overall management 1 trained nurse for medical follow-up (could also act as supervisor) 1 nutritional assistant per 30 children 2 nutritional outreach workers to follow up defaulters and carry out screening 1 cook plus assistant per 50 children 1 cleaner per 50 children 1 or more watchmen
– Therapeutic feeding centre (100 beneficiaries)	1 medical doctor (part-time) 2-3 trained nurses for overall management and medical follow-up 10 nutritional assistants (1/10 children) 2 outreach workers to follow up defaulters and carry out screening 1 storekeeper 4 cooks plus assistants 4 cleaners 1-2 watchmen
Water/sanitation programme	1 sanitation or environmental health technician for supervision (in large programmes: 1 for water supply and 1 for sanitation) number of staff required depends on the situation and the tasks to be performed
Support activities (administration/logistics)	1 general administrator accountant, secretary, administrative assistant, etc. 1 or more logistician, logistic assistants, storekeeper, purchasing officer drivers, watchmen possibly: pharmacist, mechanic and radio-operators

STAFF QUALIFICATIONS

There are two main types of staff:

– qualified staff who have been officially trained in the tasks to be performed (e.g. nurses). The curricula covered in that training and the titles received may differ according to the educational system of the country of training; and

– non-qualified personnel who have not been officially trained but who may have acquired valuable skills to perform certain tasks, either through experience and/or unofficial training.

Various categories of qualified staff are required in the two main areas of refugee health interventions:

– the health-related field: physicians, nurses, midwives, pharmacists, nutritionists, sanitation officers and other health professionals whose titles depend on the educational system of the country of training (medical assistant, health assistant, community health workers, etc.);

– support services (logistics and administration): administrators, accountants, mechanics, etc.

The categories of non-qualified staff include: home-visitors, registrars, dressers, cooks, cleaners, watchmen, casual labourers for construction facilities, etc.

Every intervention requires staff at the decisional level (e.g. programme coordinator) [2]. In the initial phase, professionals specialized in emergency intervention are required for launching programmes. These are generally experienced professionals with specific technical competence, such as medical doctors, nurses, experts in immunization, sanitation technicians, logisticians, etc.[9]. A number of relief organizations employ a pool of professionals specialized in emergency work who are available at short notice to carry out short missions. This has the advantage that right from the start there are people available who know the standard procedures for interventions and the common constraints. They are also used to working as a team and share a common understanding of refugee situations.

Human resource management

In principle, UNHCR should provide guidance in local staff management, aiming at a certain level of standardization. However, this is seldom reached in practice, or at least only at a later stage when the majority of staff have already been contracted.

LOCAL STAFF RECRUITMENT

Ideally, local staff recruitment should not start before the following tasks have been completed for each programme.

• The categories and numbers of staff required should be clearly defined, and job descriptions prepared for every staff category (see above). There is often a reluctance to spend time on job descriptions during the heat of an emergency. However, it is an essential tool for staff management, acting as the basis for preparing the profiles expected of candidates (job profile) and clearly laying out each person's tasks and responsibilities. Job descriptions for emergency interventions are generally prepared in advance. Standard job descriptions exist for some categories of staff, but they will have to be adapted to the situation, i.e. dependent on the qualifications and skills of the human resources available and the characteristics of a particular programme.

- An organization chart must be drawn up for every programme and facility (e.g. health centre). A prototype will probably be designed before recruitment begins, but will be adapted afterwards, according to the level of staff actually recruited. It should indicate the supervision system and communication flow.

- The job profile is the basic tool for effective recruitment. It describes the tasks to be performed, the diploma and level required, necessary language ability, level of responsibility, and position on the organization chart.

Local staff recruitment takes place among the refugee population and residents of the host country, and information about vacancies should be made directly available to them.

Applicants should be selected on the basis of the recruitment profile, interview and possibly testing. A first screening usually involves cross-checking the applicant's profile against the job profile. Interviews normally follow (although not for casual workers), and are mandatory for skilled staff. Tests are useful for many jobs, for example, written tests for secretaries and administrators, practical tests for different categories of medical staff, drivers, etc.

The selection procedure is usually conducted by the person in charge of the programme, while the administrative aspects of recruitment (contract, salary scales, etc.) are taken care of by the project administrator. In very large emergencies, it is recommended that human resource specialists are temporarily employed to assist the team with initial staff recruitment, organization (e.g. job description and organization chart) and training. Newly-recruited staff should sign a contract and receive a copy of their job description, if this exists on paper.

Some considerations regarding the local staff recruitment

- The question often arises as to whether refugees should be given preference for jobs over residents of the host country. The answer depends on the jobs themselves and on the local context. Consideration must be given to the possibility of national long-term programmes being harmed if competent national staff are drained from existing public services. Refugee staff have the advantage of being familiar with the culture and language of their own community. Employment also allows them to be actively involved in activities targeting their own welfare and provides them with the opportunity to acquire new skills[1,2] (see also refugee participation in Part I, *Socio-cultural Aspects*). Refugee staff should be preferred for community services (e.g. constructing and maintaining latrines, and as outreach workers for nutrition and immunization programmes, etc.) and there are a few job categories that should - whenever possible - only be filled by refugees, such as home-visitors and traditional birth attendants (TBAs)[1]. However, employing refugee workers is often a complex issue, especially on the administrative side, as described below in the section *Special issues: Refugee workers.*

There are also several advantages to recruiting staff from the host country: the host communities are more likely to accept the assistance given to refugees thereby reducing the risk of tension between them, resident staff will be less subject to pressure from the refugee community, and there is generally a greater likelihood of finding qualified staff among the host population than among the refugees (better educated refugees often have better opportunities than ending up in a camp).

- Care should be taken also to employ female staff (see *Socio-cultural Aspects* in Part I), although the socio-cultural patterns of the population must be taken into consideration. Female health staff and TBAs are particularly important for ensuring that refugee women have greater access to health services[2].

- Those involved in the recruitment process may need to consider maintaining a balance between different ethnic groups among the staff and in some situations this may be particularly important. For instance, in MSF refugee programmes in Rwanda (October 1993), staff members were originally recruited according to classical criteria - such as qualification - but it was then found that around 75% of them belonged to the Tutsi group who represented only 15% of the total population. This subsequently became the source of a major conflict with the local authorities[13]. In addition, staff attitudes towards refugee groups may be influenced by their tribal membership and become a possible source of inequities and other problems in relief assistance.

- It is particularly useful to recruit highly skilled professionals from among the local population. One advantage is that if such staff can be recruited locally, it will not be necessary to ship in large numbers of expatriates.

STAFF POLICY

A standard staff policy must be defined and formalized. This should generally cover working hours, holidays, salary scale and other material advantages, as well as warning and dismissal procedures, etc. Standardization is imperative within an agency and is facilitated when all administrative aspects of staff management are under the responsibility of the same person. Standardization is also useful between agencies, especially in regard to salary scales in order to avoid a flow of staff towards agencies paying more (as it is frequently the case with some international agencies who offer high wages).

It is important to have a knowledge of the national labour laws of the host country for deciding staff policy, particularly if legal problems are to be avoided, such as court cases over improper staff dismissal. Standard procedures are not always respected in the acute phase of the emergency because a large number of staff have to be recruited very rapidly. However, this leads to a lot of time being wasted later on trying to reorganize and bring in delayed standardization.

Contracts should take into consideration the specificity of refugee emergencies, i.e. the specific status of refugee workers, the high number of non-qualified personnel initially required, the temporary aspect of refugee programmes and the risk of unexpected events occurring, etc. This highlights the need to design contracts covering a specific service or for a set duration (see *Part III, The Post-emergency Phase*). For instance, it is useful in the initial stage of the emergency to either contract national workers on a daily basis, or give them preliminary two-month contracts until sufficient information has been gathered on labour laws in the host country. Another possibility is to first hire staff as 'volunteers' (see Table 9.1), and pay them incentives[14]. Refugees, who are often not officially entitled to sign work contracts in the host country, can be hired and paid under such arrangements (see also *Specific issues: Refugee workers*). The main types of contract and general legal principles which should be respected when hiring and dismissing staff are given in Table 9.2.

Table 9.2
Types of contracts or agreement and major principles[14]

Labour contract	Temporary contracts are advised in refugee emergencies, but they can only be renewed up to a maximum number of times (before becoming a permanent contract de facto). A probation period should be indicated (e.g. one month), during which contracts can be terminated without notice. A clause should stipulate the maximum lump sum to be paid on premature termination of contract (e.g. one month's salary).
Volunteer agreement	Takes the form of a temporary «contract» (only if permitted by the labour law of the host country). States that the person is a volunteer cooperating with the relief agency for a specific period. Compensation is through 'incentives' (e.g. payment or food-for-work). The volunteer agreement has to be signed.
For both	The contract should contain a clause stating that the agency has the right to terminate the contract or agreeing to termination if the project is forced to close. Reasons for immediate dismissal (stealing, etc.) should be indicated as well as the procedure for giving warnings. Any dismissal must respect local labour laws and be confirmed in writing.
Hiring casual workers	People hired for a short period to perform a defined task, (e.g. digging latrines), are paid by incentives. No contract is required, but a signed agreement is sometimes preferable.

A local staff salary scale must be determined, although this is complex to draw up and a frequent cause of conflict. Distinctions will have to be made between refugee and non-refugee staff (see below). Whenever possible, salary levels should take into account the local cost of living and be adjusted to inflation and devaluation. Given the heavy workload usually demanded in such situations, salaries should be high enough to ensure regular work attendance and a sufficient level of motivation. It is also important to offer attractive conditions to highly qualified staff, i.e. appropriate salary, clear responsibilities with involvement at decisional level, participation in meetings, housing for those not resident in the area, etc.

- For national staff (from the host country), the national salary scale (for state employees) may be used as a guide, but it must take into account that state employees are frequently underpaid in developing countries and their salary may be insufficient to cover the basic needs of extended families, obliging them to take on extra jobs. This scale should therefore be seen as a minimum remuneration level, and other salary scales should be looked at (e.g. private hospitals, other agencies, etc.). When national staff have to be relocated far from their home areas (sometimes necessary for qualified staff), compensation should be offered, for example, in the form of extra allowances.

- For refugee staff, there is often a debate about which salary scale to use since refugees are already supported by outside aid. Some organizations make it their policy that refugee wages should be well below the national rates (e.g. UNHCR policy)[1]. Although the material advantages received by refugees must be taken into account (especially food rations), it is recommended that significant differences should be avoided between the payments made to refugee and national staff with similar qualifications and performing the same job. Other aspects in relation to refugee staff and the issue of whether or not to pay them for community services is dealt with below under *Specific issues: Refugee workers*.

HUMAN RESOURCE COORDINATION

Staff coordination (both local and expatriate) is essential, although complex and frequently overlooked[1]. This responsibility should be assigned to one person, logically the person in charge of human resources, who should have had previous training, should be briefed for the specific situation and should receive appropriate guidelines. The principles for coordination are similar to most public health projects but they must, of course, be adapted to the emergency situation and the specific refugee context.

Main recommendations

- Job descriptions and organization charts that were drawn up at the start of operations (see above) should be regularly adapted to programme developments. Both remain essential tools throughout the programme for ensuring that the distribution of tasks is clearly understood by everyone, and are useful references in cases of disagreement[1].

- Close supervision and on-the-spot training are essential and attention should be paid to them from the beginning. New staff should be accompanied in the first days of their job and never left to fend for themselves or sent out alone into a totally unfamiliar setting. Supervision is also important to enable health teams to understand the overall relief programme from a public health point of view and the importance of every individual activity as part of the whole intervention effort[6,9].

- Communication and information-sharing are also crucial to ensure a good understanding of priorities and to maintain motivation. Regular meetings are required (at least weekly) at both general and/or sector level (health, logistics, etc.). These will help to ensure a good information exchange and regular feed-back on activities to all staff.

- Adequate working conditions should be guaranteed for all staff and the responsibility for this clearly assigned to one person. There is always a high risk that staff quickly become burned out in the emergency phase, which may lead to serious health consequences and a high staff turnover. Very heavy working hours should be avoided and a minimum of rest (e.g. 1 day per week) should be instituted, even though it might be necessary to compel staff to comply with this. Access to adequate curative care must be organized. Under particularly stressful conditions, counselling and close support for staff may have to be provided.

  Adequate living accommodation should be secured for staff not resident in the area (relocated national staff, expatriate or international staff) and include appropriate housing, safe water and food supplies. Vaccination and prophylaxis may also have to be considered.

- Security problems may arise in situations where armed conflict is the cause of internal displacement. These can affect expatriate as well as local staff, and specific measures and safety precautions should be taken. There are no standard ways of dealing with them. Every organization has its internal guidelines and procedures with which to respond and these should be in writing (e.g. evacuation plans). In principle, it is in the mandate of UNHCR to ensure the protection of refugees and relief workers. Expatriate staff should be aware that local staff may sometimes be exposed to a higher risk, as happened in refugee camps in Rwanda in 1994, where most of the local staff were killed during the genocide. This factor should be taken into account if withdrawal is being considered.

SPECIFIC ISSUES

Refugee workers

Employing refugees as staff is usually not a simple process and several aspects must be assessed beforehand to avoid subsequent problems.

1. The legal status of refugees should be checked as they are frequently denied access to legal employment by the host country.

2. Their qualifications might not be recognized by the host country: diplomas and certificates are frequently lost during displacement, training curricula are often not known outside their own country and the desire for

employment may sometimes lead to false declarations concerning qualifications.

3. The payment of refugee workers is subject to debate, as highlighted under *Staff policy*. It is not only a question of deciding whether or not they should be paid for community services, but also how to pay them: in cash (incentives) or in kind (e.g. food-for-work programmes). On the one hand, payment for community services is open to criticism because it may reduce the sense of responsibility for their own welfare. UNHCR, for instance, does not recommend payments during the first days of an emergency[1]. On the other hand, experience has shown that most refugees will not continue to work on a regular basis without some sort of incentive[3]. It must be kept in mind that there are frequent disruptions to community life, refugees are under pressure to find sufficient resources to survive and they may sometimes not understand the usefulness of some services for which they may be asked to contribute their efforts. There is thus a risk that essential jobs are not done if there is no payment for them[1]. Payment also helps refugees to start up independent economic activities and diversify their diet by making purchases on the local market, and reduces dependence on external aid. There is no straightforward solution to this dilemma. The best recommendation that can be made is to adapt payment strategies to the local context: whether or not refugees already started community services on their own initiative; whether or not there is sufficient food aid available (in addition to general ration distributions) to organize food-for-work programmes; whether or not food-for-work will provide sufficient incentive. As previously stated, a practical option is to enrol refugee workers as volunteers. This can be formalized in a signed agreement and offers compensation (payment or food-for-work). See Table 9.2.

Health workers

One of the crucial points in regard to medical programmes is to find local personnel with medical training to staff them. In situations where qualified health staff are scarce, alternative solutions must be found for responding to health needs.

- **Active recruitment of health staff from neighbouring areas**: however, this can be an inappropriate solution as it drains competent national staff from existing health services, and may harm long-term health programmes because staff may be attracted towards working in refugee projects by the higher salaries sometimes paid by relief agencies.

- **Expatriate doctors and nurses may be brought** in to provide curative care.

- **Non-qualified staff may be trained** in medical tasks: such training is necessary in most situations, but should be extended and intensified when there is insufficient staff. However, newly-trained staff should be closely supervised by qualified staff.

Health staff of the host country, frequently employees of the Ministry of Health (MOH), may be assigned to refugee health care. Specific arrangements should be discussed with the MOH: whether there should be an employment contract or written agreement with the agency, financial compensation for a higher workload to improve motivation and continuity of service, how responsibilities can be shared between the MOH and the agency (if agreed by the MOH), etc. Any such arrangements should be formalized in writing.

Expatriate staff

The role of expatriate staff in refugee programmes is a controversial subject[7].

- On the one hand, expatriates usually have no familiarity with the refugee community or the host country and their presence may prevent the development of local expertise and thus have a negative effect on the sustainability of refugee programmes in the long term.

- On the other hand, experts in emergency action are usually not available locally and as expatriates are not under pressure or at risk of intimidation from local communities or authorities, they can play a more effective role in regard to refugee protection, witnessing to what they see (témoignage) and ensuring a more equitable distribution of resources. Also, they already know the principles and working habits of the relief agencies, which facilitates starting up operations and enables everything to go ahead faster. Finally, the presence of expatriates may be necessary for ensuring continuing support from donors.

In most refugee emergencies, expatriate staff specialized in emergency operations are employed in the first stages to launch interventions (see above) and provide training; after the acute phase, their role will also cover the supervision and management of programmes, and the provision of technical assistance. Exceptions have to be made for situations where there is a scarcity of local qualified staff, and expatriates have to fill in the gaps by carrying out tasks that would usually be done by local staff (see above). It has been observed that some expatriates are reluctant to recruit local staff in sufficient numbers or to delegate tasks to them. The person in charge of human resource management should watch out for this situation and take action to remedy it.

There is no standard rule for the number of expatriate staff required in any given refugee situation since this is dependent on many different factors: the qualifications of available local staff, the stage reached in the intervention (more expatriates may be needed in the emergency phase), security conditions and the risks encountered by local staff, heightened ethnic tensions requiring a large presence of neutral personnel, etc.

TRAINING

Assessment of training needs[9,12,17]

Training becomes necessary whenever there is a discrepancy between the observed level of competence of personnel and the required level of competence to perform a job. This implies that several types of staff may require training.

- Personnel who have never had any training in the tasks they are asked to perform, which is often the case for home-visitors, sanitation staff, etc., should be taught the specific tasks that they are to perform. The job description will be the basis of the training programme.

• Some professionals may require additional training in order to perform new tasks; in emergency situations skilled staff are frequently asked to perform tasks for which they have never received any training.

• Some professionals may have to upgrade their level of performance. They may have diplomas, but their actual level of competence may be low; in many countries, training courses are very theoretical and do not provide sufficient opportunity for acquiring practical skills.

In these two last cases, the training needs of professional staff have to be carefully assessed through interviews and observation and by checking the curriculum contents of past training courses.

In regard to refugee emergency health, it is usually necessary to organize training courses on:

– conducting mass measles immunization,
– data collection,
– essential drugs and standard treatments,
– conducting surveys,
– environmental health measures,
– specific measures to take during epidemics,
– oral rehydration,
– active screening for those who are sick and/or malnourished, etc.,
– safe deliveries.

Feasibility study[12,17]

Once training needs have been clearly identified, the training that is most appropriate to the situation should be selected. This may include:

– on-the-job training (or 'bedside training' for medical staff),
– a few practical or theoretical lessons,
– specific initial training courses (ad hoc on specific topics or tasks),
– refresher courses.

The type of training selected will depend on: the number of people to be trained, the number of tasks to be taught, the optimal duration of the course, and the human, material and financial means available. These are all essential factors to consider before initiating any training programme.

During the emergency phase, it is clear that people have to be trained quickly. This implies that only a limited number of tasks should be taught and that the number of trainees should not exceed 10 per trainer. In addition, the trainers must be competent and clearly allocated for this task; space for conducting courses has to be organized, and adequate equipment and training material provided[9]. Some guidelines have been drawn up by relief agencies to facilitate the rapid training of home-visitors and other health workers on the major topics of refugee health care[4,5]. However, there are no available guidelines for using straightaway on the spot: every training course will have to be adapted to local conditions, in line with the major health problems at the time, the socio-cultural context, and the level of qualifications of the staff.

In order to ensure that there is a degree of homogeneity among staff being trained, it may be wise to select candidates according to relevant criteria, such as an ability to read and write, speak a specific language, calculate, etc. These criteria will depend on the jobs for which training is to be offered.

In addition, a training contract should be established between the training agency and the participants, stipulating the internal regulations of the programme and the commitment expected from the participants. Such contracts have the advantage of making instructors and students aware of their responsibilities, and should be established to even in emergencies.

Training may be a sensitive issue in many countries.

- Some governments do not allow refugees to be trained, especially in the health field. It is therefore essential to come to an agreement with the authorities before starting a training programme and the relevant ministries may therefore be invited to participate.

- Another sensitive issue is related to the status of refugees who have followed a training course organized by an NGO. For various reasons, such training will usually not be recognized either by the host country or by the home country. This likelihood should be clearly explained to potential trainees so that they do not build up false hopes for the future. Relief agencies working in refugee camps are not specialized training agencies and the purpose of their presence in a country is not to decide on the health policy of that country. Therefore, agencies should not be involved in any lobbying for the recognition of personnel trained in the camps and no diploma should be delivered at the end of a training course. However, a document mentioning that someone has followed a training course and is capable of performing a list of specific tasks may be very useful to that person when applying to work later on.

Methodology[9,12,17]

Teaching and assessment methods should be selected according to the main tasks to be taught, whether they cover intellectual, practical or communication skills. The importance of assessing and evaluating 'students' cannot be over-stressed; it is an incentive to learn, provides feedback on the learning process to participants and trainers, and acts as a protection against incompetent personnel continuing to practise.

It is useful to keep written reference documents on training content as references for future training activities and further evaluation.

Evaluation

Evaluating and following up on training programmes are part of the supervision process which should take place regularly in order to identify further training needs to be met through a continuing education programme.

A REFUGEE-SPECIFIC CATEGORY OF STAFF : HOME-VISITORS

Home-visitors are an essential component of any refugee programme ensuring the link between refugees and the services offered to them and conducting outreach activities in the settlement. Home-visitors should be recruited rapidly at the start of programmes (within the first few weeks) and function as a network covering the whole refugee population.

Home-visitors (HVs) should be distinguished from community health workers (CHWs) or village health workers (VHWs): CHWs are an essential aspect of (long-term) primary health care programmes in stable countries, aimed at extending health services to all communities and supporting them in solving their own health problems. CHWs are members of the community, who have received a short training on health-related matters and are already integrated into the public health system of their country[16]. HVs are also selected from the community, but only in response to a refugee crisis. Their tasks differ from those of the CHWs, and it is preferable that they do not provide curative health care. The CHWs already present in the refugee community will generally be assigned to health services (e.g. health posts) because of the health knowledge they have already acquired.

The characteristics of home-visiting programmes include the following:

- Home visitors should be selected from among the sections of the population they will care for; initially there should be 1 HV for every 500-1,000 refugees. The most important selection criteria is that they are accepted and recognized by their community, whether or not they have previous skills or are literate. Difficulties in the HV selection process arise when refugee leaders try to unduly influence it, or designate friends or relatives who may not be suitable. Care should be taken that women are among those recruited (see above, *Staff recruitment*). The number of HVs can be increased depending on how events and activities evolve.

- The main tasks to be performed by HVs are listed below (see also *6. Health Care in the Emergency Phase*).

  - **Data collection**: HVs ensure the regular collection of population figures (census, new arrivals and departures, births, etc.) and mortality figures (number and causes of deaths in the population).

  - **Active screening**: they make regular visits to shelters to screen for sick persons, malnourished children and those not immunized against measles, and refer these to health or nutritional facilities. They may also be required to screen for other problems: defaulters from particular programmes (e.g. feeding centre), vulnerable groups with specific problems, etc. In the case of disease outbreaks, this screening task will have to be reinforced.

  - **Informing the population**: they are responsible for transmitting necessary messages in regard to, for example, the availability of services, distributions that are to take place, the need to bring children for measles immunization etc. They should also conduct health education, for instance, on the use of latrines, the importance of personal hygiene, etc.

– **Assistance to other programmes**: HVs can assist in many activities: mass immunization, health posts, feeding programmes, conducting surveys, etc. However, this should not be at the expense of making home visits.

A main role of HVs is thus to facilitate the flow of information by informing refugees about relief services and informing relief agencies on refugee needs and problems.

- **Supervision and training of home-visitors**: A few HVs who demonstrate superior skills should be assigned a supervisory role; one supervisor for ten HVs. Overall supervision of the home-visiting programme should be ensured by a health professional (for instance, an experienced nurse). Frequent and regular meetings between HVs and their supervisors must be instituted from the start, on a daily basis in the initial stages. This allows HVs to make a daily report, hand over data collected, exchange information about refugee needs, etc. It also provides an opportunity for training: an initial and basic training session should be organized on the first tasks to be performed (mainly data collection, possibly active screening), and is continued through these regular meetings to cover other tasks and specific issues related to refugee programmes. The general guidelines for training in a refugee context are given above under *Training*.

- **Contact with other refugee activities**: HVs should maintain close contacts with staff working on other programmes. Collaboration with health services is particularly important: HVs should be linked to the health post to which they refer patients; the person in charge of the health post may also supervise their work and provide them with support.

Post-emergency phase

Priorities usually change after the emergency phase: some programmes may be closed down (e.g. supplementary feeding) and others may be started (e.g. EPI). Staff requirements must therefore be re-evaluated in line with new plans. Once again, job descriptions have to be written down in order to clearly identify the tasks that have to be performed.

In many situations, overall staff requirements will decrease: most of the necessary infrastructure has been set up, and a large number of staff is no longer required. Some emergency programmes employing a large number of staff will close down and, in some situations, repatriation or resettlement of refugees will begin so that the site will progressively empty. This implies that it is time to terminate the contracts of some of the local staff. This is a difficult job due both to emotional links with the staff and administrative obstacles if sufficient advance warning is not given. Ensuring appropriate contracts at the start (see above) can prevent later security and legal problems (such as court cases) and compensations for dismissal. Whenever possible, national staff should be re-employed by any partners taking over the activities they have been involved in; recommendation letters, proofs of work done and certificates for training sessions attended by previously non-qualified staff are all useful to refugees for future jobs.

Coordination is more necessary than ever at this stage in order to ensure that working methods remain unchanged and standard activities continue normally in spite of changes in staff.

Training needs must be assessed, and new training programmes may have to be organized in order to adjust to the situation[12,17]. If staff have been specifically trained to perform a very limited number of tasks during the emergency phase, it may be wise to reorganize and allow them to diversify their activities as the situation calms down. Indeed, providing a less boring job will maintain the level of employee motivation in any programme. New tasks may be added to some specific job descriptions after the completion of appropriate training courses.

Because of these new training needs, it is important not to decrease the number of expatriate staff too rapidly when the emergency phase comes to an end. However, once refugee personnel have been properly trained, it is essential to delegate tasks to them and give them opportunities and responsibilities for contributing towards the relief effort directed at their own people.

Principal recommendations regarding human resources and training

- Recruitment, management and training of human resources are essential and complex tasks that cannot be improvised. They should follow specific procedures and be supervised by experienced senior staff.

- The first step is the determination of the number of staff required, per category, based on the activities to be carried out. Then, a job description should be prepared for each category of staff, and an organization chart must be drawn up for every programme and facility. Both of these will remain essential tools throughout the programme.

- A standard staff policy must be defined in line with the labour laws of the host country. Several aspects should be addressed early on, in the emergency phase: salary scale, appropriate type of contracts, what is the legal status of refugee workers, etc.

- Several types of training are necessary in most refugee programmes, but it should be preceded by an assessment of the training needs.

- Home-visitors are an essential component of any refugee programme as they ensure the link between refugees and the services available to them. This network of home-visitors should be rapidly established in the first weeks of any refugee intervention, and requires close supervision and training.

➤ References

1. UNHCR. *Handbook for emergencies*. Geneva: UNHCR, 1982.

2. Kenez, O, Forbes Martin, S. *Ensuring the health of refugees: Taking a broader vision*. Refugee Policy Group, 1990.

3. Simmonds, S, Vaughan, P, William Gunn, S. *Refugee community health care*. Oxford: Oxford University Press, 1983.

4. Brown, M, Poeung Sam O. *Medic training manual*. Minneapolis: American Refugee Committee, 1987.

5. Médecins Sans Frontières. *Organisation d'un camp de refugiés, Module 1 Approche générale de l'organisation d'un camp*. Brussels: CRED, Médecins Sans Frontières, 1988.

6. Castilla, J. *MSF refugee camp programmes for Somalis in Kenya*. [Evaluation mission] Brussels: AEDES, 1993.

7. Refugee Policy Group. *The Georgetown Declaration on health care for displaced persons and refugees: Conclusions on progress, problems and priorities reached by an international symposium*. Washington D C: RPG, 1988.

8. Brown, V. *Evaluation des interventions en urgence de Médecins Sans Frontières*. [Internal report]. Paris: Epicentre, 1992.

9. Abatt, F R. *Teaching for better learning*. Geneva: WHO, 1980.

10. *Médecins Sans Frontières. Nutrition guidelines*. Paris: Médecins Sans Frontières, 1995.

11. Médecins Sans Frontières. *Prise en charge d'une épidémie de choléra en camp de réfugiés*. Paris: Médecins Sans Frontières, 1995.

12. Médecins Sans Frontières. *Guide pratique pour la formation des personnels de santé*. Paris: Médecins Sans Frontières, 1994.

13. Poivre, P. *La crise Burundaise et les réfugiés Burundais au Rwanda*. Case study. Brussels: Médecins Sans Frontières, 1993.

14. Médecins Sans Frontières. *Guide du personnel national*. [draft]. Paris: Médecins Sans Frontières, 1995.

15. Médecins Sans Frontières. *Conduite à tenir en cas d'épidémie de rougeole destiné aux responsables de santé confrontés à des épidémies de rougeole dans différents environnements*. Paris: Médecins Sans Frontières, 1996.

16. WHO. *The community health worker*. Geneva: WHO, 1990.

17. Guilbert, J J. *Educational handbook for health personnel*. Geneva: WHO, 1992.

10. Coordination

Introduction

Coordination is one of the top 10 priorities in a refugee situation, but is probably also one of the most neglected or least well implemented. Nevertheless, without proper coordination, any relief programme will rapidly become disastrous.

Coordination could be described as the integrated organization of the various relief activities under an accepted leadership, made effective via communication among all the partners. Integrated organization means that common goals are pursued by all partners who implement a common plan making the best possible use of all available resources. The partners in a relief programme are usually UNHCR, host country authorities, refugee representatives and non-governmental organizations (NGOs). Other UN agencies may also be involved, especially when internally displaced are concerned. Communication implies regular contacts between partners, both formal and informal. It involves information-sharing and decision-making[3]. Leadership signifies that one of the partners takes the lead in planning operations, and overall responsibility for decisions. This does not mean that the other partners have no role to play in coordination; on the contrary, good coordination is only possible if every partner is actively involved.

Although its importance is usually underestimated, coordination among partners directly influences the effectiveness of any relief work. It is particularly essential in major refugee programmes where a large number of agencies are working in the same place. Without coordination, there is a high risk that some programmes will overlap while other needs are left uncovered. This is aggravated by the seeming inability of many specialized agencies to take a broad overview of the situation. For instance, in refugee camps in Kenya in 1992, the development of programmes was hampered by the presence of multiple organizations working in the same field but with conflicting objectives, unclear tasks and poor coordination[5]. Coordination is also crucial to ensure that the policies of the host country are not overlooked in important matters such as immunization or malaria programmes. A final important aspect of coordination is that it makes it possible to deal more efficiently with security problems in unstable areas.

Coordination is required at every level: from the central level (national or regional) to the field level (refugee site). It is just as necessary in camp settings as in open situations (where refugees are dispersed or integrated into the local population). Coordination also applies to 'internal' coordination, or the coordination of activities and human resources within an organization, where the same principles may be applied. This issue is partly dealt with in 9. Human Resources and Training.

Coordination is thus an early priority in relief programmes. However, the quality of coordination has to be maintained beyond the emergency phase in order to ensure continuity despite changes in staff and any adjustments to programme objectives due to an evolving situation.

From the above, it is obvious that the coordination of refugee programmes is not easy. Relief operations are complex. Important resources are involved (staff, logistics, food and medical supplies) and there are often many constraints, such as site inaccessibility, insecurity and political obstruction. In addition, the partners may have conflicting interests or differing philosophies of work and will be reluctant to adopt common objectives. Furthermore, individual relief agencies may resist anything which is seen to decrease their power and autonomy[2].

Objectives

The main goal of refugee programme coordination is to achieve the greatest possible impact on the situation through the management and integration of relief activities.

To reach this goal, operational objectives must be set and it is therefore necessary to:
– establish clear leadership,
– create a coordinating body,
– ensure that priorities are shared by agencies,
– prevent programme duplication and ensure all needs are covered,
– rationalize services by creating common standards and using common guidelines.

Action to be taken

1. ESTABLISH CLEAR LEADERSHIP

Although leadership in coordination varies from one refugee situation to another, it is essential that relief teams understand how the responsibilities are attributed in principle.

• **The host government** always remains the final authority but may adopt various positions[1]:
  – it may itself take the lead in coordinating relief work; or
  – it may completely or partly hand over responsibility for policy and coordination to UNHCR and/or international agencies[4].

The government may coordinate through different channels:
  – a Ministry (Internal Affairs or Planning) takes the overall responsibility and designates an individual or a special unit within the Ministry. Other Ministries (Health, Agriculture or Social Welfare) will be responsible for coordinating specific sectors; for instance, the Ministry of Health (MOH) may coordinate all relief activities related to health;

– the government sometimes creates a new, autonomous body to take charge of coordination, such as a government relief committee.

In rebel-held areas, there are usually no Ministries operating and a relief branch of the rebel government may ensure the coordination of assistance. However, such bodies often have political objectives and strategies that may conflict with those of the relief agencies.

Cooperation and communication with the various levels of government should always be encouraged, and at least one government representative should attend coordination meetings. It is also useful to assist the host country to strengthen its ability to coordinate refugee assistance at central and field level[1,2].

- **UNHCR** plays a major role in the leadership of refugee relief programmes. Its mandate includes responsibility for ensuring protection and the adequate care of refugees and may also be extended to cover internally displaced populations[12]. Other aspects of UNHCR mandate are dealt with in *Part I, Refugee and Displaced Populations.*

  – at the international level, UNHCR is responsible for coordinating the provision of general assistance to refugees[2];

  – at the national and field level, the host government is normally responsible for coordinating relief efforts but often shares this task with, or hands over completely to UNHCR. At national level, UNHCR is also responsible for coordinating the response of the UN system to a refugee emergency[1].

In certain situations, UNHCR will accept the responsibility for displaced persons and for repatriation programmes. In all the situations where the coordination of assistance to internally displaced persons is not ensured by the UNHCR, this may be undertaken by another UN agency (e.g. UNICEF) or a special coordination body. In some large-scale population displacements, the UN Secretary-General may create a UN-led entity with overall responsibility for coordinating the whole UN response, as was the case in Sudan where Operation Lifeline Sudan (OLS) coordinated relief assistance[1].

- **NGOs** are usually the operational partners of UNHCR. They have an active role to play in coordination and must participate at every level of the coordination body. Their role is even more important at field level, where an NGO may take the role of lead agency for coordination (at the request of UNHCR or the host government). The lead agency should have a good overall view of a refugee situation, an understanding of how relief activities are integrated into the relevant services of the host country, and should preferably have previous experience of working in a refugee context[3].

2. CREATE A COORDINATION BODY

The creation of a coordination team or committee encompassing all partners, including representatives from government and the refugee community, is the best way to ensure coordination in most refugee emergencies. Such teams should be organized at both national and field levels[1,2].

UNHCR recommends the following[3]:

- at camp level, a camp committee should be established with 1 representative from each organization involved, chaired by a lead agency; and
- at central level, a refugee coordinator from the host government, UNHCR, or an NGO should be appointed to chair an overall coordination committee.

In large-scale relief programmes, coordination teams for each sector (e.g. health, nutrition and sanitation) may be established in addition to a central coordination committee to deal with technical issues and may play an important part in the development of standards for the delivery of assistance[1].

In the health sector, a health coordination committee will usually be set up. It is best that this committee is chaired by a refugee health coordinator, preferably assigned by one of the lead agencies, e.g. UNHCR, or by the MOH. MOH leadership has the advantage that it may facilitate the integration of the refugee health care system into the national health system once the emergency period is over[2]. WHO has the role of supporting the national MOH with technical expertise and advice. During an emergency this support may need to be reinforced[12].

NGOs arriving on a site where coordination mechanisms have not yet been set up should remedy this situation by setting up a coordination team in collaboration with the local authorities and, if necessary, one of them should lead the team.

3. COMMON OBJECTIVES MUST BE DEFINED BY THE COORDINATION BODY

After the initial assessment (see *1. Initial Assessment*), the priorities for intervention have to be determined. Clear objectives should then be established and agreed upon among partners. A plan of action to cover basic needs will be worked out as a team effort and should be made available to all concerned[1]. The coordination team should monitor the implementation of the different activities and discuss their progress at regular meetings.

In most situations, the first objectives are to immunize all children against measles and to provide sufficient supplies of water, shelters, general food rations and basic medical care. The coordination team has responsibility for dissuading agencies from starting non-urgent programmes such as schools, comprehensive family planning programme, Expanded Programmes on Immunization (EPI), etc., until the primary objectives are fulfilled.

4. THE ROLES AND RESPONSIBILITIES OF ALL PARTNERS MUST BE CLARIFIED

The tasks to be undertaken must be allocated among the agencies, as well as the areas where they will work. According to their resources and expertise, the various relief organizations will take responsibility for certain programmes (nutritional centres, measles vaccination, etc.) in defined areas (camp or sector of a camp). A clear task distribution will prevent overlaps between programmes and gaps in covering needs. This distribution of tasks should be formalized in a written agreement. This agreement may be signed by the government, UNHCR and NGOs, although this does not often happen in the emergency phase.

Experience has shown that health activities should preferably be grouped under the responsibility of one single organization in the area, in order to avoid disorganization in the health system, duplication of services and missing links in the referral system.

5. ESTABLISH GOOD COMMUNICATION CHANNELS

Information exchange is a basic condition for effective coordination. Decision-makers require information in order to decide on programmes and adapt them to changing needs. In fact, all the actors in relief programmes require information if they are to maintain a sense of involvement and motivation, and make their work more effective. Unfortunately, information does not flow easily between agencies and between the central coordination level and the field level if an efficient system of information is not established. Informal contacts and cooperation may exist but they are not a sufficient basis for decision-making and effective coordination. Communication channels should be established or strengthened, and formalized, mainly by regular meetings and reports.

Regular meetings should be organized, at both central and site level. In large programmes, general meetings should preferably be complemented by meetings at sector level (health, nutrition, sanitation and logistics). The purpose of these meetings is primarily the exchange of information in regard to different programmes and the problems encountered, enabling practical decisions to be taken: starting or ending programmes, changes in the distribution of tasks, allocation of material, etc. If meetings do not lead to action, they are a waste of time. Sector meetings will generally deal with the technical aspects of assistance; technical information will be exchanged, specific nutritional or health problems (current outbreak) discussed, and guidelines developed for the standardization of assistance. (See below *The introduction of standardized guidelines.*) It is preferable that all sectors related to health (water and sanitation, nutrition, etc.) meet regularly to agree on appropriate and integrated interventions.

These meetings must be properly organized, working to a prepared agenda and chaired by the person responsible for coordination. Minutes should be taken, and these should highlight the decisions taken: what specific action needs to be implemented, by whom, and by what date. These minutes should be distributed to all partners so as to ensure the circulation of information, to formalize discussions and to evaluate action undertaken[5]. At central level, there is a risk of meetings developing into long, crowded and unproductive inter-agency conferences. To avoid this, the agenda should be limited to essential points, and participation restricted to one person from each of the operating agencies; in large-scale emergencies where a large number of agencies are present, it may be advisable to limit the number of participants to the major operating partners. Decisions should be followed up systematically. In the emergency phase, these meetings should be held at least weekly, whereas in the post-emergency phase, monthly meetings will usually be sufficient. At field level, information exchanges are even more important as any misunderstanding will directly affect the refugee community; refugee representatives should preferably be involved at site level (see below *Camp management*)[1]. Meetings may take place twice a week, or even daily in acute or complex emergencies.

Reporting on programmes and population status should be organized and supervised by one agency at each level. The information required from each sector should be rapidly defined and standardized, and will include the information provided by the public health surveillance system (see *8. Public Health Surveillance*). Standard forms should be distributed, reports collected regularly and processed by the agency in charge; it is however essential that the persons in charge of data analysis are fully involved in drawing operational conclusions from the reports. Relevant information should then be discussed in coordination meetings. Close relationship should always be maintained between surveillance and coordination activities.

6. THE INTRODUCTION OF STANDARDIZED GUIDELINES AND POLICIES

Standardized guidelines and policies accepted by all the partners are essential to any coordinated assistance because they ensure the consistency and efficiency of programmes, and complement activities. They help avoid the chaotic delivery of assistance. For instance, this can occur when several organizations are in charge of a number of nutritional centres, using different criteria for admission and discharge[5].

Standard protocols should be used from the beginning, based on the national guidelines of the host country, or on standard international guidelines developed by international agencies such as UNHCR[1,3], Oxfam[6], CDC[7] or MSF[8,9]. Since these standard documents may not be suitable for every refugee situation, they may need to be adapted locally. This process should be monitored by the coordination team and sectoral meetings should be used to establish common policies for intervention and to discuss guidelines. For instance, nutritional policy will be defined during food and nutrition meetings so that admission and discharge criteria are consistent between supplementary and intensive feeding centres. These guidelines also serve as the basic tool of staff training. After the acute phase of the emergency, guidelines specific to the situation may be worked out in cooperation between ministries, UNHCR and implementing agencies. They may even be endorsed by the host government, as happened in Somalia (1983)[10], Cambodia (1988)[11], etc.

The value of guidelines depends on the extent to which they are used. The lead agencies and coordinators must check that protocols are being observed, being aware that local and international staff often resist using them. For instance, in Somalia, one of the first things the Ministry of Health undertook was the development of guidelines on the management of common diseases, but it took 3 years before agencies began to apply them[4].

However, it is important to maintain a flexible attitude towards standardization keeping in mind that each refugee programme and each agency will be faced with its own specific constraints and difficulties[3].

Common problems in coordination

- There are frequently delays before someone takes the initiative and responsibility for coordination. Several factors may explain this: UNHCR may arrive on the spot after delays because of security problems, diplomatic or bureaucratic obstacles; or the host authorities may not take the initiative for coordination, and NGOs completely absorbed by relief activities, may not always be aware of the need for overall coordination.

- The host government may have little involvement in coordination for many reasons:
  - the government may not see it as important;
  - there may be conflict between the government and UNHCR over leadership, especially when UNHCR is in charge of programme financing[4];
  - international agencies do not always accept the authority of Ministries which may lack emergency skills, have a weaker financial and operational capacity, and suffer from bureaucratic inertia;
  - Ministries and NGOs may have different objectives or interests;
  - there may also be conflict within the government itself, e.g. rivalry between different Ministries for control of the relief programme.

- The distribution of tasks among the agencies is often either not clear or not respected. In addition, communication problems are frequent and most people do not know who is in charge of what.

- The timetable for the implementation of programmes is frequently not respected by the partners.

- Staff turnover on-site may be rapid in terms of UN, NGO and local government staff.

Coordination in the post-emergency phase

The general mechanisms of coordination remain the same although there are some additional elements to take account of once the emergency situation is under control:

- Despite improvements in the overall refugee situation, good coordination must be maintained in order to avoid changes in programmes and strategies when relief teams or agencies are replaced.

- Objectives must be adapted, especially when refugees are likely to remain in the host country for an extended period. Self-reliance should be promoted and assistance should be more consistent with the policies of the host country. The coordinating body has a responsibility to orientate the operational partners towards these objectives.

- Effective leadership by the host country must be fostered. Host government involvement is essential for programme continuity over the longer term[2]. This is facilitated if the line ministries (health, water, etc.) have been kept fully involved from the outset of the emergency.

- Refugees should participate in the coordination process to the maximum possible extent to ensure that programmes eventually become less dependent on expatriate input.

- The periodicity of meetings and reporting may decrease to once monthly.

Principal recommendations regarding coordination

- Coordination mechanisms must be established in the early stages of assistance. Leadership has to be defined. If the initiative has not been taken by UNHCR or the host government, relief organizations must organize a coordination team and, if required, take on the leadership role themselves.

- The host government must be encouraged to participate in the coordination process; line ministries (e.g. health and water) should be involved.

- In large-scale refugee programmes, an overall coordinator is required as well as a coordination committee in each technical sector.

- Common objectives should be agreed upon and followed by all involved. Distribution of tasks must be determined among agencies, and formalized in a written agreement.

- Regular meetings and reporting must be formalized to ensure information exchange and facilitate decision-making. Sector meetings are useful for working on technical guidelines and standardization.

- Technical guidelines, standard policies (including standard data collection) will be introduced from the beginning. Their content can be better adapted to the situation after the emergency period.

➤ *References*

1. UNHCR. *Handbook for emergencies.* Geneva: UNHCR, 1982.

2. Kenez, O, Forbes Martin, S. *Ensuring the health of refugees: Taking a broader vision.* Refugee Policy Group, 1990.

3. UNHCR. *Operational guidelines for health and nutrition programmes in refugee settings.* [draft]. Geneva: UNHCR, 1987.

4. Harrell-Bond, B E. *Imposing aid: Emergency assistance to refugees.* Oxford: Oxford University Press, 1989.

5. Castilla, J. *MSF refugee camp programmes for Somalis in Kenya.* [Evaluation mission]. Brussels: AEDES, 1993.

6. Mears, C, Chowdhury, S. *Health care for refugees and displaced people.* Oxford: Oxfam Practical Health Guide No.9, 1994.

7. CDC. Famine-affected, refugee, and displaced populations: Recommendations for public health issues. *MMWR*, 1992, 41(RR-13): 1-76.

8. Médecins Sans Frontières. *Clinical guidelines, diagnostic and treatment manual.* Paris: Hatier, 1993.

9. Delmas, G, Courvallet, M, et al. *Public health engineering in emergency situations.* Paris: Médecins Sans Frontières, 1994.

10. Oxfam Refugee Health Unit, Somali Ministry of Health. *Guidelines for health care in refugee camps.* Oxford: Oxfam, 1983.

11. UNBRO. *Medical guidelines for the Thaï-Kampuchean Border.* UNBRO, 1988.

12. Refugee Policy Group. *The Georgetown Declaration on health care for displaced persons and refugees: Conclusions on progress, problems and priorities reached by an international symposium.* Washington DC: RPG, 1988

A special issue: camp management

Most large-scale refugee and displaced populations settle in areas that have insufficient resources to cope with the additional burden. They either live in open situations, hosted by the local community, or concentrated on sites where there are no pre-existing facilities to accommodate them, leading to the creation of camps (see *Part I, Refugee and Displaced Populations*).

The precarious conditions of hygiene and overcrowding in these camps, the lack of resources and the poor health status of the population, which may have travelled long distances, the disruption in their social organization, and the absence of infrastructure or services on the site, all favour the development of epidemics and high mortality. Relief assistance must be mobilized rapidly to provide water, food, shelter, health care, and implement other priorities of intervention (see *The Ten Top Priorities* in Part II). These 10 priorities cannot be achieved without effective camp management. As good camp management is not only necessary for the organization of relief programmes (especially the distribution of goods), but also to counter several risk factors for communicable diseases, it is obvious that it will have a real impact on the health status and mortality of camp populations.

Camp management covers several different areas of activity:
– the administrative organization of the camp and its population,
– organization of the site itself and the installation of the necessary infrastructure (see also *5. Shelter and Site Planning*),
– setting up a reception structure for new arrivals, including screening and registration,
– installation of an efficient and equitable system of general distributions,
– organization of staff working in different programmes (see *9. Human Resources and Training*).

In most refugee settlements, camp management falls under the responsibility of UNHCR. Health agencies are rarely called upon to perform this task, for which they are usually not prepared. However, in view of the direct relationship between management and health risks, it is in the interests of the health agencies to follow the situation very closely. If camp management activities are not undertaken, health agencies must persuade UNHCR either to take on the responsibility or delegate it to another agency (for example, the agency responsible for food distributions). In cases of internal displacement, or in refugee situations where UNHCR is not present, one of the agencies operating on site will have to take responsibility for camp management.

Camp management involves activities which are difficult to organize, which demand large resources and for which there is no ideal strategy. They may also provoke some resentment among the population, which may see camp management as a method of control rather than as a means of improving the organization of aid. A certain level of expertise is therefore necessary, and there are a number of guidelines which should be followed.

In general, one of two possible situations is likely to be encountered.

1. The refugees have not yet settled in the new camp before relief agencies arrive. In this case, everything can be organized in advance and the most efficient strategies selected: registration on entry to the site, the distribution of ration cards for each family, the most appropriate number and location of facilities, etc. Although this situation represents the operational ideal, unfortunately it is the least frequently encountered. It usually only occurs when it is decided to transfer a population to a new camp.

2. Most refugees are already established on the site and the camp therefore has to be organized within the existing framework.

In both these situations, the needs are the same, the objectives and major principles identical. The difference lies in the methods of implementation and the choice of strategies.

Reception of refugee and displaced populations

Ideally, every new arrival to a refugee settlement should pass through a reception centre where registration takes place, ration cards and a first package of goods (plastic sheeting, blankets, etc.) are distributed, medical screening is carried out, plots on which shelters can be constructed are allocated and, on some sites, space in temporary accommodation may be allotted.

However, as already indicated, in most displacement situations, the population has already settled on a site before aid could be organized or else the influx of people is so large that individual processing on entry is impossible to organize and a reception centre will only start to function later. As a result, medical screening, registration and the distribution of ration cards will have to be conducted in the settlement itself and an attempt made to cover everyone who has arrived; this is much more complex to implement.

Registration of refugee and displaced populations[1,2,4]

Registration is required for the twin purposes of protection and assistance. Registration makes it possible to identify the target population and vulnerable groups, secure basic information on individuals, allow a fair distribution system to be established through the distribution of registration/ration cards (see below) and carry out health screening in parallel[1,4,6].

Registration must therefore be envisaged right from the beginning of the relief effort, provided that the health and security situations allow it (for example, registration would not be practicable during a cholera epidemic)[4]. This task should be assigned to an agency by the coordination body; in refugee populations, it is the responsibility of UNHCR, which may prefer to delegate and supervise implementation by another partner (WFP, Red Cross, NGOs, etc.)[3,4].

There are several prerequisites for registration[4]:

- There should be a sufficient level of security and confidence among refugees to permit registration to be carried out without major problems arising[1].
- The local authorities should be informed and their authorization obtained[6].
- The refugee population should receive clear information on the benefits of registration beforehand in order to encourage their acceptance of the process[6].
- A sufficient number of personnel and logistical tools (cards, etc.) should be available to perform the task.

Although these conditions will serve to facilitate the process, failure to meet all of them should not serve as an excuse for delaying registration.

The amount of information to be collected at registration depends mainly on the time available (particularly how urgently food rations need to be distributed) and the type of data required in order to conduct relief programmes properly. Registration usually provides more accurate figures than can be obtained in the initial assessment (see 1. Initial Assessment).

The minimum information required for family registration/ration cards is:

- name of the family head,
- size of the family,
- estimate of the age/sex of family members.

Other data concerning individuals that are usually collected include[2,4]:

- names of family members (useful for protection and for tracing missing persons)[1,4],
- place of origin (useful for camp organization, identification of minority groups and planning repatriation)[8],
- membership of any specific vulnerable group (e.g. disabled, unaccompanied minor, etc.),
- shelter identification (e.g. number),
- possibly other data such as religion, language, etc.

Given that efficiency drops as the amount of information to be recorded rises, it is best to concentrate on collecting only data which is really necessary for conducting programmes efficiently[2,4].

The most practical time to register refugees or displaced persons is on arrival at the site (at the reception centre), in tandem with health screening. But in most situations (see above), another system will have to be organized to register the refugees already present on the site: several methods for doing this are described in guidelines[4,6,13].

Registration may comprise several steps[4]:

1. **Planning**: once the prerequisites are met, staff must be carefully selected, briefed and trained; the data to be collected must be determined.

2. **A first identification of refugees**: this may be required when registering a population already established on a site, so as to limit the risk of double registration. UNHCR suggests a one-day rapid identification process during which bracelets are distributed to each refugee in order to allow them to register in the next step. However, this is not always indicated or useful, and may usually be left out (especially in small camps).

3. **The registration itself**: data is collected on each person, and ration cards are handed out to heads of household.

4. **Updating registration records**: new arrivals are registered on entry, and data on the settled population (births, deaths, departures, etc.) are recorded by the person in charge of each section (see below *Administrative organization*)[2,8]. A further general registration may be advised if major population movements occur[4].

There are two common problems which may be encountered:

- **Security problems**[1]: registration is sometimes boycotted by refugee leaders or armed groups who see registration as a threat to their power (e.g. through loss of control over food distributions), or by individual members of the population, who may be suspicious about how the data will be used. For example, in a Somalian refugee camp in Hagadera (Kenya, 1994), registration had to be suspended due to hostility from the population.

- **Unreliable data**: there may be errors in registration data resulting from multiple registrations of the same family, inflation of family size, 'phantom' families (families which are invented), the sale of ration cards, registration of non-eligible persons from neighbouring areas, etc.[6,13] This may be due to: corruption among members of the registration staff, attempts by some refugees to bypass the control system and register twice or, where camps are located close to a border, non-refugees crossing over to receive ration cards to sell later.

Although they cannot entirely be prevented, these problems can be alleviated by ensuring that the population receives thorough and valid information on the aims of registration, by controlling entry into the camp during the registration process and by ensuring that registration staff (who should be recruited from outside the camp wherever possible) are properly paid[4]. Separate registration places may be indicated if different sub-groups are present in the camp. Although such problems often arise and there is no perfect system, they should not be used as an argument against undertaking registration.

Screening

A medical (and nutritional) screening system should be set up as soon as possible. The purpose of screening is to identify individuals at (health) risk within the general population and to organize appropriate responses (detection which is not followed by action is useless)[12].

Medical screening includes the following[8,12]:

– the identification of children not yet immunized against measles and their referral for vaccination (or vaccination on the spot). A mass campaign should take place at the outset of health agency involvement, and screening offers an opportunity to check vaccination status and vaccinate the unprotected (see 2. *Measles Immunization*). Vitamin A prophylaxis is often given at the same time;

– the detection of sick or injured new arrivals, who are referred to the nearest health facility;

– detection of the malnourished and their referral to a feeding centre;

– other activities may be added, depending on the circumstances; for example, referral to meningitis vaccination when there is a risk of an outbreak, or identification of pregnant women in the post-emergency phase for referral to ante-natal care.

Implementation of general screening depends on each refugee situation. As explained above, a population should be screened on entry to a camp[1,3]. For refugees already established on a site, active screening is carried out by home-visitors making regular visits to shelters (see 9. *Human Resources and Training*, and *Health Care in the Post-emergency Phase* in Part III).

Administrative organization of the camp

When a population finally arrives in a new location after the stress and upheaval of displacement, their social structures and traditional community leadership have usually been severely disrupted. Efficient camp management is facilitated by the involvement of representatives from the refugee community and a recognition of certain levels of social organization within this community. The more refugee life in the settlement differs from their former community life, the more important it is to achieve this as early as possible[1].

Refugee representatives may fulfil several roles[8]:

• They should serve as the mouthpiece of their community in their relations with local authorities, UNHCR and other agencies.

• They pass on to the population the information coming from the various agencies in regard to the organization of the camp (food distribution, health services, etc.).

• They participate in the organization of the different camp sections by showing new arrivals where to install themselves, and assisting with any necessary reorganization.

• They keep and update the population records of the refugees living in their section (i.e. births, deaths, departures and new arrivals). However, it should be borne in mind that these figures might be deliberately inflated in order to receive increased food rations; they should therefore be compared regularly with data obtained from other sources (e.g. census or data collection by home-visitors).

Administrative (or social) organization covers several aspects of camp life:

- Wherever possible, refugee households should be assembled in smaller sections of around 1,000 people, which are both geographical entities in themselves and administrative units[1,8] (see *5. Shelter and Site Planning*).

- In each section, one or two representatives should be chosen by the population to ensure that all groups within the refugee community are fairly represented and participate in relief assistance. Traditional leadership patterns should be respected whenever possible, as it is essential that these persons truly represent their community and are trusted by them. Care should be taken that different cultural and religious minorities within the population are all represented in order to avoid the exclusion of any particular group[1].

- Coordination is essential for ensuring that regular meetings take place between the refugee representatives and the different relief agencies working in the camp, in order to share information and discuss problems[7,8].

- A UNHCR presence on the spot is usually ensured by a field officer whose main role is to ensure the protection of refugees; this officer may also be available to deal with the particular problems of individual refugees (see below, *Infrastructure*)[1].

- Keeping the population well-informed is a key element in camp management and should generally be ensured via the communication systems previously described, backed up by home-visitors regarding public health information (see *9. Human Resources and Training*). It is clear that camp management would be impossible without the full cooperation of the refugees. Unfortunately, this aspect is often neglected in the emergency phase, as priority is usually given to intervention activities[1].

General distributions

Displaced persons and refugees have generally fled their homes in haste, taking with them only very few belongings. Distributions must therefore be organized to provide them with essential goods which should respond to priority needs[1]. These include:

– water containers for the storage of water in households,
– food rations,
– cooking utensils (and very occasionally, cooking fuel),
– material for the construction of shelters (local material, plastic sheeting, tents, etc.),
– soap,
– tools for building family latrines or digging waste disposal pits,
– blankets, depending on the climate,
– in certain cases, clothing, sometimes to targeted groups (pregnant women, children).

The distribution of non-food items is just as important as that of food rations, particularly as refugees who lack these essential items may sell or exchange part of their food ration in order to procure them[3].

The responsibility for general distributions should be clearly assigned to either one or several agencies. The type and quantity of items, and the agency distributing them should be clearly decided in coordination meetings. In refugee situations, where UNHCR usually takes the overall role of coordination, it may either take charge of distribution itself, or delegate the task to another organization. Distribution to displaced persons will be undertaken by a UN agency or another relief agency (e.g. ICRC, local Red Cross, CARITAS, CRS, etc.).

Organizing general distributions is a large and complex task. The major difficulties to be faced are security problems (tensions within the population, theft, etc.), shortages of supplies and/or inequities in the distributions (see also *4. Food and Nutrition*). Care must be taken to ensure that vulnerable groups have access to distributions: the elderly and disabled, orphans, single women and minority ethnic or religious groups should not be excluded, and it may sometimes be necessary to organize a separate distribution system for these groups[2].

The main conditions for a successful distribution are[1,4]:
– good organization of the distribution site, with a clearly marked route from entry through to exit, sufficient staff, a waiting time that is not too long and somebody in charge of each item being distributed[4,10];
– a good logistical system with adequate supplies, transport and appropriate storage facilities;
– registration of the population (see below);
– an effective system for informing beneficiaries of the items and quantities to be distributed, dates of distributions and how they will be effected[4,11];
– prevention of fraud, and monitoring the quantities received by individual households (e.g. food basket monitoring for food items, see *4. Food and Nutrition*)[4].

There are two main types of distribution system:
– centrally-organized distributions, where goods are distributed directly to the households and requires that registration has already taken place, and ration cards have been distributed to each family[4,6]; another option is to distribute rations to individuals, but this system places a heavy demand on logistics and is best avoided;
– community-based distributions, where goods are given to community representatives, leaders, groups of families or a group of people chosen by the community (distribution committee), who themselves undertake redistribution to households[6,16].

The implementation of an efficient and equitable distribution system generally requires the registration of beneficiaries.

The preferred system is to distribute to the heads of households or groups of families as this is often the only way to ensure reasonable equity in distributions[3,4,6]. But, when there has been no general registration, distribution to refugee leaders or representatives is the only solution and has the advantage of involving the refugees as much as possible, and respects traditional structures.

However, the redistribution of goods often poses several problems: the person in charge may give in to strong pressure, even threats, which increases the risks of non-equitable distributions (i.e. not all beneficiaries receive the amounts to which they are entitled), as the distributing agency has no control over the final destination of the goods[3]. When this happens, those who are left out are usually members of vulnerable groups such as female-headed households, the elderly and orphans. For example, a food basket study in a Rwandan refugee camp in Kahindo (Zaire, 1994) found that, although the average daily food ration was 2,118 Kcal per person, 27% of families received less than 1,000 Kcal per person whereas 8% received over 5,000 Kcal per person[14]. It is also clear that the role of food provider strengthens the leaders' control over the population and reinforces their political power. The longer this situation continues, the better organized these persons become to oppose any change in the system. Every effort should therefore be made to switch as early as possible to a household distribution system[13].

The frequency of distributions depends on the items in question; once determined, the frequency should be respected as much as possible. Food rations may be distributed weekly in the beginning due to supply difficulties or limited storage capacities[3]. Once these problems are resolved, distributions should take place twice a month for as long as the emergency phase continues, and then be reduced to once a month[10]. Daily distributions, which are impractical and difficult to organize, should be avoided. Soap may be distributed together with food rations, while blankets, cooking utensils and plastic sheeting can be distributed on a one-off basis (on entry to the camp if possible).

Distributions should take place at prepared distribution sites (see below *Infrastructure*)[4]. The circuit to be followed by the beneficiaries into, through and off the site should be clearly indicated. The UNHCR advises to establish at least 1 distribution site per 20,000 or 30,000 refugees[16].

Infrastructure

The necessary facilities must be installed rapidly in order to respond to the basic needs of the refugees and allow services to be organized. A map of the camp is essential for planning these. During the emergency phase, many facilities are organized in tents (e.g. health centres). However, given that a camp is likely to exist for several months, if not years, more durable constructions should then be built out of local materials[5] (see also *5. Shelter and Site Planning.*).

The main infrastructures must cover all the different activities to be undertaken:

- **Water and sanitation facilities**: from the outset, the number and location of facilities such as water distribution points, latrines and/or defecation areas, waste disposal pits and washing areas should be planned for all sections of the camp, and sufficient space allocated to them. A cemetery, and sometimes a morgue, will be necessary. More details may be found in *3. Water and Sanitation.*

- **Access routes**[2,5]: easy access must be ensured to all parts of the camp and in all seasons. Road layout will depend on the position of essential facilities, such as distribution areas and health care facilities. Firebreaks must be included in the plans.

- **Reception facilities**[1]: facilities for the reception of new arrivals should be located at the camp entrance and include the reception centre where new arrivals are registered and screened, and possibly collective transit shelters, which can host new arrivals for a few days until individual shelters have been organized.

- **Health and nutritional facilities**: The number and location of facilities are planned during the initial assessment period (see *6. Health Care in the Emergency Phase* and *4. Food and Nutrition*). These will include:
  - a central health facility (or health centre) usually offering in-patient care and serving as a referral centre for other facilities, located in a quiet environment (e.g. far from the market place or distribution areas), and easily accessible to all refugees; an eventual extension should be anticipated;
  - several peripheral health facilities (or health posts), dispersed throughout the camp;
  - space for meetings and training home-visitors;
  - under certain circumstances, a field hospital, which can be located next to the health centre if there is sufficient space;
  - facilities for storing drugs and medical material (pharmacy or cold store);
  - a site for an eventual cholera camp, which should be prepared for outbreaks;
  - supplementary and therapeutic feeding centres depending on the nutritional situation. These are usually located next to health facilities.

- **Distribution sites**: These sites should be fenced in, be sufficiently large, and located at a certain distance from the camp (to avoid security problems) but still easily accessible to refugees and trucks[11].

- **A central office**: This may be set up by the UNHCR to ensure an on-the-spot presence.

- **Social facilities**: Adequate space should be planned for markets, schools, religious events, leisure activities and meeting places for refugees[1,5].

➤ References

1. UNHCR. *Handbook for emergencies.* Geneva: UNHCR, 1982.
2. Simmonds, S, Vaughan, P, William Gunn, S. *Refugee community health care.* Oxford: Oxford University Press, 1983.
3. Cuny, F C. *Field management.* [draft]. Geneva: UNHCR, 1985.
4. UNHCR. *Registration. A practical guide for field staff.* Geneva: UNHCR, 1994.
5. Kent Hardin, D. *Camp planning* [draft]. Geneva: UNHCR, 1985.
6. Mitchell, J, Slim, H. *Registration in emergencies.* Oxford: Oxfam Practical Health Guide No. 6, 1990.
7. Castilla, J. *MSF-Belgique Refugee camp programmes for Somalis in Kenya.* [Evaluation Mission]. Brussels: AEDES, 1993.
8. Médecins Sans Frontières. *Organisation d'un camp de refugiés, Module 1 Approche générale de l'organisation d'un camp.* Brussels: CRED, Médecins Sans Frontières, 1988.
9. Vercruysse, V. Evaluation du programme d'urgence de MSF en faveur des réfugiés burundais. *Medical News*, 1993, 3(2): 6-10.
10. Young, H. *Food scarcity and famine: Assessment and response.* Oxford: Oxfam Practical Health Guide No. 7, 1992.
11. Perrin, P M. *Assistance médicale en situation d'urgence.* Geneva: CICR, 1984.
12. UNHCR. *Operational guidelines for health and nutrition programmes in refugee settings.* [draft]. Geneva: UNHCR, 1987.
13. Stephenson, R S, Romanovsky, C, et al. Problems of beneficiary registration in food emergency operations. *Disasters*, 1987, 11(3): 163-72.
14. Suetens, S, Dedeurdewaerder, M. Food availability in the refugee camp of Kahindo, Goma, Zaïre, November 1994. *Medical News*, 1994, 3(5): 16-22.

PART III

The post-emergency phase

Introduction

Health care in the post-emergency phase and some specific issues

Introduction

The post-emergency phase begins when the excess mortality of the emergency phase is controlled and the basic needs (water, food, shelter, etc.) have all been addressed through the implementation of the 10 top priorities (see *Part II, The Ten Top Priorities*). The commonly-used criterion indicating transition from the emergency to the post-emergency phase is, by convention, a crude mortality rate under one death per 10.000 per day, representing mortality levels close to those of the surrounding population[1]. However, the border between these two phases is not that clearly defined and the evolution from emergency to post-emergency is not unidirectional. Events may occur during the post-emergency phase, such as outbreaks of disease or a large influx of new arrivals, which create a new emergency situation. For instance, new influxes of refugees in Malawi, Sudan and Honduras have been associated with temporary increases in mortality rates[1].

The post-emergency phase ends when a 'permanent solution' is found for the refugee problem (repatriation, integration into the host country or re-settlement in a third country). The duration cannot therefore be defined. It may last for a few months or, if the situation results from causes that are complex and lasting (e.g. a protracted civil war), it may persist for many years. Long-standing refugee settlements are not exceptional: some refugee groups have been in exile for over a decade, e.g. Palestinian refugees in the Middle East. In such situations, the post-emergency phase will eventually become a chronic phase, in which refugees may progressively rebuild some kind of sustainable life in the host country.

During this phase, relief programmes have to be adapted to changing needs and constraints. The overall situation, and individual programmes require re-evaluation so that new plans can be made. Existing programmes generally need to be adapted in regard to strategy, scale and resource requirements; new programmes can be started to tackle problems that were not addressed earlier because they were not considered as urgent (or did not envolve high mortality): for instance, AIDS, mental health, etc.

Refugee situation in the post-emergency phase

The context of the post-emergency phase is complex.

- On the one hand, there is a greater stability; most problems linked to the emergency are under control, and the general welfare of the refugees has improved. A proportion of them will have started some income-generating activities: marketing, small businesses, employment with relief agencies, working for local farmers, or farming for themselves if they have access to arable land, etc.

- On the other hand, this phase is not completely stable. For example, refugees may continue to arrive, depending on the situation in their country of origin. In addition, a crude mortality rate under 1/10,000/day still represents twice the 'normal' rate for settled populations in most developing countries (mortality rates around 0.5 deaths/10,000/day)[6]; and a major proportion of the refugees are still dependent on relief aid, at least partially, particularly in regard to food[3]. Any, or a combination, of these factors may exacerbate the situation and return it once again to a state of emergency.

Consequently, a post-emergency situation should be seen as a fragile state of equilibrium which still requires vigilance and adequate input to sustain it. It should not be a signal for relaxing efforts.

In many situations, refugees are both socially and politically vulnerable; sometimes they may also have to face the hostility of the local population, especially when the standard of living among refugees due to international assistance is higher than that of the local population. Many of them remain in the social quarantine of closed refugee camps for many years[1]. In some other situations, the local authorities may fear that refugees will remain permanently and exert pressure on them to leave[7].

In more favourable circumstances, some refugee groups may slowly integrate into the host area, e.g. build houses, begin farming a piece of land, etc. This is more frequent in open situations where they have initially been hosted by the local population. However, refugees cannot become self-sufficient within just a few months and will therefore continue to need assistance for some time.

HEALTH STATUS

Disease patterns are roughly the same as those in any non-refugee population. Diarrhoeal diseases, acute respiratory infections and malaria are the major killers and the most frequently encountered health problems. Others, such as reproductive health problems, AIDS, tuberculosis, mental problems, etc, may also account for a significant proportion of morbidity and mortality[1]. In addition, epidemics of communicable diseases continue to occur: cholera, hepatitis, measles, meningitis, etc.[1] Unfortunately, surveillance tends to be less intensive in this phase, so that the beginning of an outbreak could be overlooked. However, even though the overall health situation may have improved, most refugee settlements remain at higher risk from the rapid spread of disease.

Since public health measures have normally been implemented during the emergency phase, mortality has decreased and access to health services increased; as a result, the health status of the refugees may eventually become better than that of the local population[1]. This is a difficult issue: on the one hand, it is likely that the refugee population is still more vulnerable than the more stable settled population. On the other hand, the host population has its own health needs and these may far too easily be overlooked.

NUTRITIONAL SITUATION

In most post-emergency situations, low malnutrition rates have been reported. However, high prevalence rates may still be found in some refugee populations; for instance, rates greater than 20% were found in Somalia more than 8 years after Ethiopian refugees had settled there[1]. Micronutrient deficiency disorders such as scurvy, beriberi, pellagra, and iron deficiency anaemia have been commonly reported; scurvy is frequent in camps of long standing and its prevalence increases with the length of time that refugees remain in the camps[7].

Populations totally dependent on food distributions are most at risk from these nutritional problems, because inadequacies in the food rations (in quantity and quality) continue to occur beyond the emergency phase. Furthermore, as refugees rarely have adequate access to land for farming, food self-sufficiency is rarely attained.

THE RELIEF PROGRAMMES

It may be difficult to continue to obtain the resources required to ensure that programmes are adequately maintained; foreign donor interest and relief agency support often decline dramatically once the emergency stage is over[1]. It is also noticeable that once a programme routine has been established, it can be difficult to maintain a sufficient level of vigilance; as a result, some sectors may receive insufficient attention and some needs may be overlooked, e.g. food distributions, measles immunization, public health surveillance, etc.[2]

Most programmes set up during the emergency phase need to be adjusted at this time. Many emergency activities, designed for the very short term, require large amounts of material and financial resources, and are generally not affordable in the post-emergency phase. For instance, supplying water by tankers in the initial phase is extremely expensive and should be replaced by more sustainable methods.

Relief agencies which specialized in emergency activities can start scaling down, and their programmes may be taken over by local organizations, the host government or other agencies. However, this transition needs to be properly planned, which is not always the case[3].

If the refugees' stay is prolonged into a chronic phase, long-term programmes can be started, and efforts should be made to help them decrease dependency upon relief aid.

ENVIRONMENT

The environment surrounding refugee camps may be drastically altered as natural resources are used up, leading to severe ecological problems; for instance, chopping down trees to provide cooking fuel leads to deforestation, and water sources may be exhausted, etc.[2]

Objectives of interventions in the post-emergency phase

The major objective of intervention in the emergency phase was to reduce excess mortality. Objectives in the post-emergency phase clearly differ as high mortality is no longer present. However, refugees are still at a higher health risk than stable populations. The main aims should therefore be to consolidate the situation and help refugees to cope with the new environment.

In summary, this means:

– consolidating what has already been achieved: low mortality, good nutritional and health status, etc.;

– preparing for possible new emergencies: a major disease outbreak or a large influx of new arrivals, etc.;

– achieving a certain level of sustainability: reducing assistance in line with decreased needs, encouraging better use of local resources, training, etc.

General interventions in the post-emergency phase

Programmes and strategies should be adjusted at the beginning of this phase. A re-evaluation of the situation will allow new priorities to be identified, activities to be planned for longer periods (e.g. 6 months) and new objectives to be defined.

In practice, the 10 top priorities developed during the emergency phase remain an appropriate framework for the post-emergency phase, but the strategies and means employed will aim further into the future and be easily managed with local resources. Furthermore, other health programmes may be undertaken to respond better to problems that were only partially addressed in the emergency, such as AIDS, maternal care, mental health, etc.

Some specific issues must be considered:

• **Health screening**: health screening should continue for newcomers, coupled with measles immunization[3]. Although influxes are mostly small, screening should still receive adequate attention.

• **Health care programmes**: this topic is described in the chapter *Health Care in the Post-emergency Phase*, on page 249.

• **Surveillance**: surveillance and programme monitoring remain essential tools now more than ever (see *8. Public Health Surveillance* in Part II). They follow health trends, give warning signs and provide decision-makers with information to allow them to react promptly when necessary[2]. A major goal is to give warning of any outbreak of disease as soon as it occurs. Any relaxation of effort in regard to data monitoring should be avoided. The minimum set of indicators monitored in the emergency phase should continue to be followed in the post-emergency phase[2].

Nevertheless, certain aspects need to be reconsidered:

– The surveillance system should be adapted to changes in the health situation and services provided. Other diseases (e.g. sexually transmitted diseases - STDs) and new activities (e.g. Expanded Programme on Immunization - EPI) should now be monitored as well. However, the surveillance system should not be overloaded by the collection of non-essential data, i.e. data that are not used in decision-making.

– The frequency of reporting may change from weekly to monthly.

– The surveillance system should take into account the national health information system (HIS), although bearing in mind that this may be inadequate and lack the particular sensitivity to new trends required in any refugee situation. A compromise should be reached on this with the national health authorities because, in most cases, the refugee surveillance system will eventually be integrated into the HIS of the host country.

• **Food and nutrition** (see *4. Food and Nutrition* in Part II): it is still very important at this stage to monitor the adequacy of food rations in regard both to quantity and quality: nutritional value of the food basket and micronutrient contents, frequency of distributions, availability of food on the local market, etc. The nutritional status should be monitored, and micronutrient deficiencies should be detected as early as possible. The need for continuing feeding programmes should be re-evaluated: these will usually be scaled or closed down once malnutrition is under control. Where land is available, refugees should be supported in farming activities by, for example, distribution of seeds and tools.

• **Water and sanitation** (see *3. Water and Sanitation* in Part II): ways must be found to ensure a durable water supply using less expensive material and aiming at methods that can easily be maintained by local resources (e.g. hand pumps). Arrangements for the disposal of excreta must be improved and the building of family latrines should be promoted. Hygiene within the camp should be encouraged, both generally and at a personal level. Health education in regard to hygiene measures can now be given more attention.

• **Human resources** (see *9. Human Resources and Training* in Part II): task distributions and job descriptions, which were clearly defined during the emergency phase, should now be re-evaluated in line with new plans, which will often indicate a reduction in staff (especially non-qualified staff). Training for local staff should be emphasized and an increasing number of tasks delegated to them[2].

• **Coordination** (see *10. Coordination* in Part II): it is important that the continuity and quality of all activities remain constant despite changes in staff, modifications in relief programmes, and new agencies coming in to take over some responsibilities. The standardization of programmes and protocols that have been developed during the emergency must be maintained, although the standards need to be revised[2]. The coordinating body should supervise the hand-over of programmes between agencies. The involvement of local health officials in decision-making is more necessary than ever.

Programmes other than public health measures will be undertaken. Some of them aim at enhancing self-sufficiency among the refugees via the promotion of income-generating activities, gardening projects, etc. They could include education programmes, programmes to address environmental damage (e.g. reafforestation), etc. However, such programmes do not fall within the range of this book.

References

1. Toole, M J, Waldman, R J. Prevention of excess mortality in refugees and displaced populations in developing countries. *JAMA*, 1990, 263(24): 3296-302.

2. Moren, A, Rigal, J, Biberson, P. Populations réfugiées. Programme de santé publique et urgence de l'intervention. MSF-F, Epicentre. *Rev Prat*, 1992, 172: 767-76.

3. Mears, C, Chowdhury, S. *Health care for refugees and displaced people.* Oxford: Oxfam Practical Health Guide No. 9, 1994.

4. Médecins Sans Frontières. *Organisation d'un camp de réfugiés, Guide opérationnel pour la phase d'urgence.* Brussels: CRED, Médecins Sans Frontières, 1988.

5. Nieburg, P, Person-Karell, B, et al. Malnutrition-mortality relationships among refugees. *J Refugee Studies*, 1992, 5(3/4): 247-56.

6. CDC. Famine-affected, refugee, and displaced populations: Recommendations for public health issues. *MMWR*, 1992, 41(RR-13): 1-76.

7. Allen, T, Morsink, H. *When refugees go home.* UNRISD, Africa World Press, 1994.

Health care in the post-emergency phase and some specific issues

Introduction

The re-evaluation carried out at the beginning of the post-emergency phase will help determine new health care priorities (see *The Post-emergency Phase: Introduction*).

The health services already set up during the emergency phase (mainly curative care and measles immunization) usually need to be re-oriented and probably reinforced during the post-emergency phase.

This is a convenient time to work on improving the quality of health care as the emergency phase focused mainly on the quantity. Studies of current activities, such as vaccine coverage survey, drug consumption study, etc., will help to target the main weaknesses.

Training and supervision of health staff can receive more attention. The standardization of medical activities should be improved at this point; standards usually need to be adapted to and, if possible, linked with national standards.

Other health care programmes can now be started in line with the health needs identified during the re-evaluation, the resources available and the overall level of stability. These may include the following:

- other child health activities, such as an Expanded Programme on Immunization (EPI);

- comprehensive reproductive health services that include ante-natal, delivery and post-natal care, family planning, prevention and treatment of sexually transmitted diseases (STDs) and HIV/AIDS, etc. (see *Reproductive health in the post-emergency phase*, page 252).

• The relevance of starting a tuberculosis treatment programme should be carefully evaluated, as several prerequisites must be in place, such as stable conditions overall, and a certainty that adequate and strict patient follow-up can be ensured (see *Tuberculosis Programmes*, page 275).

• Programmes covering other health problems that were not amongst the priorities in the emergency phase, such as AIDS and sexually transmitted diseases (STDs), mental health, chronic diseases, etc. should be addressed as required by the situation (see *HIV, AIDS and STD*, page 265 and *Psycho-social and Mental Health*, page 286).

Some of the programmes implemented in the post-emergency phase should have been prepared during the emergency phase and may even have begun operating at a basic level.

In the post-emergency phase, it is crucial that the health agencies take the local population into consideration. Their health status and needs should be assessed. In principle, the level of health care to be provided to refugees should be comparable to the levels that the local population is entitled to receive. However in practice, it is difficult to avoid differences in quality between refugee health services and those available to the local population. The best option is to give support to rehabilitating the health system in the host area. Indeed, where possible, the relief health programme may be incorporated into a programme of assistance to the local health district. This should result in improving the overall standard of health in the local population, and facilitate the integration and acceptance of refugees among them.

The likely evolution of the refugee problem should always be taken into consideration in the planning.

For example:

- If repatriation is expected to take place in the near future, some long-term programmes (e.g. treatment of TB patients) should not be launched or, if already underway, should not admit any new cases; a medical screening should be planned before departure.

- If refugees are to remain and integrate into the host community, plans should be made to integrate refugee health services into the host country's national health programme. This requires that refugee health care is progressively adapted to fit in with national policies; for instance, the number of refugee facilities generally needs to be reduced (as the population to be covered by one facility is generally smaller in refugee situations) and integrated into the district health service.

The following sections of this chapter cover some specific issues that take on greater importance during the post-emergency phase:

- Curative health care

- Reproductive health care

- Child health care

- HIV, AIDS and STD programmes

- Tuberculosis programmes

- Psycho-social and mental health

Curative health care

In general, most of the curative health services set up in the emergency phase are maintained and some are reinforced. Usually, the 4 levels of health services are retained (referral hospital, central facility, peripheral facilities and home-visiting) but may need to be adapted, e.g. some facilities might close down when the workload of curative care has decreased (see *6. Health Care in the Emergency Phase* in Part II).

- Preventive activities (e.g. EPI) should be fully integrated with curative activities into existing health facilities (health centres and health posts).

- When the activities previously mentioned (see *Introduction* to Part III) are to be implemented, these should be launched and integrated into existing facilities: treatment of STDs, chronic diseases, tuberculosis programme, etc. (see relevant chapters). Specific staff training will be required as well as additional drugs, as the limited list of essential drugs established during the emergency will generally not be sufficient to conduct these further activities.

- The curative health system will have to be adapted to the host country's health system. National guidelines and health policies should be followed wherever possible, if they are suited to the refugee context.

- Improvements in the quality of curative care generally require further staff training in diagnosis and treatment, e.g. the rational prescription of drugs, nursing techniques, etc. Basic laboratories may be installed in some of the health facilities to help in improving diagnosis.

- In countries where patients pay for health care, it is a difficult issue to decide whether a financial contribution towards curative care should be requested from refugees (preventive care should remain free of charge) and, if so, when this should be introduced. Health management experts usually have to be brought in to assess the best policy in this context, based on the level of self-sufficiency reached by the refugee population and what they can afford to pay, etc. However, any eventual payment system should be introduced gradually and with flexibility as sudden changes in their situation may affect the refugee's access to curative health programmes.

- The role of home-visitors should also be re-evaluated with regard to the tasks they perform and whether or not their numbers should be increased or decreased. In most situations, they will become more involved in promoting community awareness and participate in health education, etc.

- Home-visitors still have a special role to play in reaching high risk groups, and active screening.

Reproductive health care
in the post-emergency phase

Introduction

Reproductive health (RH) is a part of general health that has to do with the reproductive system, its functions and processes; reproductive health care comprises those activities that contribute to reproductive health and well-being[1].

Although the target group is made up of both women and men, women are specifically targeted as they bear the greatest burden of reproductive ill-health. RH care in the post-emergency phase covers a wide range of activities such as[1]:

– antenatal care, delivery care and postnatal care (safe motherhood),

– family planning,

– dealing with the consequences of sexual violence,

– prevention and treatment of sexually transmitted diseases (STDs), and HIV/AIDS,

– other RH issues such as care after unsafe abortions, female genital mutilation, and other harmful traditional practices.

In the emergency phase, RH-related activities are limited to a minimum package of activities, which is described in chapter *6. Health Care in the Emergency Phase* (Part II). Correct implementation of the complete package of RH activities requires important investments, both in terms of human and financial resources, and is therefore not a priority in the emergency phase. At that stage the relief effort focuses on reducing high mortality and resources cannot be diverted from the priority requirements of the emergency phase.

In the post-emergency phase, once high mortality rates are under control and basic needs properly addressed, complete and integrated RH services can be planned, and the necessary resources allocated[2]. It is important that RH-activities are properly integrated into all the preventive and curative health care services in order to increase their efficiency and impact.

A comprehensive field manual on reproductive health in refugee situations has been produced by collaboration between several health agencies, and can be used as a reference[1].

Some considerations in regard to reproductive health care planning

- RH programmes do not require separate facilities: RH activities should be integrated into the other activities already established in the health facilities, especially at the peripheral level. These services must be easily accessible to the target groups. Apart from integrating with existing health activities and facilities, it is also essential to liaise with any existing social community, or other services (e.g. education and protection). The latter very often includes liaising with other NGOs and agencies.

- Special attention should be paid to the referral system, which must be a coherent one as it is an essential element in linking detection with action. Indeed, it is senseless to carry out screening for health problems and detecting risk factors if no appropriate action can be undertaken subsequently. Emergency referral procedures need to be put in place as early as possible.

- Involvement of the target groups (women, men and young people) in the planning phase should routinely be undertaken. This ensures that the reproductive health activities meet the needs as identified by them. Special attention must also be given to serving adolescents, as they are often especially at risk, have specific RH needs and are not always easy to reach.

- The availability of human resources differs from one setting to another, but it is always preferable to train and employ female health workers as they communicate more easily with the target groups. To extend coverage among women, at least some of these should be recruited from amongst traditional birth attendants (TBAs) in the community as they are already experienced in maternal and child health, and are likely to be trusted.

- Home-visiting linked to RH programmes is also essential in the post-emergency phase as it makes for greater coverage and increases the possibility of reaching high-risk families and individuals not attending the clinics[3].

- Often, the local population living in the area where the refugees have settled do not have access to the services offered to refugees, and consideration should be given to extending these services (e.g. family planning) to the local population.

Reproductive health care

ANTENATAL CARE, DELIVERY CARE AND POSTNATAL CARE

In most developing countries, maternal mortality is a problem, although the magnitude is not always recognized. WHO estimates that the mortality rates per 100,000 live births are approximately 640 for Africa, 420 for Asia and 270 for Latin America. Up to 80% of these maternal deaths are due to only a limited number of causes, many of which are preventable. The main causes of maternal mortality are obstructed labour, haemorrhage, infection, toxaemia (hypertensive pregnancy disorders), complications of unsafe abortion and anaemia. Women in refugee camps may face increased risks in pregnancy because of a variety of additional factors such as malnutrition, mental trauma or violence[4].

A significant proportion of maternal mortality can be avoided by a combination of adequately organized antenatal, delivery and postnatal care aiming at the detection and treatment of these problems. This is as valid for refugees as for any other population group although the conditions that prevail in a refugee setting make the problem harder to tackle. Although referral is likely to be easier from a practical point of view as the patient requiring treatment will never be very far from a health care facility, security problems and cultural traditions complicate referrals. It is therefore essential:

– to provide for obstetric emergencies. A proportion of minor obstetric emergencies may be dealt with on site (e.g. retention of placenta, infections, etc.) in the health centre or in the hospital, if there is one. In regard to major obstetric emergencies, suitable surgical facilities are usually not provided in the camp itself; the nearest surgical facility should be identified and transport organized for prompt referrals;

– to identify staff that may be available in the refugee population: nurses, midwives, trained TBAs, etc. Experience has shown that TBAs can play an important role in a refugee setting and therefore it is extremely important to identify them and provide them with the means for carrying out 'clean deliveries'. This includes providing refresher courses, supervision and delivery kits.

In circumstances where there are many TBAs present, a careful selection should be made. For instance, in the Somali refugee camps in Kenya in 1993, the TBAs that carried out most deliveries and those most accepted by the community were selected. Although they did not necessarily all provide the greatest quality of care at the beginning, the programme proved successful once they were included in the existing Mother and Child Health programme and supplied with delivery kits. Regular opportunities for training and discussion were provided when the TBAs went to their base health facility to re-supply their kits after each delivery.

Antenatal care

In a refugee setting, antenatal care should cover the following:

– identification AND referral for adequate treatment of high risk pregnancies,

– identification AND referral for adequate treatment of complications,

- prevention, screening and treatment of anaemia (iron and folic acid supplementation),
- immunization against tetanus.

Other activities can be included, depending on the situation:

- chemoprophylaxis for malaria when this is indicated, i.e. basically when refugees coming from a non-endemic area are settled in an endemic area. However, even in this situation, chemoprophylaxis is debatable because of the poor compliance frequently encountered (see section *Malaria control* in Part II);
- administration of other micronutrients if needed: iodine, vitamin C, etc.;
- supplementary food ration whenever indicated by the nutritional situation;
- screening for maternal syphilis (using simple RPR card test) and treatment.

- The frequency of antenatal check-ups should be decided in line with the overall workload and the resources available in the camp. It is recommended that each pregnant woman is seen at least twice during her pregnancy, with extra check-ups if needed (high risk pregnancies).

- A referral system must be established and adequate care provided for women at risk, i.e. all essential obstetric care, including surgery, anaesthesia and blood transfusions, must be available at hospital level (on-site or nearby).

- Immunization against tetanus should be carried out in line with EPI policies; ideally all women aged 15-44 years should be immunized, not only pregnant women. The age limit should be lowered if it is common in the specific refugee population for girls under 15 to become pregnant.

Delivery care

As far as the place of delivery is concerned, recommendations are similar to what is appropriate in other settings:

- women who are not at risk can usually deliver at home, with the help of trained TBAs if there are any; the TBAs should have delivery kits to ensure safe deliveries and know the risk factors for early referral to the nearby health centre;
- women at risk should be referred to a health centre with competent staff who can supervise labour;
- basic surgical facilities (caesarean section, anaesthesia, transfusions, etc.) should be accessible; whenever located outside the refugee site, transport should be provided.

Postnatal care

- There should be at least one check-up after delivery, preferably before the 4th week. This check-up also provides an opportunity to give vitamin A prophylaxis to protect the infant up to the age of 6 months and to discuss aspects of contraception[5].

- In the postnatal period, it is essential to promote exclusive breast-feeding. Indeed, breast-feeding is even more important in a refugee camp than in other settings because of the greater risk of diarrhoea (weaning practices), among other reasons[3].
- In some situations, lactating women may be admitted into a blanket supplementary feeding programme (see *4. Food and Nutrition* in Part II).

FAMILY PLANNING (FP)

It is widely accepted that reproductive health, both in women and men, is very much threatened in a crisis situation such as a refugee camp. Normal social patterns are disrupted; there is an increase in sexual violence, promiscuity (both of which often lead to unwanted pregnancies), unsafe abortions and sexually transmitted diseases (STDs), etc. In such situations, a family planning (FP) programme can therefore have broader objectives than would normally be the case. Apart from responding to a need for spacing/ limiting births, it also addresses unsafe abortions through a reduction in the number of unwanted pregnancies, and providing information about STDs, and referring cases for treatment.

Including these issues in an FP programme may eventually result in improvements in the maternal and infant morbidity and mortality rates[6].

When to start a family planning programme

Apart from emergency contraception which should be made available right from the start (as part of the RH activities in the emergency phase), a complete FP programme is started only later as it requires an intensive use of resources and specific follow-up. However, some contraceptive supplies should be made available for women who may request them. For instance, some refugee populations may have a high acceptance rate of contraception prior to displacement (e.g. Bosnian and Chechnyan women). Certain conditions must be met before FP implementation can be considered; no comprehensive programme should be undertaken unless[5]:

- the situation is stable and the emergency phase is over (crude mortality rate below 1/10,000/day);
- refugees are expected to stay in the camp for at least another 6 months;
- the necessary resources are available;
- there is a demand for contraception within the population AND this need has been thoroughly assessed.

Other important aspects to consider are:

- the acceptability of such a programme by other organizations working in the camp (especially any local groups of the host country);
- the extent to which the continuity of the programme can be guaranteed (e.g. the person put in charge should remain in the camp for at least 6 months).

These conditions highlight the need to properly assess the situation and the level of demand among the refugees before starting up any FP programme. Policies of the host country should be taken into account.

Implementation

When the basic conditions are met and it is decided to launch an FP programme, the steps to be followed are no different than for any other FP programme. These can be summarized as follows:

- Assess whether the refugee population has been exposed to a FP programme in their home country.
- Decide on the role of the national FP organizations of the host country and how to collaborate with them.
- Estimate the potential demand overall and the specific demand for contraceptives.
- Plan stocks of contraceptives.
- Plan the number of sites and staff that will be required, decide where and when FP consultations will be carried out, select the methods to be offered, plan the protocols to be used during the FP consultations, prepare a monitoring system, estimate the workload to check if the programme is feasible.
- Plan an information campaign (targeted at women and men).

Some of the points mentioned above merit special attention.

- It is essential that the methods offered are carefully selected, taking into consideration the level of knowledge and preferences in the population. No new methods should be introduced in a crisis situation.
- Adequate training for staff involved in the programme is paramount and should not only cover technical aspects (e.g. methods and protocol) but also the human relations aspect with regard to attitudes and behaviour.
- Providing information is crucial if the programme is to reach the target population.

For several reasons, it is recommended that the programme starts modestly. First of all, a small programme allows for close monitoring of and support to local staff. Second, the large-scale use of information campaigns and TBAs can turn women away from using the services in order to avoid becoming known as contraceptive users.

SEXUAL VIOLENCE

Violence against refugee women, including sexual violence, is seldom reported because of the pain and shame felt by the victims and their fear of being stigmatized. Nonetheless, those involved in working with refugee women know it is a significant problem and an important (political) issue with regard to the protection of refugees.

There are some practical measures that can be implemented both to prevent and to respond to sexual violence, and health agencies can certainly play a role in this; these include the provision of medical, psychological and social care to sexually-abused women, and raped women and men.

When dealing with rape, health professionals should take care to:

- Provide medical attention that may be needed: counselling and psycho-social support, pregnancy and STD detection, possibly STD treatment, emergency contraception and possibly abortion.

- Where appropriate, complete a medical certificate: this transforms the act from a personal harm into a crime that can be punished[7]. This certificate needs to be filled out by a physician following a prescribed format (a standard form exists). It is up to the victim to decide whether or not to use this certificate; health workers may report to UNHCR on her behalf, if the victim agrees.

Some guidelines have been developed for the prevention of sexual abuse and care of sexually-abused women in refugee situations[9]. Responding to the urgent needs of women who have been sexually abused and violated requires a multi-disciplinary approach, and may also be part of the FP programme.

In addition to direct sexual violence, other forms of sexual intimidation are frequently encountered in refugee situations. These aspects are dealt with in the *Socio-cultural Aspects* in Part I. For instance, it is obvious that refugee women who are unable to feed, clothe and shelter themselves and their children, will be much more vulnerable to manipulation and to physical and sexual pressures in order to obtain such necessities[8].

PREVENTION AND CARE FOR SEXUALLY TRANSMITTED DISEASES, INCLUDING HIV/AIDS

Activities in this area aim at preventing and reducing the transmission of STDs and HIV as well as providing care for those infected. STDs and AIDS are among the problems targeted in reproductive health, but they embrace also other aspects, such as blood transfusion safety and protection of health staff. All issues of STD and AIDS control in refugee populations are dealt with in a separate chapter: *HIV, AIDS and STD*.

OTHER REPRODUCTIVE HEALTH ISSUES

Abortions can be either spontaneous or induced, the latter can be either legal or illegal. Where illegal, the abortions carried out for unwanted pregnancies are very often unsafe. Whatever the law of the host country, the health services must be able to deal with the often life-threatening consequences of incomplete and/or septic abortions.

Amongst RH issues, one may have to deal with female genital mutilations, or other traditional practices affecting the reproductive health status of women. These practices should not be supported by health personnel, and the health facilities must be ready to deal with the often serious health consequences (e.g. complicated deliveries) of this practice.

🖎 References

1. UNHCR. *Reproductive health in refugee situations. An inter-agency field manual.* Geneva: UNHCR, 1995.
2. Donnay, F. *La planification familiale en pratique.* [draft]. Brussels: Médecins Sans Frontières, 1996.

3. Simmonds, S, Vaughan, P, William Gun, S. *Refugee community health care.* Oxford: Oxford Publications, 1983.

4. Mears, C, Chowdury, S. *Health care for refugees and displaced people.* Oxford: Oxfam Practical Health Guide No. 9, 1994.

5. Gillespie, S, Masson, J. *Controlling vitamin A deficiency.* ACC/SCN State-of-the Art-Series, Nutrition Policy. Discussion Paper No. 14, 1994.

6. Walker, B. *Women and emergencies.* Oxford: Oxfam Focus on Gender, 1994.

7. Saulnier, F. *Manuel de droit humanitaire.* Paris: Médecins Sans Frontières, 1993.

8. Tomasevski, K. *Women and human rights.* London: Zed Books Ltd, 1993.

9. UNCHR. *Sexual violence against refugees. Guidelines on prevention and response.* Geneva: UNHCR, 1995.

Child health care in the post-emergency phase

Introduction

The normal conditions of a refugee camp (overcrowding, inadequate food supplies, disruption of family life, etc.) mean that children in the under-five age group are more at risk of developing health problems, and therefore under-five mortality rates may be very high. Services targeted at children should aim at preventing illness and nutritional deficiencies, and ensuring early diagnosis and adequate treatment for health and nutritional problems. The under-fives should be targeted for most preventive activities and children up to 15 for curative activities. Every possible means should be employed to ensure that these target groups are reached.

Consequently, as the same 5 major killers are at play (measles, diarrhoeal diseases, malnutrition, acute respiratory infections and malaria – in affected areas), the activities in the post-emergency phase are basically the same as those in the emergency phase and aim to reduce excess mortality brought about by these health problems[1]. The main difference in intervention lies in the immunization of children: it is limited to measles immunization during the emergency phase, but afterwards it involves the implementation of a complete EPI.

The essential services to be provided for children are:
– paediatric curative care (or clinics for the under-fives) which also includes identification and referral of sick children;
– early detection of malnourished children and referral to relevant nutritional services;
– therapeutic and supplementary feeding programmes wherever indicated;
– immunization in line with EPI recommendations;
– usually, vitamin A supplementation; supplementation with other micro-nutrients if indicated.

The first 3 activities are covered more fully in the chapters *6. Health Care in the Emergency Phase* and *4. Food and Nutrition* in Part II.

Considerations with regard to planning

- All programmes targeting children must be properly integrated into all the preventive and curative health care services in order to increase their efficiency and impact. This is especially important at the peripheral level (i.e. health posts, about 1 per 5,000 population). Furthermore, it is essential to ensure they are always easily accessible to the target group.

- From the beginning, every effort should be made to also address the health needs of women, preferably on the same day and at the same place. For example, a mother who comes to the health post for medical care for her sick child should be enrolled in an antenatal care programme if she is pregnant, her child should be vaccinated if necessary, etc.

- Apart from integrating with existing health activities and facilities, it is also essential to liaise with any social or other services for children that may exist outside the health sector; for instance, a good starting point for an EPI programme could be a well-functioning supplementary feeding programme.

- Attempts should be made to reach all under-fives, although it is sometimes recommended to only target the under-twos when resources are limited[2,3].

- Home-visiting linked to child health activities is also essential in the post-emergency phase as it makes for greater coverage and increases the possibility of reaching children at high-risk, and/or not attending the clinics, and can also assist in providing services at home[4].

- Often, the local population living in the area where the refugees have settled do not have access to the services offered to refugees, although their own living conditions may be poor. Extending such services - e.g. EPI - to the local population will have to be studied carefully. There is no general rule; each decision will depend on the individual situation.

Health care activities

PAEDIATRIC INTEGRATED CURATIVE CARE

These services will already be set up in the emergency phase and should continue in the post-emergency phase. Basic curative care includes the early diagnosis and treatment of common childhood conditions such as: diarrhoea, acute respiratory infections (ARIs), measles, malnutrition, malaria, skin conditions (e.g. scabies) and anaemia (see chapters *7. Control of Communicable Diseases and Epidemics* and *4. Food and Nutrition* in Part II, and appendix 4).

EXPANDED PROGRAMME OF IMMUNIZATION (EPI)

In the emergency phase, the only immunization indicated is vaccination against measles. In the post-emergency phase, a complete EPI programme should be implemented as part of the overall health programme; ideally all necessary immunizations should be administered to all children in the relevant age groups.

However, as a complete EPI requires significant human, material and financial resources (vaccines, cold chain, etc.), certain conditions must be met before implementation should be considered[3]. An EPI programme can be undertaken when:

- the population is expected to remain stable (say for at least 6 months);
- there are adequate resources (human and material) to ensure implementation;
- the programme can be integrated into the national immunization programme of the host country.

Principles of EPI activities in refugee settings

• Any EPI carried out in a refugee setting should come within the framework of the national EPI programme wherever possible; the health authorities of the host country should be contacted prior to setting up an EPI.

• The recommended vaccines to be administered, in addition to measles, are DTP (diphteria, tetanus, pertussis), polio and BCG. Depending on the specific situation and national EPI strategy, other vaccinations may also be included, e.g. yellow fever and hepatitis B.

• Age group: see Table 1. Most vaccines should be administered before children reach the age of five[3]; however, there are some exceptions to this in regard to measles vaccination (see *2. Measles Immunization* in Part II):

  – the age limit is lowered to 6 months in all refugee settings; children vaccinated prior to 9 months should receive a second dose on reaching 9 months;

  – the upper age limit, which was raised to 12-15 years in the emergency phase, may be brought down to 5 years providing an adequate vaccine coverage has been attained. However, if a measles outbreak occurs, children up to 12-15 years will be included as well.

Table 1
The target age groups for EPI programmes[3]

VACCINE	TARGET AGE GROUP
Measles	6 months - 5 years
DTP	6 weeks - 5 years
Polio	at birth - 5 years
BCG	at birth

However, following the national EPI policies of the host country may entail certain difficulties in conducting EPI on a refugee site:

– very often, EPI policy in the host country is to vaccinate children up to the age of 2 years, rather than 5 years (or even 15 years for measles)[3]. This issue must be negotiated with the authorities;

– in an open situation, where refugees are integrated into the local population, immunization should be extended to local residents. This is usually not the case in a closed refugee camp, where local residents are unlikely to be included in any EPI carried out by relief agencies working in the camp.

Operational aspects of EPI programmes

From an operational point of view, EPI should follow the same principles wherever it is carried out. However, some aspects are specific to the refugee situation.

• Responsibility for each aspect of the immunization programme must be explicitly assigned to the agencies and individuals involved.

- If an effective local immunization programme exists in the host country, it should be possible either to use the local cold chain facilities or to give some assistance towards upgrading these. If there is no local immunization programme or cold-chain facility, special arrangements will have to be made (see also *2. Measles Immunization* in Part II).

- Proper immunization records must be kept; individual immunization cards - preferably EPI cards - must always be issued, and a register or tally sheet should be used to record the doses administered.

- Often, documents related to previous vaccinations (health or EPI cards) have been lost or left behind, and the vaccination status of children is not known. The general recommendation is to consider those with an unknown vaccination status as unvaccinated, even if the refugees come from a country with a high vaccination coverage. There is no danger in vaccinating twice.

- 'Missed opportunities' for vaccination should be limited as much as possible: each opportunity (e.g. each contact made in regard to any form of health care) should be used to check the vaccination cards and administer vaccines whenever indicated. However, depending on the context, the advantage of vaccinating at every opportunity must be weighed against the cost of wasting vaccines before deciding on this.

- Strategies for increasing vaccine coverage are relatively easy to implement in refugee settings. For example in Gode (Ethiopia) in 1994, a supplementary feeding programme was started for all children under five and a mobile EPI team visited the different distribution centres on a regular basis to administer vaccines.

- The way EPI is implemented will depend very much on the particular situation. For example, in El Wak (Kenya) in 1993 no EPI programme was implemented because the conditions were not met. However, 3 rounds of mass vaccination targeting the under-fives, coupled with blanket supplementary feeding, were carried out before refugees returned home.

OTHER PREVENTIVE ACTIVITIES TARGETED AT CHILDREN

Vitamin supplementation

(see *4. Food and Nutrition - Nutrient deficiencies* in Part II)

Vitamin A deficiency is likely to occur in any refugee or displaced population and is known to increase morbidity and mortality rates, particularly in the case of measles. Vitamin A should always be distributed to all children aged between 6 months and 5 years (or even 15 years) of age[5].

This vitamin A distribution can be made through child health activities. However, there is a risk that repeated doses may result in overdosing as children may receive vitamin A during the measles campaign, in supplementary feedings, during regular MCH visits, etc. It is therefore essential to decide on a policy of distribution which avoids repeated doses and always registers when a child receives a dose of vitamin A (e.g. on the vaccination card).

Apart from vitamin A, other micronutrients may be required: vitamin C in case of scurvy, iodine in areas where goitre is endemic, etc.

Screening for malnutrition

(see *4. Food and Nutrition* in Part II)

It is essential to detect children with nutritional problems early on as malnutrition is a major cause of mortality among children. For screening purposes, it is recommended to use the mid-upper arm circumference measure (MUAC), which is a quick way of identifying children at risk. Referral to feeding programmes must be organized in line with MUAC cut-off points and the criteria selected[6]. The time and resources devoted to malnutrition screening will depend on the degree to which malnutrition is a cause of mortality.

Routine growth monitoring does not generally have a place in the services provided to refugee children. Such growth monitoring ('road to health' charts) presents several disadvantages: it is very time-consuming, difficult and seldom correctly done, and it is not useful for nutritional surveillance. In the specific context of a refugee setting, MUAC is preferred for regular screening and, when coupled with the prompt referral of the acutely undernourished, is far more effective.

➥ References

1. Toole, M J, Waldman, R J. Prevention of excess mortality in refugees and displaced populations in developing countries. *JAMA*, 1990, 263(24): 3296-302.

2. Mears, C, Chowdury, S. *Health care for refugees and displaced people*. Oxford: Oxfam Practical Health Guide No. 9, 1994.

3. CDC. Famine-affected, refugee, and displaced populations: Recommendations for public health issues. *MMWR*, 1992, 41(RR-13): 1-76.

4. Simmonds, S, Vaughan, P, William Gun, S. *Refugee community health care*. Oxford: Oxford University Press, 1983.

5. Gillespie, S, Masson, J. *Controlling vitamin A deficiency*. ACC/SCN State-of-the Art-Series, Nutrition Policy. Discussion Paper No. 14, 1994.

6. Médecins Sans Frontières. *Nutrition Guidelines*. Paris: Médecins Sans Frontières, 1995.

HIV, AIDS and STD

Introduction

Refugees and displaced populations have regularly been the subject of debate in regard to acquired immune deficiency syndrome (AIDS) over the past few years. In the refugee context even more than elsewhere, AIDS and HIV seropositivity pose a serious problem with regard to human rights. Within a group which is already endangered by poor sanitary conditions and an unstable political climate, the protection of individuals affected by HIV will become even more important. The medical and psycho-social management of the disease, and how to prevent it, remain difficult issues in the refugee context.

It is important to acknowledge that, from an epidemiological point of view, no study has indicated that refugee or displaced persons have a higher risk of contracting AIDS, and no specific measure, discriminatory or otherwise, is justified in relation to them[1]. On another side, there is obviously no evidence that refugees are at a lower risk than others of AIDS/STD, and all efforts should be undertaken to decrease the risk of HIV transmission.

There are a number of constraints - political, humanitarian and medical - which are specific to such situations: the presence of acute health problems, frequent breakdowns in the normal systems of blood screening and universal precautions, social, political and cultural disruption, the difficulties for planning medium and long-term programmes, the large number of operating partners, limitations in regard to human and material resources, etc. These constraints should however not be used as an excuse for not tackling AIDS in refugees, but rather implies that this problem deserves special attention in this context.

UNHCR, WHO, the International Organization for Migration and some other NGOs have established guidelines for dealing with this issue, based on 3 main principles[1,2,3,18,21].

These cover:

– respect for ethical rules, involving the protection of individual and refugee rights,
– prevention of virus transmission, within health services, and within the community,
– medical and psycho-social management of the disease.

Ethical considerations in regard to HIV and AIDS

By definition, a refugee is usually an 'uninvited guest' in the host country, and is often considered more or less undesirable. The status of displaced persons, victims of civil wars or ethnic persecutions, is seldom better, particularly as there is no international convention regarding protection for them, or defining their specific rights (see *Part I, Refugee and Displaced Populations*. Experience shows that at first, these populations are almost always the objects of suspicion in regard to health issues, communicable diseases in particular: they may be suspected of introducing certain epidemic diseases into the host country, of destabilizing an already precarious health situation, or of receiving better assistance than the local population. Refugees are therefore singled out as the suspected source of disease by the local community, and health data may be manipulated and used as a political weapon against them.

Although the concentration of people in precarious situations such as refugee camps does facilitate the spread of many epidemics, there is no convincing argument that AIDS is one of them. However, in these circumstances more than elsewhere, individuals who are HIV-positive or have fully developed AIDS may be exposed to discriminatory measures, whether for cultural or other reasons, even within their own community. This may result in basic rights being denied: *non refoulement* (i.e. the right not to be prevented from entering a country to seek refuge: see *Introduction*), freedom of movement, the possibility of resettlement in a third country, access to health care, and fundamental individual human rights.

Such discriminatory measures should always be condemned and prevented wherever possible. Everything should be done to minimize the risks: strict adherence to the rules of medical ethics is the best guarantee for protecting patients, both at the individual and collective level.

The important ethical rules to respect include the following:

- Strict confidentiality, whatever the circumstances, is the primary condition for preventing or significantly reducing the risk of discrimination. All staff involved in testing, patient information and counselling, must be made very aware of this. Attention should also be paid to the difficulty of ensuring confidentiality in refugee settings, because of the conditions of crowding and lack of privacy.

- The rapid test for HIV screening is primarily indicated for ensuring the safety of blood transfusions and does not enable an actual diagnosis to be made (more specific tests would have to be carried out). Blood donors should not be informed that their blood will be tested for HIV unless the following 3 conditions can be met: proper laboratory confirmation is available, and information and effective psychological support can be provided both pre- and post-testing. Unless all 3 conditions can be met, anonymous unlinked testing must be the rule[6].

- HIV testing for individual diagnosis should be avoided unless conditions are strictly met: the patient is properly informed and has given consent, strict confidentiality is guaranteed and comprehensive management of the patient can be ensured, i.e. appropriate psycho-social support and counselling as well as curative care (see also under *Management of AIDS patients* below). The same principles must obviously be respected if testing is requested voluntarily by the patient. The use of rapid HIV tests in order to arrive at a presumptive diagnosis ('just to get an idea') is never justified and cannot be condoned.

- Mass screening must be avoided at all costs for the same reasons as those indicated in regard to individual testing[1]. Surveys conducted for epidemiological monitoring or research should generally be avoided in the refugee context, unless their usefulness has been debated and an agreement is reached between the partners involved - national programme officers of the host country, representatives of international organizations (UNHCR, WHO), NGOs, and the refugee community. Such surveys must not have any hidden agenda and they must never represent a risk either to individuals or to the community as a whole.

- In addition to the problems linked with testing, it is essential to ensure that HIV-positive and AIDS patients have a constant right of access to health care. UNHCR recommends that refugees should benefit, if possible, from the same treatment level as that offered in the host country[1]. Any measure leading to their ostracism from health services must be strictly avoided; for example, the isolation of AIDS patients in in-patient wards is not justified, assuming that the basic rules of nursing hygiene are always respected for every patient (see below).

Prevention of HIV transmission

THE MAIN WAYS OF VIRUS TRANSMISSION

1. **Sexual intercourse**: infected genital secretions are the major transmission route. Heterosexual transmission prevails in most tropical areas and is increasing everywhere else. Some specific groups at higher risk have been identified (prostitutes, individuals with a high number of sexual partners, etc.) but the whole population is at risk. The presence of a sexually transmitted disease (STD) considerably increases the risk of transmission during unprotected sexual intercourse.

2. **Blood**: the main contamination routes are either through the transfusion of infected blood, or injection using infected and unsterilized reused materials, e.g. needles. Contamination by these routes remains frequent in most developing countries due to poor health care hygiene and a lack of blood-screening tests, the unnecessary and even abusive use of blood transfusion and injection practices (within the health services or by unsupervised traditional practitioners) and often, inadequately trained medical staff. Surgery and other invasive procedures are also significant sources of contamination.

3. **Transmission from mother to child**: this may occur during pregnancy, at birth or, less frequently, through breast-feeding; in developing countries, 20% to 30% of the children born to HIV-positive mothers are themselves infected.

THE PREVENTION OF TRANSMISSION

There are some well-known preventive measures which can be taken against the two main routes of HIV transmission. However, in developing countries, there is so far no affordable measure that can be taken to prevent transmission from mother to child.

In relation to HIV transmission through breast-feeding, current data from areas where infectious diseases and malnutrition are the causes of death, indicate that infants who are not breast-fed run a particularly high risk of dying from these conditions. Therefore, to date, breast-feeding should remain the standard advice in these settings, because its benefits generally outweigh the possible risk of transmission[18].

Measures aiming at the protection of patients and medical staff against accidental infection in health facilities (iatrogenic transmission) are imperative, and are included in the priorities of the emergency phase, whatever the circumstances (see *6. Health Care in the Emergency Phase* in Part II)[18]. Staff should be aware that this iatrogenic transmission can simply be prevented by respecting the universal precautions in health care settings. The AIDS virus is not transmitted any more easily by these routes than are many other pathogenic agents such as hepatitis B/C, tetanus, etc.

Protecting patients and reducing the iatrogenic risk

- Transfusions[4,5,6]

  Even with correct blood screening, there still remains a residual risk of infection in areas of high HIV prevalence which cannot be ignored (0.2% to 1%), and transfusion of contaminated blood infects the recipient in at least 90% of cases. The improper use of transfusions is frequent in most countries and it is therefore essential to limit these to the minimum. Practical measures include[18]:

  – strict indications for the use of transfusions: any transfusion that is not strictly indicated is contraindicated, and should be limited to life-threatening circumstances, and when no other alternative is possible;

  – training medical staff to recognize and treat severe anaemia, as well as in the use of blood substitutes whenever possible;

  – the selection of blood donors case by case, after exclusion of all individuals at risk (as it is generally impossible to set up a blood bank in refugee settings);

  – when transfusions are really necessary, they should be safe: all blood samples must be screened before transfusion, with no exceptions, using rapid HIV screening tests. The proper use of these tests and their quality should be checked regularly;

  – transfusion procedures must be clearly defined and standardized[6].

  Technical details on the use of transfusions and substitutes are available in several reference documents[6,13,14,15].

- Proper disinfection, sterilization, and disposal of medical waste

  The fundamental rules of hygiene are of primary importance, and should be strictly applied as soon as health services are implemented. These include strict procedures for the disinfection and sterilization of re-usable material, and the proper disposal of medical waste, including incineration; staff should be given proper training in these procedures early on. In the first stage of the emergency phase, before training can be organized and sterilization material made available, single-use materials should be employed, especially for injections, as is done for instance, in mass immunization campaigns. These rules must be observed in all health facilities and by all staff members, whatever their proximity to patients; they are described in several manuals (see also *3. Water and Sanitation* in Part II)[4,5,7,8,9,17,18]. Particular attention should be paid to ensuring a sufficient supply of all the required materials (needles, syringes, gloves, disinfectants, etc.).

- Limiting the number of injections

    Although frequently regarded by patients and many prescribers as a very valuable form of treatment, the use of injections must be restricted to a basic minimum (emergency or specific indications) and should not take place outside health facilities. Staff must be educated on the risks incurred.

PROTECTION OF STAFF

From the outset of an emergency, detailed information must be given to all staff members working in health facilities (medical and other), in regard to the necessary precautions for reducing the risk of accidental contamination. These precautions are described above.

It is important to insist on the use of gloves for any direct contact with blood and body fluids, the correct use of needles and cutting instruments, and the measures that should be taken immediately upon accidental exposure. It should also be pointed out, however, that the risk of contracting HIV from an infected patient is very low, and that respecting these simple rules reduces the chances to almost nil.

PREVENTION OF HIV TRANSMISSION WITHIN THE COMMUNITY

In refugee settings, specific programmes to prevent HIV transmission within the community are limited by certain constraints, particularly in the emergency phase:

- During this phase, most human and material resources are directed towards dealing rapidly with those acute health problems that are responsible for the highest proportions of excess mortality (see *Introduction* to Part I). Therefore AIDS is usually not perceived as a priority requiring immediate action.

- Health education programmes requiring long-term involvement are difficult to implement in this context. Medical personnel are usually not sufficiently trained in this, and retraining requires a longer-term investment and specific expertise.

- There is an lack of information on the epidemiology and management of AIDS in refugee camps and in crisis situations. Frequently ignorance of the cultural context limits the implementation and impact of preventive programmes.

- Preventive programmes targeted at specific risk groups would be difficult to conduct: these groups are not known at the outset and are difficult to identify due to the problems connected with screening and preserving anonymity that have already been mentioned.

However, none of these constraints should be used as an excuse for doing nothing. Some preventive measures can be taken.

- Promoting safer sex and making condoms available

    In the emergency phase, a health education programme on HIV transmission and prevention will not usually be considered a priority, but some simple messages could certainly be communicated to the community. Condoms should be made available, at least in health facilities, and on a larger scale if there is a demand from the population (for instance, in tandem with mass immunizations, food distributions, etc.). Since the use of condoms by a population depends largely on cultural and religious taboos and previous experience, there is no standard rule in regard to this; for instance, condoms should not be promoted where their use is not acceptable to the population.

    In the post-emergency phase, a more extensive programme can be considered. It requires liaison with the national AIDS programme of the host country and the other agencies involved (UNHCR and other NGOs). Health education within the settlement and access to condoms should be undertaken step by step, and in accordance with the recommendations of the national AIDS programme of the host country. HIV/AIDS programmes in refugee populations should ideally aim to provide a level of health education and condom distribution at least similar to that of the national programme in their country of origin. In general, a system of condom distribution should include the following[18]:

    – condoms and appropriate instructions for their use should be available with passive distribution on request of health facilities;

    – when possible, condom distribution can be extended to community agents (e.g.home-visitors), shops, local groups, etc.;

    – promotion through campaign-like activities may be used as opportunities to spread information;

    – condoms should ideally be made available to the host community as well, as contacts between the refugee and local populations are likely to occur.

    It is essential that the strategies of HIV prevention are adapted to the particular situation. For instance, in the Benaco refugee camp (Tanzania, 1994), one agency decided to make condoms more available and accessible to the Rwandan refugees by distributing them through 'non-traditional' outlets such as shops, boutiques, and social events (e.g. football matches); this strategy was selected because AIDS awareness among the Rwandan population was already very high, and there was already a demand for condoms[12].

- Control of sexually transmitted diseases (STDs)

    The adequate treatment and prevention of STDs is an important aspect of AIDS control. In the emergency phase, STD patients can receive basic treatment in the health services as for any other health problems. In the post-emergency phase, it is often necessary to put more effort into STD prevention and treatment.

Appropriate and effective STD case management requires the following[18]:

- training of health care workers on the syndromic approach to STD management;
- standardization of case management, and introduction of guidelines. Flow charts for diagnosis of syndromes facilitate STD diagnosis and treatment, and can be obtained from the WHO[16]:
- consistent availability of appropriate drugs and condoms.

The question as to whether specialized STD clinics should be organized, or whether treatment could be provided in normal consultations (out-patient department – OPD), is still under discussion. Some guidelines recommend setting up STD clinics in areas where there is a high prevalence of STD and HIV infections, indicated on the basis of the number of consultations for STDs[5]. The advantage of such a system is that it provides more privacy, better management of these diseases by staff who have been specifically trained in STD management, together with appropriate advice on personal STD prevention (safe sex measures). However, patients attending such services risk being labelled as STD-infected and discriminated against as a result, and setting up such additional facilities demands additional resources.

In refugee settings, it is generally preferable to integrate the management of STDs into normal curative care in order to avoid discrimination against these patients. However, it is important to organize services that are user-friendly, private and confidential, and this may require special arrangements within the health services[18]. For instance, privacy during consultations may need to be improved, and separate consultations for men and women may have to be organized. In situations where easy access to OPD services cannot be provided or where policy calls for it, separate STD consultations could be organized. Condoms should, of course, be available at this level.

Management of AIDS patients

THERAPEUTIC ASPECTS

AIDS is a chronic disease for which there is presently no cure. Specific treatments have only very limited effectiveness, and their high cost is an important obstacle to their use. A large part of the morbidity and mortality linked with AIDS is due to infections for which specific, and effective treatment is possible, even when only limited means are available. Appropriate treatment of the most common infectious complications results in a significant reduction in the suffering of these patients and may lengthen their lives. Such treatment should be provided as soon as health services are in place, as part of normal curative care.

Whenever it becomes feasible, usually after the emergency phase, health workers should be specifically trained in the management of HIV-associated diseases. The detection of cases on clinical criteria is sufficient for case management, and diagnostic procedures should be kept simple. Guidelines for the clinical management of these patients through simple flow charts adapted to each health care level have been developed and published by WHO, and some national programmes[10,11,19].

Treatment of serious complications arising from AIDS (severe opportunistic infections and tumours) is symptomatic and palliative, and patients should be given appropriate psychological support (as for any serious disease in the terminal phase). Referring AIDS patients to local health facilities, which are generally unable to provide a better quality of diagnosis and treatment, should be avoided[1].

Tuberculosis and malnutrition

Tuberculosis, which is often associated with HIV infection, and malnutrition, are frequent in refugee and displaced populations and their clinical features frequently overlap those of AIDS. HIV testing in patients with these diseases is not justified, particularly as treatment will not be modified whether they are HIV-positive or not.

If a tuberculosis programme has been set up, treatment with thiacetazone should be avoided if at all possible, because of the more frequent and severe cutaneous reactions in HIV patients, especially in areas where there is a high HIV prevalence[19].

Vaccination

All vaccines included in the Expanded Programme on Immunization (EPI) remain to date indicated for HIV-infected children, whether symptomatic or not, except BCG which is contraindicated in patients with clinical AIDS because of the risk of serious systemic BCG infection. WHO recommends, however, that all new-born babies in areas of high tuberculosis prevalence receive BCG vaccinations.

SOCIO-PSYCHOLOGICAL SUPPORT AND COUNSELLING OF THE PATIENT

Social support, psychological support and advice on prevention are key elements in the management of HIV-infected or AIDS patients. These various activities require specific expertise, substantial means, and a sufficient knowledge of the cultural context.

Programmes aiming at social and material support are not likely to be implemented in the emergency phase since they can only be considered as part of a comprehensive AIDS control programme. In the post-emergency phase, and depending on the circumstances, it may be possible to use locally-trained specialists and to start a more active programme.

Specialized NGOs and the social services of organizations like UNHCR may offer a great deal of help. However, this kind of programme is very difficult to implement in the context of displaced populations, because of the unstable background to the situation and the existence of more urgent or severe health problems. Nevertheless, any qualified health staff should be able to provide patients with advice on preventive measures, and give them psychological support following a minimal training.

Principal recommendations regarding HIV, AIDS and STD

- AIDS management and control is difficult everywhere, but even more so among refugee or displaced populations because of the specific constraints inherent in such situations. However, special attention should be paid to the correct use of basic and easily implemented measures; simple, universal precautions and blood screening are already very efficient and constitute the mainstay of the intervention.

- In the emergency phase, the protection of individual rights, prevention of the HIV iatrogenic transmission, and protection of health staff constitute the minimal measures to be taken by everyone involved in medical activities. Basic treatment of STDs and the common infectious complications arising from AIDS should be ensured as part of normal curative care from the beginning; condoms should be made available to individuals requesting them.

- In the post-emergency phase, depending on the circumstances, certain other interventions may be considered. These must always be well planned, taking account of the cultural context, the national AIDS programme of the host country, and agreed upon by the various partners involved and refugee community representatives.

References

1. UNHCR. UNHCR *Policy and guidelines regarding refugee protection and assistance and Acquired Immune Deficiency Syndrome (AIDS)*. Geneva: UNHCR, 1988. UNHCR/IOM/70/88, UNHCR/FOM/63/88.

2. WHO. *Migration Medicine*. A seminar of the International Organization for Migration co-sponsored by the World Health Organization, 6-9 February 1990, Geneva, Switzerland. Papers 3.4, 3.6, 3.8, 3.9.

3. Refugee Policy Group. *Summary of discussion, Meeting on refugees and AIDS, held September 18, 1989, Washington, DC*. Washington, DC, RPG, 1989.

4. WHO. *Detailed Guidelines from WHO on prevention of HIV infection*. Geneva: WHO, 1986. WHO/CDS/AIDS/86/1.

5. Lamptey, P, Piot, P. *The Handbook for AIDS prevention in Africa*. Durham: Family Health International, 1990.

6. Médecins Sans Frontières. *La pratique transfusionnelle en milieu isolé*. Paris: Médecins Sans Frontières, 1997.

7. Médecins Sans Frontières. *L'hygiène dans les soins de santé en situation précaire*. Brussels: Médecins Sans Frontières, 1996.

8. Renchon, B. *Manuel d'utilisation des désinfectants. Principes directeurs du HCR pour le choix et l'utilisation des désinfectants.* Geneva: HCR, 1993. HCR/GEN/1993/MISC/13.

9. WHO. *Guidelines for the nursing management of people infected with human immunodeficiency virus (HIV).* Geneva: WHO, 1988. WHO AIDS Series, 3.

10. WHO.*Guidelines for the clinical management of HIV infection in adults.* Geneva: WHO, 1991. WHO/GPA/IDS/HCS/91.6.

11. WHO. *Guidelines for the clinical management of HIV infection in children.* Geneva: WHO, 1993. WHO/GPA/IDS/HCS/93.3.

12. A first AIDS work with refugees. *AIDS Analysis Africa*, 1995, 5(1): 10-11.

13. WHO. Global blood safety initiative. *Guidelines for the appropriate use of blood.* Geneva: WHO, 1989. WHO/GPA/INF/89.18. WHO/LAB/89.10.

14. Denantes, C, Le Floch, A. Stratégies transfusionnelles post-opératoires. *Développement et Santé*, 1994, 113: 4-13.

15. WHO, Global blood safety initiative. *Use of plasma substitutes and plasma in developing countries.* Geneva: WHO, 1989. WHO/GPA/INF/89.17.

16. Global programme on AIDS. *Management of sexually transmitted diseases.* Geneva: WHO, 1994. WHO/GPA/TEM/94.1.

17. Global programme on AIDS. *Preventing HIV transmission in health facilities.* Geneva: WHO, 1995. GPA/TCO/HCS/95.16.

18. *Reproductive health in refugee situations. An inter-agency field manual.* Geneva: UNHCR, 1995.

19. Global programme on AIDS. *AIDS care handbook.* Geneva: WHO, 1993. WHO/OPA/IDS/HCS/93.2.

20. Brady, B. Controlling STDs/HIV within dynamic refugee settings. *Refugee Participation Network*, 1995, 20: 26-9.

21. UNHCR, WHO, UNAIDS. *Guidelines for HIV interventions in emergency settings.* Geneva: UNAIDS, 1996.

Tuberculosis programme

Introduction

Tuberculosis (TB) remains a major public health problem throughout the world, especially in developing countries (see Table 2)[1]. The tubercle bacillus infects one third of the world's population and tuberculosis is the primary cause of death from a single pathogen in adults[9]. Poor living conditions, overcrowding and malnutrition favour the spread of the disease. The prevalence of tuberculosis is increasing world wide, mainly due to deteriorations in socio-economic conditions in several countries, ineffective treatment programmes and the spread of the human immuno-deficiency virus (HIV). The emergence of multi-drug-resistant tuberculosis, mainly due to inadequate or incomplete treatment, also poses a serious threat for the future.

Table 2
Incidence of smear-positive tuberculosis in developing countries, 1985-90[2]

Area	Incidence rate (per 100,000)
Sub-Saharan Africa	117
North Africa and Western Africa	54
Asia	79
South America	54
Central America and the Caribbean	54
Total	**79**

Most of the world's refugees are found in African and Asian countries, where the estimated incidences of smear-positive pulmonary tuberculosis are the highest (see Table 2). In addition, risk factors for TB transmission such as overcrowding, malnutrition and poor hygiene are intensified in refugee settlements. The loss of community structure, the lack of regular access to health care, malnutrition and psychological shock have also been described as factors increasing the transmission[16,17]. However, evidence of an increasing TB transmission in refugee settings has not been documented so far[8]. Tuberculosis generally becomes more evident after the emergency phase, when the major killer diseases are under control (see *Introduction* to Part III). It can then become a significant cause of adult death as occurred in Somali camps in 1985 where it was associated with 25% of all deaths among those over 15[11].

TWO CASE STUDIES IN REFUGEE SETTINGS

Table 3
Results of a TB programme in Karen refugees camps, Thailand, 1985-92[5]

No.	Cured %	Completed %	Death %	Failure %	Defaulters %	Others %
288	80	6	5	2	7	0.7

The TB programme in Thailand (see Table 3) was characterized by very strict management, good coordination and total patient compliance. Cases were all admitted as in-patients to a centre where living conditions were acceptable for the duration of the treatment. This was possible as all patients came from a closed refugee camp and their absence therefore had little economic effect on them or their families.

Table 4
Treatment outcome of sputum-positive patients
in the refugee camp of Hagadera, Kenya 1992-1994[3,4]

	No.	Cured %	Completed %	Death %	Failure %	Defaulters %	Transferred %
Evaluation 1	90	26	37	11	11	13	12
Evaluation 2	98	72	3	1	3	16	4

- **The first evaluation** covered patients enrolled in programmes from 11/92 up till 31/7/93, and revealed very poor results in terms of patient outcome; strict recommendations were then made in regard to programme management.

- **The second evaluation** concerned quarterly cohorts of patients enrolled after improvements in the programme, covering the second quarter of 1993 to the first quarter of 1994. Results indicated an improvement but the cure rate targeted had not yet been reached (see below *Objectives*)[3].

The treatment of tuberculosis, though theoretically simple and very effective (95% of patients can be cured with adequate treatment), demands technical knowledge and long-term commitment. In refugee settings, TB programmes have had different degrees of success: very positive results have been reported in camps with good access to the population, where adequate patient follow-up and compliance to treatment was ensured; while in other situations, badly-managed programmes have shown very poor results.

The dilemma of tuberculosis treatment in refugee settings

In refugee settlements, health workers are frequently confronted with patients affected by tuberculosis and have to decide whether to start a treatment programme or not; this is not an easy decision to make. The dilemma of tuberculosis control in such settings stems on the one hand from the ability of chemotherapy to decrease transmission and successfully treat patients, and on the other hand from the considerable problem of ensuring regular and prolonged treatment in a transient population[8].

- On the one hand, health workers are keen to treat TB patients for several reasons[8,15]: refugee populations may be at high risk of infection; tuberculosis is a deadly disease if left untreated; the treatment is very effective in preventing TB deaths and is one of the most cost-effective interventions; patient follow-up and compliance to treatment may be facilitated by good access to populations in camps, due to 'confinement' conditions in some closed camps. In addition, prolonged crisis and long-standing refugee settlements are increasingly observed, and TB may arise as a significant problem in these populations. There is therefore often heavy pressure to start such a programme, not only from the health staff but also from the host country's health authorities, donors and refugees themselves.

- On the other hand, TB programs on refugee sites may easily fail for several reasons[8,14,15]: the difficulties of ensuring treatment compliance in highly transient populations, whose mobility is unforeseen (relocation in other sites, repatriation); short-term mandates of most relief agencies, resulting in insufficient commitment in terms of time and resources,and lack of experience in supervising lengthy therapy; frequent security problems which may aggravate the usually poor compliance and lead to the withdrawal of health agencies; limited financial resources in the post-emergency phase and high cost of (short-course) treatment; the desire of providing no better health services to refugees than those available to local citizens.

Health workers should be aware that ineffective programmes may do more harm than good as inappropriate treatment affects both the patient and the whole community for two reasons[1,8,15]:

1. It may prolong infectiousness beyond the natural course, which means that a good number of sputum-positive patients will survive longer, although not cured, and will continue to spread the infection; this will further increase TB transmission throughout the community.

2. It can help create and spread multi-drug resistant bacilli.

Objectives of tuberculosis treatment programmes

As was previously stated, a TB programme is, in theory, relatively simple. It consists of a proper microscopic diagnosis, treatment (chemotherapy with 3 to 4 drugs) over a 6-month period or longer, and an appropriate follow-up. However, in practice, such a programme is difficult to manage as it requires sustained supervision and monitoring (see below) and the length of treatment in itself is an important obstacle to patient compliance. Once a programme is started, case detection and management must be properly conducted.

TB programmes directed at refugees generally have the overall objective of reducing the morbidity, mortality and transmission of the disease[1,6]. Reducing the transmission requires early detection and proper treatment of patients with positive sputum, which are the most contagious cases and also those at most risk of dying. Therefore, the overall objective is met by giving priority to the treatment of patients with positive sputum.

In addition, TB programmes should aim at curing a high proportion of all detected smear-positive patients (see below). High cure rates can only be obtained through good quality programmes; in terms of public health, cure rates lower than 60% to 70% render programmes almost useless and may even be harmful for the community.

The major objective of a refugee TB programme is to achieve a minimum cure rate of 85% for smear-positive patients passively detected[1]. Passive case finding must be the rule until very high and sustained cure rates have been achieved over a long period; then active case finding can be organized.

Note that WHO has defined the following targets for global TB control to be achieved by the year 2000:
– to cure 85% of detected positive smear cases, and
– to detect 70% of all existing cases.

Minimum conditions for starting a TB programme

The first principle is that no harm should be done, either to the individual or the community (see above). The International Union against Tuberculosis and Lung disease has stated that if you cannot ensure that a patient will be treated properly, you must carefully consider whether it is ethical to treat such a patient at all[12].

Before considering whether or not to initiate a TB programme, 3 absolute conditions must be present[1]:

1. The basic health priorities must have been adequately addressed and the health situation must be under control. A TB programme cannot take place in the emergency phase when resources have to be devoted to more urgent needs.

2. The implementing organization must guarantee a long-term commitment of at least 1 year (12-15 months) from taking on the first case. This implies that the agency in charge is not only prepared to stay for at least 12-15 months, but can also secure the input of sufficient resources to carry out such a programme during this period.

3. The population is expected to remain stable so that TB patients will be able to complete their treatment. Usually the time refugees will remain on a site can only be guessed at: the camp may suddenly be closed down, plans for relocating or repatriating refugees may be drawn up but deadlines are frequently not respected, the security situation might deteriorate, etc. Here again, the 'life expectancy' of the settlement should be at least 9-12 months.

This means that both the stability of the refugee population, and the commitment of the implementing agency need to be assessed before taking any decision in regard to a TB programme.

These conditions also imply that there are certain circumstances which definitively prevent the implementation of a refugee tuberculosis programmes:

Absolute contraindications to initiating a tuberculosis programme in a refugee setting

- Emergency phase following the population displacement
- Open warfare or significant insecurity
- Very unstable population (e.g. nomadic, or population moving up and down a border area)
- Major health problems not correctly addressed (e.g. serious disease outbreak)

Once the decision to start a TB treatment programme has been taken, a number of requirements will have to be met before the programme can be implemented.

- Clear protocols or guidelines referring to all aspects of the programme should be prepared: case definition, possible outcomes, treatment regimens including specific cases (relapse, treatment failure and defaulting), data collection, and evaluation.

- Monitoring and evaluation must be organized from the beginning, with all the required forms for registration and data collection made available (laboratory register, patient identity card, TB treatment card, TB register, etc.).

- A proper laboratory with well-trained staff is indispensable; the quality control of slides by a reference laboratory must be ensured.

- Sufficient supplies of drugs, laboratory items and food supplements must be secured for the estimated number of patients.

- The programme should be supervised by one person, preferably a medical doctor, and in each treatment site a person should be designated to be responsible for TB treatment.

- Everything possible should be foreseen for ensuring the best possible level of compliance, and a system for tracing defaulters through the home-visitor network should be set up.

- The proposed refugee treatment programme should be discussed and agreed upon with national authorities. A general principle, recommended by the UNHCR, is to strenghten the national tuberculosis programme in the area, in order to help them to cope with the increased number of patients to treat, if this is feasible[1]. In practice, this strategy can be followed in open situations, but in camp settings, a specific TB programme needs to be set up within the camp as part of the health care activities[1]. The same is true as regards internally displaced people living in an area which is not controlled by a government. In any case, there needs to be excellent collaboration and coordination between NGOs involved in tuberculosis treatment, and the TB control programme of the host country[1,15].

Essential elements in the implementation of TB programmes

CHEMOTHERAPY

Short-course chemotherapy, using directly observed therapy, is the recommended treatment for refugees and displaced populations[1,15].

Short-term treatment with 4 drugs achieves very good cure rates, diminishes the risk of drug-resistance, and improves compliance by reducing the length of treatment. It also reduces the number of failures and the risk of relapses, and thus the need for expensive retreatment schemes[2]. The only disadvantage seems to be its cost, but operational studies have concluded that it is more cost-effective than longer-course treatment (lower cost per patient cured and lower cost per death averted). This type of treatment may be difficult to establish in some countries whose national programmes still resort to older and longer regimens. In such cases, every effort should be made to promote the short-course regimen with the authorities, or a different regimen must be introduced for the refugees since these need adequate treatment in the shortest possible time[1].

A six-month regimen is preferred because the uncertainty of the duration of the present situation makes it urgent that treatment is completed as soon as possible, in case refugees are forced to move[1]; but in very stable refugee situations, when the national programme policy of the host country recommends an eight-month regimen, this scheme could be adopted. Whenever possible, the use of thiacetazone should be avoided because of its side-effects on HIV-positive patients (see further)[18]. The directly observed therapy - or DOT - refers to the system in which each dose of medication adminis-trated to the patient is observed by the health staff to ensure that it is taken and swallowed. The DOT, which is currently recommended by the WHO, must be adopted in refugee situations because it is the best way to deal effectively with an unstable population. It should be supervised by qualified staff[1,15].

MEANS OF ENSURING A GOOD LEVEL OF COMPLIANCE

A good level of compliance is mandatory in order to achieve a high cure rate, and all possible measures should therefore be taken to ensure that patients receive treatment daily throughout its duration.

Such measures include[2,5,8,14]:

– directly observed therapy, administrated daily,

– hospitalization if required,

– special housing if required (TB units),

– treatment free of charge,

– use of incentives, such as food supplementation,

– early tracing of defaulters, using home-visitors,

– informing patients about the disease and the consequences of interrupting treatment,

– developing a good and trusting relationship between staff and patients and between staff and supervisor,

– other measures adapted to the situation: the requirement for a signed contract between the patient and the TB programme is currently recommended[1]; a reimbursable deposit has been requested in some refugee camps (e.g. Thailand refugee camps).

SUPERVISION

Supervision should be carefully organized from the start of the programme. This should include technical supervision of the staff, laboratory and data collection. Particular attention should be paid to the relationship with patients. The supervisor, who should have a public health approach and be well informed about the principles of TB control, will be responsible for final decisions on diagnosis and treatment, and should be assigned for at least 6 months.

MONITORING AND EVALUATION

All the necessary elements for adequate data collection must be in place and implemented from the very beginning. A strict registration system should be organized with proper forms to be used in all the facilities concerned (out-patient department, in-patient department and laboratory). The same definitions - preferably the standard international definitions - for identifying disease, categorizing patients, and determining the outcome of treatment should be used throughout the programme[19]. Standard surveillance information can be given in the routine surveillance report, but this is not sufficient for a proper monitoring of the programme.

Evaluation is an on-going process for allowing the early identification of any problems occurring in the programme and the implementation of necessary solutions. A tuberculosis programme must be evaluated in regard to its ability to cure positive smear patients and not simply its capacity to treat them[7]. This also means that patients who have completed their treatment should not automatically be considered as cured. Case findings and treatment outcomes must be reported on a quarterly basis following the cohort analysis method[6]. WHO considers that, 'Cohort reporting is the best way to accurately assess the quality of treatment, treatment services, case management and, indirectly, staff performance, because it gives the basis for calculating the proportion of patients cured (numerator) out of the total registered for treatment (denominator) in a given period of time: cure rate'[6].

> **Evaluation is crucial and has to be organized from the start:**
>
> **No evaluation, no programme.**

When to stop a TB programme in a refugee setting

A TB programme should be stopped when[1]:
– the minimum requirements are no longer being met (or were never met),
– the cure rates are too low (e.g. below 60% or 70%),
– the defaulting rate is too high,
– population displacement is foreseen (closure of the camp and relocation or repatriation),
– the withdrawal of the implementing agency is foreseen.

Where population movements or the departure of the implementing agency are foreseen, the admission of new cases should be stopped in time to allow all patients to finish their treatment (for instance, 8 months before the date of departure where treatment lasts for 6 months). If repatriation is intended, it is usually unrealistic to expect that patients will be able to complete treatment after repatriating, as it is unlikely that there will be a national programme functioning in the home country; in any case, patients will have other priorities when they first return. The agency in charge of a TB programme should also take into account that there is little likelihood of another agency taking over the programme, since different agencies have different priorities in regard to intervention.

Specific problems in regard to TB programmes

• When no refugee tuberculosis programme can be implemented - for instance because the requirements are not met - patients should be transferred to the existing TB programme of the host country. Tuberculosis treatment should never be started on an individual basis.

• When patients have previously been under treatment elsewhere: they should be transferred into the existing programme if there is one, or complete their treatment under individual follow-up. However, this is a rather rare event.

• When patients repatriate spontaneously while still under treatment (see Part IV): they should be considered as defaulters. High defaulting rates are one of the main reasons for discontinuing a programme.

TUBERCULOSIS IN CHILDREN

TB is often suspected when children do not gain weight despite appropriate intensive feeding. It is known that TB and malnutrition are linked: malnutrition predisposes to TB and TB results in malnutrition. Clinical features in children are not specific and diagnosis is difficult because children do not produce sputum. This also means that they do not spread the disease. There are two possibilities:

• If a tuberculosis programme exists, diagnosis will be made after a nutritional assessment and follow-up to rule out nutritional problems as cause of the absence of weight gain, AND a good medical assessment to rule out all other possible medical causes. A score system, despite its limitations, can be a helpful tool[1,20].

- If there is no tuberculosis programme in the refugee site, no specific treatment will be given; there cannot be any 'small TB programme for children' in a refugee situation.

TUBERCULOSIS AND HIV

(see *HIV, AIDS and STD* above)

Immuno-deficiency due to HIV considerably increases the risk of developing clinical tuberculosis. Recent studies suggest that between 5% and 10% of persons co-infected with HIV and *Mycobacterium tuberculosis* will develop tuberculosis each year, compared with less than 0.2% of persons infected with *Mycobacterium tuberculosis* but not HIV[9,10]. The HIV epidemic has and will continue to have a tremendous impact on tuberculosis infection.

Nevertheless, whether patients are HIV-positive or not, early diagnosis and treatment of smear-positive cases remains the first priority in the fight against the spread of TB. There is no difference in the treatment given to HIV-positive or -negative patients; the same short-course chemotherapy and treatment schemes should be applied (with the exception of thiacetazone which should be excluded in any case).

HIV testing of TB patients is not justified and even useless since it would not change anything with regard to treatment (same treatment for HIV-positive and -negative patients). Furthermore, HIV testing can be detrimental to HIV-positive patients: they may well have difficulty in coping with the knowledge of their HIV status - since HIV counselling is rarely available - and they will be at risk of being rejected or driven out of the community if their HIV status is known (and confidentiality is extremely difficult to achieve in such conditions)[13].

SPUTUM-NEGATIVE PULMONARY TUBERCULOSIS AND EXTRA-PULMONARY TUBERCULOSIS

Since these patients are not contagious, their treatment is not considered a priority (see above). Enrolling too many of them in the TB programme would only be to the detriment of the main priority which is to cure all smear-positive cases. In case of life-threatening conditions, the decision to enrol them in the programme should be taken on an individual basis by an experienced medical doctor supervising the programme; strict protocols, adapted to the local circumstances, should be applied in order to decide on the admission of smear-negative cases (e.g. start first with antibiotic treatment for pulmonary smear-negative cases). The proportion of non-smear-positive patients under treatment should be kept low: for instance, it can be decided that the percentage of non smear-positive patients should not exceed 20% of the total number of cases under treatment (non-smear-positive cases are patients with pulmonary TB and negative smears, or patients with extra-pulmonary tuberculosis).

DIAGNOSIS POSSIBILITIES

Sputum examination is the best way to detect smear-positive patients (the main target of the programme), to follow-up their response to treatment and to decide whether or not they are cured. X-rays or cultures are usually not used in refugee settings since they are not necessary for a TB treatment programme, are seldom available on refugee sites, are difficult to interpret, and will not have any impact on transmission (TB patients who could be only detected by culture or X-ray are not likely to be contagious). Other diagnostic tests (PPD or BCG tests) are less reliable than direct microscopy for detecting smear-positive patients, and are not advised.

PREVENTION AND BCG VACCINATION

BCG vaccine provides a high degree of protection against serious forms of disease in children (miliary tuberculosis and tuberculous meningitis). It is thus strongly recommended that BCG is included in the Expanded Programme of Immunization (EPI) as soon as this starts in the refugee settlement. Whether or not it protects against other forms of tuberculosis in children or protects adults is still largely a matter of debate[2]. BCG vaccination is recommended for all infants at birth or as soon as possible after birth, unless they present clear signs of immuno-deficiency (e.g. clinical AIDS)[2].

Preventive chemotherapy (e.g. with isoniazid) should not be undertaken in refugee settlements since it does not contribute in decreasing the transmission, good compliance is difficult to achieve, the high burden of organizing it outweighs the benefits, and the emphasis should rest exclusively on curing smear-positive patients passively detected[1,2].

Principal recommendations regarding TB treatment programmes in refugee settings

- A TB treatment programme should not be undertaken in a refugee population, unless:
  - the emergency phase is over and major health problems are under control;
  - the agency in charge can guarantee a long-term committment of at least one year;
  - the refugee population is expected to remain stable;
  - there is no significant insecurity.

- A number of technical requirements must be met before the programme can be implemented: clear protocols and guidelines are developed, monitoring is organized, a proper laboratory is ready, there is a sufficient supply of drugs and other material, etc.

- The treatment should be based on:
  - passive screening,
  - focus on smear-positive TB patients, diagnosed by direct microscopic examination,
  - directly-observed, short-course chemotherapy, daily administered,
  - all measures to ensure a good compliance,
  - evaluation by quarterly cohorts.

✎ Key reference

1. Interagency working group on tuberculosis and refugees. *Guidelines for tuberculosis control among refugee and displaced populations* [draft]. Geneva: UN, 1996.

Other references

2. Murray, C J, Styblo, K, Rouillon, A. Tuberculosis in developing countries: burden, intervention and cost. *Bull IUATLD*, 1990, 65(1): 6-24.

3. Sang Richard, K A, Varaine, F. *Assessment of the tuberculosis control programs in the refugees camps of Kenya. Report on a consultation for the Kenyan Ministry of Health.* [Internal Report]. Paris: Epicentre, 1994.

4. Van Gorkom, J, Riviera, A. *Report of a visit to Hagadera, Ifo and Dagahaley on the 10 and 11 January 1995.* [Internal Report]. Brussels: Médecins Sans Frontières, 1995.

5. Bradol, J H, Carr, E., Naw Kri, M, Rigal, J. Treatment results of 288 smear-positive TB patients, Karen refugees, 1987-1992, Thailand. *Medical News*, 1993, 2(4): 10-13.

6. WHO. *Framework for effective tuberculosis control.* Geneva: WHO, 1994. WHO/TB/94.17.

7. Paquet, C. Evaluation of tuberculosis control programmes, quarterly cohort method. *Medical News*, 1993, 2(4): 14-16.

8. Rieder, H L, Snider, D E, Toole, M J, Waldman, R J, et al. Tuberculosis control in refugee settlements. *Tubercle*, 1989, 70(2): 127-34.

9. Dolin, P J, Raviglione, M C, Kochi, A. Global tuberculosis incidence and mortality during 1990-2000. *Bull. WHO*, 1994, 72(2): 213-20.

10. Narain, J P, Raviglione, M C, Kochi, A. HIV associated tuberculosis in developing countries: epidemiology and strategy for prevention. *Tub Lung Dis*, 1992, 73: 311-21.

11. Toole, M J, Waldman, R J. Prevention of excess mortality in refugees and displaced populations in developing countries. *JAMA*, 1990, 263(24): 3296-302.

12. *Tuberculosis guide for low income countries.* Paris: IUATLD, 1994.

13. Temmerman, M, Ndinya-Achola, J, Ambani, J, Piot, P. The right not to know HIV-test result. *The Lancet*, 1995, 345(8955): 969-70.

14. Sukrakanchana Trikham, P, Puechal, X, Rigal, J, Rieder, H L. 10-year assessment of treatment outcome among Cambodian refugees with sputum smear-positive tuberculosis in Khao-I-Dang, Thailand. *Tub Lung Dis*, 1992. 73: 384-87.

15. Porter, J, Kessler, C. Tuberculosis in refugees: a neglected dimension of the 'global epidemic of tuberculosis'. *Trans Roy Soc Trop Med Hyg*, 1995. 89(3): 241-2.

16. Spinaci, G, De Virgilio, M, Bugiani, D, Linari, G, Bertolaso. Tuberculin survey among Afghan refugee children. Tuberculosis control program among Afghan refugees in North West Frontier Province Pakistan. *Tubercle*, 1989, 70:83-92.

17. Miles, S H, Maat, R B. A successful supervised outpatient short-course tuberculosis treatment program in an open refugee camp on the Thai-Cambodian border. *Am Rev Respir Dis*, 1984, 130: 827-30.

18. Harries, A D, Maher D. *TB/HIV: A clinical manual.* Romano Canavese, Italy: WHO, 1996.

19. WHO. *Tuberculosis Programme. Managing tuberculosis at district level. A training course.* Geneva: WHO, 1994.

Psycho-social and mental health

Introduction

In refugee health care, in particular during the emergency phase, there is usually a tendency to focus entirely on the physical needs of refugees: the provision of food, water, medical care, etc. But even in the post-emergency phase, it is only rarely that attempts are made to address the psycho-social problems of refugees, despite obvious awareness of the traumatic experiences many of them have been through[5]. There are multiple examples of refugee health programmes where this aspect has been totally neglected. For instance, the training of health staff does not usually address the fact that many patients' complaints might have a psychological rather than a purely medical origin.

However, it is important that attention should be paid to the psycho-social needs of refugees. First of all, in order to survive, refugees have to be active enough to take advantage of the services offered; some of them may be too traumatized to react in this way and will require assistance. Secondly, once physical survival is assured, many people may start to show physical or psychological symptoms that are rooted in their traumatic experiences[2]. A programme that addresses this problem, but also aims at preventing longer-term, or even permanent damage, will require planning and this should ideally begin during the emergency phase.

Although more attention has been given to the psychological condition of refugees over recent years, concrete interventions with proven results are still hard to find. Only rare examples have been described and there is no generally recognized or ideal design for psycho-social and mental health programmes. Effective strategies have not yet been defined. As a result, the strategy proposed in this chapter is still at the stage of a pilot project. It is a community-based approach, integrated into the overall refugee assistance programme, based on actual field experience.

Background to psycho-social and mental health problems

In a refugee crisis, large numbers of people are driven from their homes. Most of them flee to save their lives. When the displacement is due to conflicts, many of them may have witnessed atrocities or themselves been victims of violence; some of them may have participated in that violence. All have lost homes, at least temporarily, and very often relatives, friends and neighbours. They have fled from a critical situation, endured a journey that was a traumatic event in itself, and now have to face a new kind of life in a refugee settlement, where they have to find the energy to make a new start; for some of them, this may be a repeat experience.

At the same time, both individuals and the community-at-large have to find ways of coping with recent events. What happens to the orphans and the elderly? Can widows organize themselves? Is the community still organized according to traditional structures or is there a new social structure for the situation? Does it dictate where each family should settle and towards which individuals or networks they must now demonstrate loyalty and support in order to survive? How should the dead be buried? If large-scale killing was the reason behind the displacement, is revenge to be taken immediately or will it be postponed? Can new neighbours be trusted? And what about all the people who are missing?

Refugees have to quickly find their way among the relief programmes that may be available; they have to learn how to get ration cards, where to settle, where to get water and firewood, etc. Every family has to 'get organized': find a way to divide tasks such as looking after children, fetching water, food, wood and material to build a shelter, devise some kind of income-generating activity so as to be able to acquire food to back up insufficient rations, etc.

A part of the population, who are not able to benefit from relief programmes because they are simply too depressed and too emotionally affected to care at all, may vanish even before an initial assessment is conducted in the settlement. These individuals may have become trapped in a vicious downward spiral: grief creates apathy, and they are too numb and listless to attend food distributions; lack of food then makes them vulnerable and this in turn increases their sense of complete hopelessness and eventually leads to death.

This may only be the situation for a relatively small group, but there are likely to be very many others who will internalize their grief, (and become 'worried sick'), but do not know why they have headaches, stomach-aches or suffer from insomnia. If they do know, fear of the worst stigma - being pointed out as 'a crazy person' - makes them keep their real worries to themselves as they stand silently in line for the out-patients department. They may eventually develop health problems which are frequently hard to tackle and become a burden for the future - not only on themselves, but on their families and on the community.

In conclusion, refugees are by definition groups of people who have frequently lived through trauma which they may still be experiencing in the refugee situation. Although refugee emergency programmes usually only give priority to the provision of basic needs, a substantial group within the population may require additional support in order to benefit from the resources and services provided. But in any case, some kind of support will be required for the population-at-large in order to prevent psychopathologies developing and the unnecessary medicalization of psycho-social problems. It is therefore to the benefit of the whole community, not just the individuals concerned, that support is given to help them develop ways of coping adequately with what they have lived through. This will strengthen the community, which is essential for its survival in the future. Within the cross-cultural realm of refugee situations and relief programmes, it should be noted that individual healing depends on a social context in which the traumatized are enabled to make themselves known and seek help. It is this socio-cultural setting which determines not only how trauma and symptoms are defined, but also how they should be dealt with.

Epidemiology

It is recognized that under normal circumstances, about 20% of people who have undergone traumatic experiences require therapeutic help in order to come to grips with the new situation[1]. In refugee situations, where the circumstances are definitely not normal, this percentage can be expected to be much higher.

The most common psycho-social symptoms and signs that are observed in refugees across different cultures include:

– anxiety disorders,

– depressive disorders,

– suicidal thoughts and attempts at suicide,

– anger, aggression and violent behaviour,

– drug and alcohol abuse,

– paranoia, suspicion and distrust,

– somatic presentation of psycho-social problems and hysteria,

– insomnia.

It is important to make a distinction between psycho-social problems and psychopathology. The type of intervention described below is directed towards the detection, prevention and management of psycho-social problems. In every population, there will be psychiatric patients who might have similar symptoms to those mentioned above. However, psycho-social intervention is not directed at a specific group of psychiatric cases within the population, but at the population as a whole through implementing preventive activities. Such a community-based approach targets the large numbers of people with psycho-social problems; although there may be a parallel spin-off effect that reaches some of the more urgent psychiatric problems.

The main problem is the distress experienced by the survivors of traumatic events. Although depressive reactions are often found in such people, a recognized, specific syndrome, known as post-traumatic stress disorder (PTSD) has been described and is frequently encountered in a number of different societies. However, whether PTSD can be used as a universally applicable diagnosis remains questionable. Typical PTSD signs and symptoms might have different meanings within different cultural contexts and, conversely, other cultures may display different signs and symptoms indicating post-traumatic disorders.

Some knowledge of anthropology is therefore essential for arriving at a diagnostic interpretation of the signs and symptoms recorded, and also for adapting methods to help the healing process. One of the central concepts of trauma theory is a search for meaning, and this is important for constructing a new way of viewing the world and reconstructing basic assumptions to live by.

The cultural background and its importance

It is therefore necessary to adapt any general model of intervention to traditional beliefs, customs and social settings, and this requires a certain level of input from the refugee population. On the one hand, existing material developed for training community workers in effective mental health interventions can be used[2]. On the other hand, this material needs to be adapted through a constant dialogue and exchange of experiences and ideas with individuals and staff from the refugee community. The ways in which a community reacts are very much culture-bound and these patterns need to be understood: how it shows distress, how grief and bereavement are dealt with, and the patterns for the somatic translation of psycho-social problems.

The resources that are available in the community should be identified. On the organizational level, most preventive work is in fact social work and a mental health intervention conducted within a refugee setting should aim at bridging the gap between health programmes and social services, which will have the additional benefit of increasing the outreach capacity of both activities. On a more practical level, the customary ways of coping should be identified, including the availability of traditional healers, the religious and social support network, mourning rituals, etc.

Assessing this socio-cultural context is not necessarily as time-consuming as may appear at first glance. In addition to a vast body of anthropological literature, rapid appraisal techniques have been developed which, if applied by experienced social scientists, can lead to appropriate intervention for helping people cope with their trauma.

Description of interventions

The objectives of a psycho-social intervention are three-fold:
– to offer support to those who cannot cope with their traumatic experiences or psycho-social problems in the current situation,
– to prevent psycho-social problems from being treated as medical ones, resulting in an irrational use of health care facilities,
– to prevent psychopathologies developing.

In the first phase of an emergency situation, the refugee population requires all its time and energy to survive. Every defence mechanism will be mobilized in order to continue functioning at this survival level. At this time, the essence of a psycho-social intervention is therefore to mobilize social mechanisms within the community to help individuals and families cope with events; it is particularly important to reach the most vulnerable people.

In a later phase, although the community overall may have established a basic degree of order and routine, nevertheless, there will still be a substantial group of people showing persistent emotional problems or psychopathology as a longer-term effect of their traumatic experiences. At this time, a more therapeutic approach is required.

THE FIRST PHASE

In this phase, intervention aims both at identifying the most vulnerable people who are unable to cope, and at mobilizing social support within the community while reinforcing the normal coping mechanisms. In addition, the goal is to prevent psycho-social problems from becoming medical ones, by providing knowledge about normal and pathological stress reactions to the population at large. The activities described below can be undertaken at this stage.

However, there have been very few experiences of psycho-social interventions so early on, and these possibilities can only be offered as suggestions:

- Information should be gathered about customary ways of showing stress, coping mechanisms, cultural approach to psycho-social issues and the social support structures that may be used to deal with psycho-social needs. This type of information generally requires an anthropological assessment.

- Short information sessions to increase awareness should be provided for staff working in the community (e.g. home-visitors, health workers, social workers, if any, etc.) in order to assist them to identify through active screening those people who are unable to cope, or even survive, on their own; they may sometimes also be able to identify and refer psycho-social problems or major psychopathologies. If feasible, they may also mobilize the mechanisms of the social network in order to provide help for those who are at risk.

- Health staff should be trained to identify different ways in which mental distress may be expressed (e.g. somatically, or via aggression and behavioural problems), so that they will know that such cases should be referred to existing social networks, or eventually to psycho-social services, rather than prescribed medication.

- The population should be made generally aware of the possible existence of such problems and of normal and pathological reactions to stress.

- Other organizations involved in refugee assistance should be informed of the importance of psycho-social issues.

THE SECOND PHASE

In the second phase, intervention aims at offering therapeutic activities or treatment to people suffering from persistent emotional problems or psycho-pathologies. Here again, there are no standard guidelines or general consensus on the methods to be used and the actions described below are examples of what may be developed.

- Groups of psycho-social workers may be trained to provide emotional support. These groups should be formed from workers who are also members of the community and who have already shown sensitivity in their work with regard to psycho-social problems (e.g. health workers, home-visitors, etc.). A training curriculum may be partly composed of existing material and partly developed in the field in line with the cultural patterns. The subjects covered may include recognizing major psychopathologies, the indications for medical referral, individual counselling techniques, forming and conducting counselling groups, relaxation exercises, etc.

- Therapeutic activities may be offered to groups, preferably whose members have a natural link, such as groups of women, children, the elderly, or religious groups.

- Medical treatment in health facilities may be offered to individuals, when indicated. However, this requires that health staff receive further training in identifying and treating major psychopathologies (e.g. PTSD, depression, anxiety disorders and psychosis).

Conclusions

Preparations for a psycho-social programme should start in the emergency phase. It is necessary to take time to become acquainted with the socio-cultural setting, to select a first group of people to work with, to learn from these people and to train them. The most vulnerable people will vanish first. It is important to make people working in the refugee community aware of how psycho-social problems can be identified, and particularly how to deal with these problems. It has been found that community workers in many refugee situations, themselves part of the refugee population and having to deal with the same traumas, tend to ignore cases which look complicated and emotionally difficult. If a psycho-social programme succeeds in improving an understanding of these problems among the population, the community as a whole will benefit. The community itself will be reinforced by bringing groups of health workers and social workers from different programmes closer together.

◥ References

1. Kleber, R J, Brom, D. *Coping with trauma. Theory, prevention and treatment.* Amsterdam: Swets & Zeitlinger, 1992: 27

2. WHO. *Mental health care in developing countries: A critical appraisal of research findings.* Geneva: WHO Tech Rep Ser No. 698, 1984.

3. Marsella, J, Bornemann, T et al. *Amidst peril and pain. The mental health and well being of the world's refugees.* Washington DC.: American Psychological Association, 1994.

4. Hiegel, J P. Psycho-social and mental health needs of refugees experience from SE Asia. *Trop Doctor*, 1991, 21 (Suppl 1): 63-6.

PART IV

Repatriation and resettlement

Repatriation and resettlement

Introduction

Repatriation (the return of refugees to their own country) is a key element in the process of restoring that country to a situation of stability. Indeed, whatever lies at the root of the refugee problem (war, drought, ethnic violence or a combination of factors), repatriation is often essential if peace and development are to be guaranteed in the home country. In any case, life as a refugee is a life on hold, and refugees usually want a solution that allows them to return home, and take control over their own lives. It must be stressed, however, that repatriation is not always the ideal solution. Indeed, it is only one of 3 possible 'permanent solutions' for refugee populations and not the natural outcome of all refugee situations. The other two solutions are integration into the host country or reinstallation in a third country.

The number of situations where repatriation is a major issue, and the number of refugees repatriating, are on the increase. For example, between 1970 and 1993, some 3.5 million refugees have been repatriated in Africa alone[1]. NGOs, including health agencies, are called upon to participate in the repatriation process, and have an important role to play in terms of monitoring and providing assistance. It is therefore important that health agencies have a basic understanding of the overall repatriation process as well as the specific related aspects and problems that commonly arise.

Contrary to most popular beliefs, repatriation is much more than just a journey back home. It is a process, often complex, which also encompasses political, social and economic reintegration into the home country. Repatriation is also often used and influenced by political interests (e.g. elections). It is important to know this, so that assistance focuses on sustainable reintegration and not only on promoting the return of refugees.

The resettlement of internally displaced persons back to their home areas involves the same issues as the repatriation of refugees. However, this type of return movement is more difficult to monitor and assist, and UNHCR is not usually involved.

Deciding to return home

ORGANIZED VERSUS SPONTANEOUS REPATRIATION

All refugees have a right to return home to their respective countries of origin. Repatriation should always be voluntary - at the freely expressed will of the refugees themselves. Nevertheless, there is an important distinction to be made between ORGANIZED and SPONTANEOUS repatriation.

- **Spontaneous repatriation** occurs when refugees make their own decision to return home. Assistance may be provided to facilitate the return and thereby influence the decision to repatriate, but there is no systematic participation of NGOs or UNHCR in the process.

- **Organized repatriation** refers to an overall programme designed to actively promote and 'stimulate' voluntary repatriation, and is planned by the body responsible for refugee welfare (host government or UNHCR). When conditions are considered to be acceptable for return, repatriation is organized by agencies or governments rather than by the refugees themselves, and large-scale programmes are usually implemented to assist the mass movement of refugees. Refugees are required to participate systematically in repatriation programmes. They must register and hand back their refugee status; in return, they often receive a substantial relief package. The support provided will often include transportation, food assistance and a resettlement package.

Organized repatriation is not the norm. It occurs less frequently than spontaneous repatriation and it is estimated that only 10% of repatriations took place through organized programmes over recent years[1].

It should be emphasized that over the past few years many spontaneous repatriations or resettlements took place to an area that is still in conflict. This probably reflects a refugee choice for the lesser of two evils when conditions in the area of asylum are worse than those of the home country (conflict, drought or discrimination). In these situations, it may be very difficult to provide assistance to refugees, due to problems of security or accessibility[4]. As UN agencies are usually not involved in this kind of repatriation, NGOs may be the sole agencies providing assistance.

WHEN AND HOW REFUGEES DECIDE TO REPATRIATE

It is important to understand that the decision to repatriate, and when and how to do so, is complex and based on many factors which relate primarily to current living conditions and future expectations for both the country of asylum and the country of origin[1,2,3].

- In the country of asylum (host country), these factors include: the level of (in)security, the type and quality of services provided (health care, food distributions, etc.), the time already spent in exile, the degree of integration, and the pressures exerted on refugees by local authorities, political and other organizations (including UNHCR) to encourage them to leave. A major factor is the degree to which refugees are in a position to determine their own lives.

- In the country of origin (home country), the main factors to be taken into account are: the possibilities for rebuilding a sustainable level of existence, the level of (in)security, such as the presence of mines or the demobilization of warring factions, the political situation (e.g. scheduled elections), the degree of social disruption in the home area, the type and quality of services and assistance provided, especially when compared to those provided in the asylum area, the availability of land for agriculture, the availability of, and access to water, and the degree of cultural and emotional attachment to the land.

- The physical conditions under which the return will take place also have to be taken into account in determining its feasibility:
  - whether transportation is available,
  - whether the way back is accessible and safe,
  - whether basic needs (water, food and shelter) will be provided on the way.

The timing of the return home is crucial, particularly the timing of the agricultural season; refugees will try to repatriate so as to be able to build shelters and clear land in time for planting crops (at least in agricultural areas). However, other time factors may also be important, such as returning in time to lay claim to vacated lands and participate in elections.

'PUSH' AND 'PULL' FACTORS[1]

Although refugees may have some economic activities in the host country, they are often largely dependent on international aid or help provided by the local population. Assistance to refugees is sometimes reduced in an attempt to push refugees to leave the host country: for example, 'push factors' may include the gradual phasing out of food distributions and a reduction in some of the services provided.

On the other hand, 'pull factors' tend to attract refugees back to their home environment. These may include improved land access, the right to vote in elections, a reasonable level of infrastructure (road and health services), farming prospects, improved security and protection, etc.

'Pull factors' aim to reduce the apparent hostility of the home environment and increase the prospects for establishing a viable existence that makes returning attractive. 'Push factors' aim to reduce the viability of remaining in the host area by reducing the support provided, thus forcing people to return. Repatriation should only be encouraged when conditions in the home areas are safe. In most situations, assistance should focus on improving conditions in the home area. Such 'pull factor' activities will ensure there is a better appreciation of the conditions in the home area and provide for sustainable return. Forcing refugees out of asylum areas by reducing services neither constitutes a voluntary decision to return home nor does it encourage the likelihood of reintegration in the home area. The risk is that a former refugee population may simply become a large destitute population in the home country. 'Push factors', therefore, can almost never have any ethical justification.

Returning home

REPATRIATION IN SEVERAL STAGES

It is rare that repatriation is simply a journey from a refugee camp to the home in which the refugee used to live. The return usually takes place in stages, particularly during a spontaneous repatriation. In the first stage, some people may return to investigate the conditions for return. In the second stage, a few stronger family members - mainly young males - may return to prepare land and create conditions for the return of the rest of the family. Many repatriations thus involve some members returning and starting farming or economic activities while still maintaining links with the host area. It may be necessary for some family members to remain in the refugee camps to look after the sick and vulnerable during the early phases of return, and to continue to receive food and other assistance. Only when conditions are ready for a fully sustainable existence will the whole family repatriate.

SOCIAL AND ECONOMIC REINTEGRATION

Repatriation also encompasses reintegration, or the resettlement of refugees into their home areas and the rebuilding of their social and economic activities. This economic reintegration is a key element for a successful repatriation. The presence, or absence, of the conditions for reintegration is usually a major issue for refugees in deciding to return.

It may be difficult to reach a successful social and economic reintegration depending on a variety of factors:
- the economic situation in the home area, such as potential for agriculture, commercial activity, access to credit, entitlement to land, etc.;
- the length of time spent in exile, due to effects on education and language, loss of skills, changes in socio-cultural habits, etc.;
- personal skills, including those acquired when in exile;
- the political, social and economic systems and eventual changes in these systems;
- the level of assistance provided to returnees and whether this can ensure their survival until self-sufficiency is attained;
- development activities.

VULNERABLE GROUPS

(see *Socio-cultural Aspects* in Part I)

Some groups of refugees are at greater risk of not surviving the return home or the difficult period of re-integration. This is especially true for female-headed households, which often form a large proportion of refugee populations, especially when civil war was the cause of displacement. There is a variety of reasons why female-headed households are more vulnerable: alienation from the traditional social system, psychological trauma due to loss of family members or possible violence including sexual abuse, economic dependency, male-oriented economic opportunities and poor access to resources, especially land, etc. Other vulnerable groups include the elderly, the malnourished, the sick (see below), orphans, and the disabled.

Vulnerable groups are often the last to repatriate and may have special needs during the journey (e.g. transportation and health care). Relief agencies should identify which groups are likely to be the most vulnerable during the repatriation process and implement special programmes to support them. Any repatriation plan must therefore give priority to the reintegration of vulnerable groups.

Assisting return

PLANNING FOR REPATRIATION AND REFUGEE PARTICIPATION

It is up to refugees to decide for themselves when it is time to go home, but external assistance can play a crucial role in creating the conditions that encourage return. Planning for repatriation should begin as early as possible so that when the political and security conditions for return are in place, physical and economic barriers do not prevent it. This planning is usually coordinated by international organizations - mainly UNHCR in the case of refugees - and the host government, in close cooperation with refugee and other agencies involved in refugee assistance. Health agencies are generally called upon to participate in such planning.

Planning for repatriation requires an understanding of the potential living conditions for the refugee population, the agricultural timetable, and what needs have to be met in order for them to survive and rebuild their lives. The refugees themselves are the experts on these issues so it is essential to encourage their participation in the planning process and work with them to establish:

– the minimal conditions necessary before repatriation can occur,
– the risks to be faced and the main obstacles to returning home,
– whether there are specific events for which they want to return,
– which periods of the year are the best times to return,
– how the refugees will make the return home and what support should be provided,
– the minimum requirements for getting restarted and the best ways of assisting,
– who are the most vulnerable and what their special needs are.

GENERAL ASSISTANCE TO REPATRIATION

Repatriation assistance should address many aspects. It should aim at improving the situation in the home area (minimizing the constraints on returning home) and facilitating the return process while, at the same time, continuing to provide adequate levels of support in the country of asylum.

Refugees make the decision to repatriate on the basis of information regarding the situation in the home area, which they receive via several sources: rumours, first-hand accounts from friends and relatives who have gone back to assess the situation, propaganda and political messages. They will always have some news of home, but this information may be biased or distorted. NGOs and UN relief agencies - especially those working on both sides of the border - may have a very important role to play in facilitating the transmission of information to refugees. Updated information should ideally be made available on a regular basis. Visits to their homeland by refugee community leaders in order to assess the situation could be facilitated. Refugees often express a clear need for this kind of 'official information'[5]. Health agencies should at least provide information on health and nutritional services, the presence of mines, water supply, etc. (see below *Health assistance to repatriation*).

Relief agencies involved in repatriation generally provide support for the return and reintegration. This may include[1]:

– provision of a repatriation package adapted to local needs, either before departure or upon arrival (i.e. seeds, tools, food, blankets and sometimes cash);
– provision of food aid at the reception site. In principle, rations should cover the period from return until returnees are producing their own food;
– the organization of transit and reception centres, to provide temporary shelter and basic services during the repatriation process;
– securing access to water at the reception site (e.g. installation of hand pumps);
– rehabilitation of the infrastructure in home areas (health facilities, schools, roads, etc.);
– witnessing and monitoring security abuses, etc.

HEALTH ASSISTANCE TO REPATRIATION

Health assistance should be provided before, during, and after repatriation.

Before repatriation

Careful planning must begin a long time before repatriation is to take place. Health interventions must be undertaken both in the departure area (host area) and the reception area (country of return).

• In the departure area

Phasing out health assistance to refugees (see above 'Push factors') is almost never justified and medical services must be available until every refugee has left, particularly as the last to leave are usually those with the greatest health needs: women delayed by childbirth, malnourished children, the elderly, and patients with chronic illnesses[5]. However, the level of activity and the capacity of health services (e.g. number of beds) may gradually reduce in line with the decreasing refugee population, but a minimum level of curative activities must always be available.

Special attention should be paid to any medical contraindications to repatriation as there are several health conditions which may prevent the return of refugees.

• Epidemics of communicable diseases with high mortality, such as cholera or shigellosis. Affected individuals are often too weak to travel; if they do, they may spread disease to a larger population.
• Pregnant women close to delivery (i.e. in the last weeks of pregnancy), and women who have just delivered.
• TB patients should be strongly advised not to leave the site before completing their treatment (see below).
• The same applies for very sick patients and severely malnourished children who may not survive the journey. Such patients should remain in the hospital or therapeutic feeding centre until they have recovered.
• Other vulnerable groups, such as the elderly, unaccompanied children, the disabled and patients with chronic illnesses are not real medical contra-indication to repatriation. However, they should only return when adequate conditions have been ensured (see above), and in assisted convoys.

If there is a TB programme in the camp, it is recommended to stop admitting new cases at least 8 months before the date foreseen for repatriation (if on a short course). Indeed, patients should ideally complete their treatment before repatriating (see *Tuberculosis Programmes* in Part III). It is usually unrealistic to expect that patients will be able to continue their treatment after they return home because there will rarely be a TB programme capable of ensuring an adequate follow up for them (there is often no functioning national programme), and patients are generally preoccupied by other priorities when they first return.

It can, however, happen that repatriation begins before all TB patients have completed their full course of treatment. They should then be persuaded to postpone repatriation until treatment has ended, although it is often very difficult to convince them to do this. Every effort must be made to ensure that these patients are fully aware of the seriousness of the disease, the consequences of defaulting, and the schedule they must follow to complete the treatment; for example, information sessions may be organized with family members also invited to attend[7]. They should be given all the necessary documentation in regard to their health status and treatment.

Immunization campaigns can be organized to maximize coverage before departure. Expanded Programmes on Immunization (EPI) in the home area will often lack resources and may be unable to cope with the influx of returnees. The first campaign should be launched at least 3 months before the repatriation period begins and be followed by 2 other campaigns for subsequent doses. Immunization campaigns also provide a good opportunity to screen children for malnutrition (by the mid-upper arm circumference measure - MUAC) and provide vitamin A supplementation. All malnourished children should be enrolled directly in nutritional programmes and mothers should be encouraged to keep children in the centres until they are strong enough to travel.

Health screening should take place before departure but this may depend on the form of repatriation (i.e. it is more difficult to plan when repatriation is spontaneous). However, caution should be taken to avoid screening being misinterpreted by refugees as a coercive measure; they should therefore be informed why it is being done.

The objectives of screening are[5,6]:

– the identification of vulnerable persons such as the sick, malnourished children, pregnant women, mothers with new-born babies, the elderly and the disabled;

– the education, referral and correct management of these vulnerable groups: information should be provided on the need to remain under treatment (for malnutrition and TB), the consequences of deciding to return, and the special programmes available to assist them during return;

– the identification of individuals who need to be referred to health services in their home area (they should receive a referral letter in the language of the home country);

– measles immunization: screening provides an opportunity to identify children who have not yet been immunized.

Other measures may be included in screening procedures but these largely depend on the national policy of the home country. Mandatory HIV testing has been decreed by the governments of some countries, but an HIV-positive result may mean the refugee is denied the right to return home. There is no public health justification for such practices, which are rejected by the UN and many NGOs[7]. All agencies should refuse any request to screen for AIDS and should lobby against mandatory testing (see *HIV, AIDS and STD* in Part III).

In areas where there are specific health risks (e.g. trypanosomiasis), it may be necessary to organize specific screening of all candidates for return so that those infected can be treated.

- In the country of origin

The Ministry of Health (MOH) of the home country and the health agencies working in the area must be contacted well in advance. This is important for several reasons:

- They can provide information with regard to the organization of the national health system, national health policies (e.g. EPI schedules, TB treatment, etc.) and the health and nutritional services available in the return area.

- If a good link is established, they can act as referral centres for patients, i.e. those with chronic illness, (e.g. diabetes), in order to maximize their continuity of care.

- It enables them to set up a coordination system for harmonizing assistance to returnees[5,6].

- It provides an opportunity to discuss the possibilities for integrating refugee health staff into national services.

Refugees need to know what services will be available to them in the home area, and what the requirements are for participating in these. It is therefore of paramount importance that the information collected in regard to services and programmes is passed onto the refugee[6,7,8,9].

Very often, health facilities in the home area require some level of rehabilitation. The requirements may range from basic repairs or the expansion of capacity (drug supplies, equipment, staff or the building itself), to building entirely new structures to cope with the influx of returnees. Rehabilitation should ideally be completed before repatriation begins. UNHCR may provide support to such projects (through funds for 'Quick Implementation Projects')[9].

If transit or reception centres are organized to assist the repatriation process, health posts provided with basic equipment should be set up along the transit route to ensure medical assistance for the returning population.

During repatriation (including arrival)

Special arrangements must be made to ensure that the basic needs of refugees are met during transportation. When refugees are transported in convoy (e.g. organized by UNHCR), some medical staff with basic equipment can accompany them to ensure health care, at least for the vulnerable groups. In many cases, refugees, including the elderly, the sick and small children, will often have to walk the whole way home carrying considerable quantities of possessions. It may therefore be essential to set up special way stations to provide food, water, temporary shelter, health care and a resting place. Vulnerable groups may travel in separate vehicles and receive special attention.

Screening for health problems may be organized where returnees arrive (in reception or transit centres) in order to:
– identify sick or wounded people and refer them for treatment;
– identify cases of a specific disease for referral to special programmes (e.g. trypanosomiasis);
– sometimes administer compulsory vaccines (e.g. yellow fever);
– facilitate contact between returnees and the nearest health service.

After repatriation

The restoration/rehabilitation of the health care system in the home country is essential[1]. In many instances, the refugees' home area has been devastated by a war that destroyed health facilities, disrupted public services and led to the departure of health staff. The home government will often lack the financial and human resources to restore these services. Assistance is required for the entire population affected by the war and to improve conditions for the return of the refugees.

• Health facilities, whether first-line facilities or referral facilities, will require reconstruction, upgrading and/or expansion. There is most often a need to rehabilitate buildings, replace basic equipment and supply drugs and medical materials. Drugs must also be supplied to treat chronic patients under treatment referred from host areas. Storage and transport facilities may also have to be provided.

• The rehabilitation of health services should start by reinstating adequate curative services. Once these are functioning, integrated and preventive services should be re-introduced or upgraded.

• Technical assistance is frequently required, particularly for refresher training courses and staff supervision. In addition, it is often necessary to assist in decisions on health policies (e.g. therapeutic standards and health information systems), facilitate the restoration of decision-making bodies, such as district health teams, and assist in restarting important vertical programmes (e.g. EPI and AIDS control).

When assistance is provided to rehabilitate health systems, two principles must be kept in mind:

• Health care systems should be designed to benefit ALL the local inhabitants and should not discriminate between returnees and the resident population[10]. This means that, in most countries, returnees will have to pay for health care and the level of amenities will usually be inferior to that provided in refugee settings.

• Assistance towards the rehabilitation of health care obviously requires good collaboration with the local health authorities. Health agencies that provided health care in refugee settings should be careful not to impose the same model of emergency health assistance onto the home area[11].

A good health surveillance system is essential for monitoring both the health and nutritional status of returnees and residents, and should take into account the increased population figures. In any situation where there is a large and sudden influx of returnees, everyone (both residents and returnees) may be exposed to higher risks of malnutrition and transmission of infectious diseases. Reasons for this include the limited availability of drinking water and food which have to be shared by all, food insecurity, increased population density and crowding, poor sanitation, etc. Health surveillance should cover the following aspects:

- Monitoring diseases: the surveillance system should follow existing national recommendations; MOH leadership and good coordination among partners are necessary conditions for success. Regular data collection is more difficult than in refugee settings as population figures are generally not exact, the population may be dispersed over large and inaccessible areas, health services may be more spread out and less regularly supervised, and staff may lack proper training. Nevertheless, it is important to monitor the status of the population at risk and detect and react to any outbreaks of disease promptly.

- Monitoring mortality figures via outreach workers is difficult to implement in an open situation.

- The nutritional status of both returnees and residents is particularly at risk as the food supply suddenly needs to feed a larger population. This risk is compounded if there are large influxes during periods of very low food availability ('hungry seasons'). High rates of acute malnutrition in both refugees and the resident population are frequently recorded in the early stages of repatriation[9,12,13]. Food production, market prices and other indicators of the food security situation should be assessed regularly and it may be necessary to conduct nutritional surveys if there are indications that the situation is deteriorating.

Specific nutritional programmes may be required during periods of acute food scarcity until agriculture can be expanded and populations become self-sufficient.

Returning health staff should be redeployed to locations in the home area whenever possible to respond to the lack of health staff. However, the MOH of the home country may not recognize their qualifications.

- Refugee health staff officially trained in the home country (previous to the refugee exodus) should generally not meet this problem.

- Refugees who received official training through the MOH of the host country may encounter problems in having their qualifications recognized by home country authorities. This will occur when the curriculum of the host country differs widely from that of the home country. UNHCR and health agencies should try to help solve these problems (i.e. by negotiations and conversion courses) before repatriation begins.

- Non-qualified staff who followed unofficial training sessions organized by relief agencies should have been informed before undertaking training that this training is generally not recognized by the home country MOH, in order to avoid false expectations (see *9. Human Resources and Training* in Part II).

COORDINATION

The complexity of a repatriation process is obvious. Repatriation is:

– a multi-sectoral process,

– involving important factors in regard to timing,

– dependent on a good flow of information,

– covering issues which transverse national borders.

Good coordination between the various organizations involved, the host government, the home government and the refugees themselves, is absolutely essential in assisting repatriation. It should ensure efficient monitoring of the population movements and their needs[1]. Coordination is also required to ensure that there is a good information flow, that conditions for repatriation are met, that policies and protocols are harmonized, and that assistance programmes are designed to respond to needs as they arise in ways that fit into the local context.

There are several aspects to promoting good coordination (see *10. Coordination* in Part II). For example, it is essential that meetings take place regularly among all the partners involved, including those operating in the refugee site and in the return area. Radio communications are also essential in order to inform other partners of refugee movements and developments.

➥ *References*

1. Allen, T, Morsink, H. *When refugees go home.* UNRISD, Africa World Press, 1994.

2. Makanya, S T. *Survey on information needs among Mozambican refugees in Malawi, July 1993.* [Internal Report]. Save The Children Fundation, 1993.

3. Médecins Sans Frontières Mozambique. Movement of people. Mozambique, 1993. *CIS Bull Bimonthly,* 1993, 12: 36-9.

4. Opondo, E O. Refugee repatriation during conflict: Grounds for scepticism. *Disasters,* 1992, 16(4): 359-62.

5. UN Kenya. *Plan of action, Mandera District.* Nairobi: UN Discussion Paper, 1993.

6. Gezelius, K. *Proposed guidelines for repatriation of Somalian refugees, health aspects, April 1993.* Nairobi: UN, 1993.

7. UNHCR. *Policy and guidelines regarding refugee protection and assistance and Acquired Immune Deficiency Syndrome (AIDS).* Geneva: UNHCR, 1988. UNHCR/IOM/70/88.

8. Myers, G W. Reintegration, land access and tenure security in Mozambique. Médecins Sans Frontières. *CIS Bull Bimonthly,* 1993, 15: 36-40.

9. UNHCR. *The state of the world's refugees - in search of solutions.* Oxford: Oxford University Press, 1995.

10. UNHCR. *Repatriation plan for Afghanistan.* Interim report on repatriation planning for Afghan refugees. Geneva: UNHCR, 1989.

11. Médecins Sans Frontières Ethiopia. *Health care assistance to the displaced and resettling populations in Eastern Haraghe and Dire Dawa regions, Ethiopia.* [Narrative report]. Brussels: Médecins Sans Frontières, 1993.

12. Holt, J, Lawrence, M. *An end to isolation. The report of the Ogaden needs assessment study 1991.* London: Save the Children Fundation, 1991.

13. UNHCR, Division of International Protection. *Voluntary repatriation: International protection.* Geneva: UNHCR, 1996.

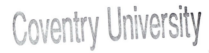

APPENDICES

1. Initial assessment form

2. Needs in vaccine and equipment in mass immunization campaigns

3. Minimal micronutrient requirements

4. Communicable diseases of potential importance in refugee settings

5. Examples of surveillance forms

6. Examples of graphs used in surveillance

1. Example of initial assessment form

Site : ....

Dates : ....../ ...../ ..... – ....../ ...../ .....

Realised by : ....

Method :
1) Cartography/mapping
2) Sample (clusters), 30 clusters of 30 households
3) Other sources of information : WHO and UNHCR

Results :

	Observed	Theoretical
Total number of refugees	55,423	–
% of under-fives	14.5%	20%
% of 6 – 59 months having a W/H < –2Z score	15.5%	< 5%
Number of deaths/10,000 persons/day in the past week	6	< 1
• Cause of death :		
Measles	35%	–
Diarrhoea	25%	–
Malnutrition	22%	–
Acute respiratory infections	5%	–
Malaria	0%	–
• Cases of epidemic diseases :		
Cholera	NO	
Shigellosis	NO	
Meningitis	NO	
Measles	YES	
Daily ration available in kilocalories	1.500 Kcal	2.100 Kcal
Average number of litres of water available/person/day	5 litres	20 litres
Number of persons per latrine	45	20
% of persons sleeping under shelter	50%	100%
Number of doctors	3	
Number of nurses	6	
Number of logisticians	1	
Number of sanitation officers	1	
Number of community health workers	28	

2. Needs in vaccine and equipment in mass immunization campaigns

Needs in vaccines

The number of doses is calculated based on:
– the size of the target population,
– the target coverage,
– the proportion of vaccine lost during a mass campaign: 15%,
– the reserves to be held in stock: 25%.

How to calculate the number of doses of measles vaccine necessary for a given population		
Total population	50,000	
Target population 6 m - 15 years (45% of total)	50,000 × 45%	22,500
Coverage objective 100%	22,500 × 100%	22,500
Number of doses to administer	22,500	22,500
Including expected loss of 15%	22,500 / 85%	26,470
Adding reserve of 25%	26,470 × 125%	33,088
To order	34,000	

Needs in equipment

INJECTION MATERIAL AND EQUIPMENT

Only disposable injection material should be used, and the golden rule 1 injection = 1 sterile syringe + 1 sterile needle must be respected. The quantity of other equipment required (trays, kidney dishes, etc.) depends on the number of operating teams. A safe system for the disposal and destruction of used material (e.g. incinerators) is essential.

COLD CHAIN EQUIPMENT

(see table on page 311)

The vaccines must be stored at 2°-8°C (or frozen for a longer time in central vaccine stores for measles vaccines). However, it should never be thawed and refrozen more than 3 times. The cold chain must be assessed before vaccines are ordered: the storage capacity of existing refrigerators and freezers, the energy source (electricity, gas or kerosene) and transportation equipment. Each main immunization site should ideally have a vaccine storage facility.

Cold chain material for immunization:		
Material	**Purpose/indications**	**Remarks**
Transport material:		
– cool-boxes (Electrolux type RCW 12 or 25) RCW 12: RCW 25:	transport of vaccines, refrigeration 5-7 days stores 3,000 doses, 14 ice packs stores 7,300 doses, 24 ice packs	
– vaccine carriers (1.7 litres)	transport of vaccines, refrigeration 18 hours	contain 4 ice packs
– ice packs	keep temperature in cool-boxes/ vaccine carriers and on vaccination table	twice the number actually in use at one time is needed (alternate between use and freezing)
Cold storage equipment:		
– refrigerators	storage of vaccines (5,000 doses in 22 litres)	install 2-3 days before vaccines arrive
– ice liners	storage of vaccines when electricity not available 24 hours a day	may require only 6-8 hours power per day
– freezers	ice packs	should freeze ice packs as soon as installed; well before vaccination
Monitoring equipment:		
– thermometers	monitor temperature in each appliance	
– refrigerator control sheet	monitor temperature in refrigerator	
– monitoring sheet	to indicate temperature of refrigerator	repeat twice daily

LOGISTICAL EQUIPMENT

Material such as ropes, tarpaulins, megaphones and stationery will also be required for organizing the vaccination site.

REGISTRATION MATERIAL

Individual vaccination cards (either national EPI cards or those provided with the kits) should be prepared for issuing to each child. Vaccination registers are not necessary; tally sheets are preferred (for each vaccination session and at each site.

3. Minimal micronutrient requirements

Nutrient	Daily recommended allowance per person
Vitamin A	1717.0 IU
Vitamin B1	1.1 mg
Vitamin B2	1.1 mg
Vitamin C	27.0 mg
Vitamin D	10.0 mg
Vitamin PP	15.0 mg
Iron	22.0 mg
Iodine	0.5 mg

Source: UNHCR Food Aid & Nutrition Briefing Kit. Minimal allowances have been calculated by aggregating age-specific FAO/WHO RDAs and are based on a typical developing country demographic profile.

4. Communicable diseases of potential importance in refugee settings

Meningitis

Hepatitis

Viral haemorrhagic fevers

Japanese encephalitis

Typhus fever

Relapsing fever

Typhoid fever

Influenza

Leishmaniasis

Plague

Human african trypanosomiasis

Schistosomiasis

Poliomyelitis

Whooping cough

Tetanus

Scabies

Conjunctivitis

Dracunculiasis or Guinea worm

Meningitis

INTRODUCTION

Large outbreaks of meningitis are exclusively due to meningococcus (*Neisseria meningitidis*). More than 13 serogroups of meningococcus have been isolated, and differ in epidemic potential: only serogroups A, B and C can cause outbreaks[2,5]. The serogroups are divided into serotypes, sub-types and clones[8]. Ninety percent of the outbreaks are due to meningococcus serogroup A. Serogroup B (in Europe and South America) generally causes only sporadic cases or small outbreaks; serogroup C has been responsible for a few outbreaks in Africa, Asia and South America. *Haemophilus influenzae* and *Streptococcus pneumoniae* are other frequent causes of sporadic meningitis cases, and other etiologic agents can also be found.

Traditionally, most meningitis outbreaks occurred in the region described as the 'meningitis belt' in sub-Saharan Africa. Outbreaks used to occur every 8 to 12 years and stopped at the onset of the rainy season[5]. However, epidemiological patterns have changed since the 80s, and outbreaks increasingly occur in African countries located outside the meningitis belt. This change may be due to the arrival of a new clone (*Neisseria meningitidis* serogroup A clone III-1), climate changes or increased mobility of the populations, including refugee movements[2,8,15]. It is now reported that epidemics occur at any time of the year and in any region[9,10,15].

Outbreaks of meningococcal meningitis have been frequent in refugee populations (see Table 4.1), and were mostly due to the serogroup A[4,5,7,13]. Overcrowding, poor hygiene, and sometimes limited access to medical care are contributing factors[5]. The outbreak will generally not be confined to the refugee or displaced population, but will be widespread throughout the whole area. Although some areas are considered to be at higher risk, meningitis outbreaks could be expected in any refugee setting, and early detection is essential to undertake prompt action[4].

DESCRIPTION OF EPIDEMICS

The population at risk is classically the age group below 30, in which 80% of cases usually occur. Nevertheless, during recent epidemics caused by meningococcus A clone III-1, high attack rates and case fatality rates were reported in those aged above 30 years (Uganda and Burundi, 1992)[1,10]. The overall attack rate usually ranges from 10 to 1,000 per 100,000, and varies widely[2]. A wide variability in weekly attack rate has been reported as well: an average of 60 cases per 100,000 inhabitants with a range of 30-630 cases per 100,000[3]. The case fatality rate (CFR) without appropriate treatment is estimated at 70%. With treatment, the average CFR usually varies from 5%-15%[2].

Outbreaks usually last 10-14 weeks, but can vary from 4 to 20 weeks. The peak is normally reached 4 weeks after the onset (range from 2 to 8 weeks)[3].

Table 4.1
Reports of meningitis outbreaks in refugee or displaced populations

Place	Attack rate (per 100,000)	CFR (in %)	Duration (in weeks)	Immunization campaign
Thailand, Sakaeo, 1980[5]	130	28	18	Not reported
Sudan, Abyei, 1989[6]	110	8	7	Yes, week 3
Ethiopia, Gode, 1993[7]	187	11	5	Yes, week 2
Guinea, Gueckedou, 1993[9]	98	15	14	Yes, week 13
Zaire, Goma, Katale, 1994[13]	137	3	around 7	Yes, week 5

PREVENTION

Vaccines are currently available for serogroups A, C, Y, W135, as either monovalent or polyvalent preparations; new vaccines, e.g. against serogroup B, are being developed[2]. The protection is 90% effective 5 to 7 days after injection in the age group above 2 years, but significantly declines after 3 years, after which the protection drops to 66% in the age group above 4 years, and disappears in the younger[5].

Routine vaccination of refugees during non-epidemic periods is probably not cost-effective since it requires huge resources, would divert efforts from other activities, and the duration of protection is short[4,5]. However, if there is strong evidence of an impending outbreak, vaccination could be undertaken without waiting for the first case to appear[2,7].

SURVEILLANCE

Meningitis surveillance should always be part of the routine surveillance system to detect the emergence of an outbreak and initiate control measures at the earliest possible time[5]. A standard case definition should be established early. Lumbar puncture is necessary to confirm the diagnosis, and identify the meningococcus in the first suspected cases (see below *Outbreak identification*)[2,4,5]. It must be remembered that diagnosis based on clinical grounds does not differentiate serogroup A meningococcal meningitis from other causes of sporadic meningitis[4].

Case definitions have been proposed by WHO[2], CDC[1], and MSF[1]. The most appropriate case definition should be selected in accordance with the context. The case definition recommended by the WHO is given below.

Case definition for bacterial meningitis[2]

Suspected case [a]	Children under 12 months	Children above 12 months and adults
	– fever	– sudden onset of fever
	WITH	WITH
	– bulging fontanel	– stiff neck
		AND/OR
		– petechial or purpural rash

Probable case [b]	– suspected case
	WITH
	– turbid CSF (with or without Gram stain)
	OR
	– ongoing outbreak
Confirmed case [c]	– suspected or probable case
	AND
	– either positive CSF antigen detection (positive latex agglutination test)
	OR
	– positive culture

According to the WHO:
[a]: *Often the only diagnosis that can be made in peripheral health facilities*
[b]: *Diagnosed in health centres where lumbar puncture and CSF examination are feasible*
[c]: *Diagnosed in well-equipped hospitals*

The number of cases should be followed closely, and the data to be collected for each patient should include: age, sex, current residence, date of onset, mode of diagnosis (clinical only/with turbid CSF/confirmed by laboratory), treatment received, outcome, immunization status and date of immunization[1,2,5]. The number of cases per 100,000 refugees per week should be computed and be compared to the epidemic threshold (see below). Age of cases is needed to determine the age groups at highest risk (at whom eventual vaccination may be targeted)[2,5].

OUTBREAK IDENTIFICATION AND CONTROL

Outbreak identification

If an outbreak of meningococcal meningitis is suspected, priority should be given to the determination of the aetiology and serogroup, since establishing the presence of serogroup A or C is crucial for the planning of immunization (see below)[2,5]. Laboratory testing should therefore be performed on the first suspected cases of meningitis (around 10), and may be done using a rapid test (latex agglutination test of CSF). This test should be available in all refugee programmes in areas at higher risk, and does not require specific skills. Confirmation by culture is more difficult to obtain in the field - the meningococcus is extremely fragile - but can be important to determine antibiotic resistance patterns[2].

It is not possible to define an epidemic threshold that can be used universally to identify an outbreak, due to wide variations in incidence rates according to season, geography, age etc.[4,5] Epidemic threshold should therefore be adapted to the specific refugee setting. In a large refugee population (over 30,000 persons), it is generally recommended to use an epidemic threshold of 15 cases/100,000 persons/week during 2 consecutive weeks[2,12]. Other thresholds should be used in a few specific situations:

- In smaller populations - under 30,000 persons - this general threshold is difficult to apply because of random fluctuations: 2.5 for instance, in a camp of 10,000 persons, only 2 cases per week (i.e. 20 cases/100,000/week) during 2 weeks would lead to declaring an outbreak. In these situations, the traditional threshold of 2 consecutive doubling of meningitis cases from 1 week to the next over a three-week period may be used (e.g. week 1: 3 cases, week 2: 6 cases, week 3: 12 cases)[4,5].

- In very large populations, the general threshold of 15 cases/100,000 persons /week may not be suitable because a low overall attack rate may obscure high rates within smaller population groups[2].

- In a refugee settlement located next to an area where an epidemic has been declared, the threshold of 5 cases/100,000/week is used[2,12].

- In urban settlements, the threshold of 5 cases/100,000/week can also be used[9].

Once an epidemic is confirmed, mass immunization and treatment of cases must be rapidly organized[5].

Mass immunization campaign

A mass immunization campaign can be effective in controlling outbreaks caused by meningococcus A and C, but it will only have a substantial impact on the course of the outbreak when implemented rapidly after the onset of the outbreak. According to some authors, it should be implemented within the first 4-8 weeks[5]. However, recent experiences suggest that this delay might be too long to allow protective levels of antibodies[13].

Mass vaccination is not recommended if it is definitely too late and the epidemic curve is clearly decreasing. The appropriateness of a mass vaccination campaign during the emergency phase when a high mortality is present, or when resources are scarce, should be questioned: an alternative strategy may be to limit intervention to active case detection and early treatment[13]. When an outbreak occurs in the meningitis belt due to a classical clone (i.e. other than the clone III-1), the proximity of the rainy season might also lead to a decision not to undertake mass immunization (see *Introduction* above).

Immunization should not be limited to the refugee population but should cover the whole area affected, as well as the surrounding areas. The same holds, of course, for open situations; where refugees are living in the local community. The target age group should in principle be decided on the basis of the age-specific attack rates, but it is preferable to consider the mass vaccination of the entire population above 6 months. However, if resources are limited, it may be necessary to restrict vaccination to the age groups most at risk, i.e. those aged from 6 months to 30 years (73% of total population)[1,2].

Good organization is crucial for a mass immunization campaign[1]. Recent campaigns conducted in Burundi (1992), Guinea (1993), and Zaire (1994) showed that an immunization team, composed of around 20 members, can vaccinate 350-600 people per hour (see appendix 2)[10]. Immunization should start with those in the centre of the outbreak and include all contacts.

Surveillance during an outbreak

After an outbreak has been confirmed, surveillance efforts should be increased to detect new cases; a case definition based on clinical signs (preferably with visual inspection of the CSF) is usually appropriate[2,4,5,12]. Weekly compilation of cases enables a drawing of the epidemic curve.

Information on the vaccination status of cases enables an estimation of the vaccine efficacy (see further details under *2. Measles Immunization* in Part II).

Treatment

Early case finding via home-visitors is important in order to ensure prompt treatment; suspected cases should be referred to the central health facility or the hospital. If laboratory facilities are available, treatment should not be delayed until laboratory results are known[5].

The isolation of patients is useless because the disease is mainly transmitted through healthy carriers, but it may be necessary to set up specific temporary treatment units to cope with a large number of patients[5].

In outbreaks, the most cost-effective and practical treatment is a single dose IM of chloramphenicol in an oily suspension (long acting), administered on admission[1,5,11]. This antibiotic is also effective against other bacterial agents causing meningitis, and may then be useful in emergency settings as a first-intention treatment of other meningitis[14].

Chemoprophylaxis

During outbreaks, WHO no longer recommends mass chemoprophylaxis or chemoprophylaxis for meningitis contacts[2].

✎ Key references

1. Médecins Sans Frontières. *Conduite à tenir en cas d'épidémie de méningite à méningocoque.* Paris: Médecins Sans Frontières, 1993.
2. WHO. *Control of epidemic meningococcal disease. WHO practical guidelines.* Lyon: Editions Fondation Marcel Mérieux, 1995.

Other references

3. Flachet, L, Boelaert, M, Henkens, M, Rigal, J, Barret, B, Varaine, F, Moren, A. *Intervention en cas d'épidémie de méningite: indications et limites. Etudes des interventions réalisées par MSF, 1985-91.* Journées scientifiques 1991-1992. Paris: Epicentre, AEDES, Médecins Sans Frontières, 1992.

4. CDC. Famine-affected, refugee, and displaced populations: Recommendations for public health issues. *MMWR*, 1992, 41(RR-13): 1-76.

5. Moore, P S, Toole, M J, Nieburg, P, Waldman, R J, Broome, C V. Surveillance and control of meningococcal meningitis epidemics in refugee populations. *WHO Bull*, 1990, 58(5): 587-96.

6. Boelaert, M. Experience with meningitis epidemics in Africa. Analysis of MSF-B reports. *Medical News*, 1992, 1(1): 11-15.

7. Ritter, H, Henckaert, K. *Narrative report: Meningitis epidemic in Gode, Ogaden, Apr-Jun 1993.* [Internal report]. Bruxelles: Médecins Sans Frontières Ethiopia, 1993.

8. Moore, P S, Reeves, M W, Schwartz, B, Gellin, B G, Broome, C V. Intercontinental spread of an epidemic group A Neisseria meningitidis strain. *The Lancet*, 1989, 2(8657): 260-2.

9. Varaine, F, Ott, D, Haba, P. *Epidémie de méningite, Haute Guinée et Guinée Forestière, avril 93.* [Rapport interne]. Paris: Epicentre, 1993.

10. Varaine, F. *Rapport narratif des activités réalisées par Médecins Sans Frontières au bénéfice des populations victimes de l'épidemie de méningite - Burundi 1992.* [Rapport interne]. Paris: Epicentre, 1992.

11. WHO in collaboration with CDC, CRED and FINNPREP. *Emergency preparedness and reponse: Rapid health assessment in meningitis outbreaks.* Emergency Relief Operations, 1990.

12. Moore, P S, Plikaytis, B D, Bolan, G A, Oxtoby, M J, Yada, A, Zoubga, A, Reingold, A L, Broome, C V. Detection of meningitis epidemics in Africa: A population-based analysis. *Int J Epidemiol*, 1992, 21(1): 155-61.

13. Haelterman, E, Boelaer, M, Suetens, C, and al. Impact of a mass vaccination campaign against a meningitis epidemic in a refugee camp. *Tropical Med and Int Health*, 1996, 1(3): 385-92.

14. Pecoul, B, Varaine, F, Keita, M, et al. Long acting chloramphenicol versus intravenous ampicillin for treatment of bacterial meningitis. *The Lancet*, 1991, 338(8771): 862-6.

15. Meningococcal meningitis. *Wkly Epidemiol Rec*, 1995, 70(15): 105-7.

Hepatitis

Viral hepatitis include several distinct infections (hepatitis A, B, C, D, E), which share similar clinical presentations but differ in aetiology, epidemiology, prevention and control[1]. Hepatitis is not among the most common diseases reported in refugee and displaced populations, but has emerged as a serious problem in camps in the Horn of Africa (Kenya, Somalia, 1985-1991): outbreaks were caused by a non-A, non-B hepatitis virus, later identified as hepatitis E, and associated with an inadequate water supply[15]. Other types of hepatitis are also encountered in refugee settings. Although the impact of hepatitis on refugee health is not likely to be significant in emergency situations, it should be considered as a serious potential problem.

SURVEILLANCE

Example of case definition for hepatitis (all types included)[2]:

Any acute onset of jaundice preceded by nausea, vomiting or anorexia, with or without fever, and no history of recent treatment with drugs causing jaundice[2].

A case definition should be included in any refugee surveillance system. As diagnosis is only clinical in refugee situations, it should be taken into account that other potentially serious diseases can present as clinical hepatitis. Therefore, a sudden rise in fatal presumed 'hepatitis' cases should make health staff suspect yellow fever (as the bleeding tendency is not always present).

Table 4.2
Characteristics of hepatitis[3,4]

Hepatitis	Transmission	% Symptomatic cases	Mortality	% Chronicity
A	faeco-oral	< 20% infants > 75% adults	low	no
B	parenteral perinatal sexual	10-25%	high	10% adults 90% new-borns
C	parenteral	5-10%	moderate	over 50%
D	with hep. B	unknown	high	80%
E	faeco-oral	unknown	high in pregnancy (low in others)	no

Hepatitis A (HA) and Hepatitis E (HE)

Hepatitis A occurs worldwide. In developing countries where sanitation is poor, infection is common and occurs at an early age; adults are usually immune[1]. Hepatitis A is a potential problem in large concentrations of people with overcrowding, inadequate sanitation and water supply[1]. Many infections are asymptomatic, and recovery without sequelae is the rule. Case fatality rate (CFR) is low - under 0.1% - but severity increases with age (CFR of 2.7% in those above 50 years)[1].

Outbreaks of hepatitis E occur primarily in areas with inadequate environmental sanitation. Hepatitis E outbreaks have been reported in refugees in the Horn of Africa with attack rates ranging from 6-8% (Somalia[5], Ethiopia[6,7] and Kenya[1]), and were all associated with a very poor water supply. The clinical picture is similar to that of hepatitis A; CFRs are also similar, except in pregnant women, where it can reach up to 20%[1,3,6].

SURVEILLANCE

In addition to the hepatitis surveillance previously described, hepatitis E should be suspected if fatal cases seem to cluster among pregnant women. The first suspected cases should be confirmed by serology[9].

PREVENTION

Preventive measures mostly involve ensuring an adequate water supply and good sanitation. An effective vaccine exists for hepatitis A, in a three-dose schedule. Vaccination is not used as an outbreak control measure, because protection against clinical infection is only obtained 30 days after the first dose, the vaccine is expensive, and the disease is not severe and cures spontaneously[1,10]. It is however recommended for the protection of health staff. For hepatitis E, no vaccine exists and immunoglobulins are not effective. Health staff are at risk; careful hand-washing after every contact with a patient is mandatory[1].

CASE MANAGEMENT

Treatment is purely symptomatic.

Hepatitis B (HB), Hepatitis C (HC) and Hepatitis D (HD)

Hepatitis B is a leading cause of death in adults because of the sequelae of chronic hepatitis: cirrhosis and liver cancer[16]. Although hepatitis B virus is found in all populations, the frequency of infections and of the carrier state has striking geographic and ethnic variability; the prevalence of chronic infection in the population ranges from 0.1 to 20%[11]. In Southeast Asia and sub-Saharan Africa where HB is highly endemic, over 8% of the population are carriers, and 15%-25% of chronic carriers eventually die of liver cancer or cirrhosis. Approximately 90% of infants infected at birth become chronic carriers[1]. Transmission is mainly parenteral, sexual and foeto-maternal, but faeco-oral transmission is possible, as well as transmission via bites, wounds, etc. Blood transfusion and the use of inadequately sterilized syringes and needles has played a major role in transmission worldwide. In refugee settings, transmission may increase due to the relaxation of sterilization measures, and emergency transfusion of unscreened blood[1].

Since it was identified in 1989, hepatitis C has been found in 0.5%-8.0% of blood donors worldwide. The infection is chronic in most infected persons, and may lead to cirrhosis and liver cancer[12].

Hepatitis D can only develop in persons co-infected by the hepatitis B virus, and is thought to be transmitted in the same way - although foetal-maternal transmission is much rarer[1]. Diagnosis is confirmed by serology.

PREVENTION AND CONTROL MEASURES

The prevention of sexual and parenteral transmission basically involves the same recommendations as for the prevention of HIV transmission[13]:

- Safe injection practices are essential everywhere. Sterilization (e.g. ebullition for 20 minutes) inactivates the hepatitis virus.

- Strict transfusion criteria must be followed (see *HIV, AIDS and STD* in Part III). Hepatitis B screening before blood transfusion (rapid test) should obviously be carried out in countries where it is a national health policy to do so (e.g. Kenya). In regard to other areas of high endemicity, the decision to screen depends on the material and human resources of the health facility. It is particularly important to screen blood used for transfusions in children, since they are less likely to have been exposed to previous infection, and therefore have a lower level of protection. Although excluding all hepatitis B carriers would make blood donors more difficult to find, the risks involved should be weighed up carefully before deciding on screening[13].

- Screening test are also available for hepatitis C virus, but are not likely to be available in refugee settings[1,12].

Immunization against hepatitis B gives 95% protection (with 3 doses). Routine immunization of infants against hepatitis B is currently being implemented in highly endemic areas; WHO has recommended to introduce this vaccine into the national immunization programmes of all countries by the year 1997[16]. Immunization schedules in refugee populations should follow the EPI policy of the host country. The vaccine doses should be timed to coincide with visits required for other childhood immunizations[11]. Of course, all preventive measures against hepatitis B cover against hepatitis D.

No vaccine against hepatitis C has yet been developed[12].

🕮 References

1. Benenson, A. *Control of communicable diseases manual.* 16th edition. Washington DC: American Public Health Association, 1995.
2. Médecins Sans Frontières. *Surveillance in emergency situations.* Amsterdam: Médecins Sans Frontières, 1993.
3. Zuckerman, A J. Hepatitis E virus. The main cause of enterically transmitted non-A, non-B hepatitis. *Br Med J,* 1990, 300: 1475-6.

4. Reconnaitre et traiter les hépatites virales. *Prescrire*, 1994, 4(145): 653.

5. CDC. Enterically transmitted non-A, non-B hepatitis: East Africa. *MMWR*, 1987, 36: 241-4.

6. CDC. Update: Health and nutritional profiles of refugees – Ethiopia, 1989-1990. *MMWR*, 1990, 39(40): 707-17.

7. Toole, M J, Bhatia, R. A case study of Somali refugees in Hartisheik A camp, Eastern Ethiopia: Health and nutrition profile, July 1988-June 1990. *Jour of Refugee Studies*, 1992, 5(3/4): 313-26.

8. WHO. *Immunization policy*. Geneva: WHO, 1993. WHO/EPI/GEN/1993/rev.2.

9. Dawson, G J, Chau, K H, Cabal, C M, et al. Solid-phase enzyme-linked immunosorbent assay for hepatitis E virus IgG and IgM antibodies utilizing recombinant antigens and synthetic peptides. *J Vir Methods*, 1992, 38: 175-86.

10. Simmonds, S, Vaughan, P, William Gunn, S. *Refugee community health care*. Oxford: Oxford University Press, 1983.

11. WHO/EPI. *Hepatitis B vaccine. Attacking a pandemic*. EPI update. Geneva: WHO, 1989.

12. Genetic diversity of Hepatitis C virus: implications for pathogenesis, treatment, and prevention. Report of a meeting of physicians and scientists, Royal Free Hospital and School of Medicine, London. *The Lancet*, 1995, 345(8949): 562-6.

13. CDC. Recommendations for preventing transmission of human immunodeficiency virus and hepatitis B virus to patients during exposure-prone invasive procedures. *MMWR*, 1991, 40(RR-8): 1-9.

14. Fournel, O. Quelques aspects du risque infectieux transfusionnel en France et dans les pays de l'Afrique sub-saharienne. *Cahiers Santé*, 1991, 1: 53-8.

15. CDC. Famine-affected, refugee, and displaced populations: Recommendations for public health issues. *MMWR*, 1992, 41(RR-13): 1-76.

16. Hepatitis B. Global control of hepatitis B virus infection. *Wkly Epidemiol Rec*, 1989, 64: 288-90.

Viral haemorrhagic fevers

Viral haemorrhagic fevers (VHF) are caused by a number of different viruses (see Table 4.3), some of which are associated with arthropods - known as arthropod-borne virus or ARBO-virus - and rodents, but may also infect humans. These viruses mostly cause mild infections, but they are all capable of causing severe and fatal disease, and some of them have led to devastating epidemics in some areas[4].

Each distinct VHF is characterized by its own specific clinical profile, and all of them have a clinical profile in common, consisting of fever and a bleeding tendency, with the risks of developing severe haemorrhage and severe shock[1]. These diseases can cause significant public health problems because of their high epidemic potential, high case-fatality rates - the highest being 50%-80% for Ebola fever - and the difficulties met in treatment and prevention. They thus warrant strict safety procedures[1].

The occurrence of each VHF tends to reflect some geographic distribution pattern (distribution of its natural host), and under normal circumstances, infection is most often acquired in endemic areas. Some VHF, e.g. Ebola and Lassa fever, are at high risk of transmission in health facilities (i.e. nosocomial transmission): in Africa, VHF transmission has often been associated with the re-use of unsterilized needles and inadequate barrier nursing precautions; several VHF have been identified when they caused hospital outbreaks[7,8]. Airborne transmission involving humans has not been documented so far, but is still considered as a possibility in rare instances (such as patients with pulmonary involvement)[8].

The major haemorrhagic fevers causing epidemics are listed below in Table 4.3. Yellow fever and dengue are usually more frequent, but other VHF should never be excluded in an emergency context.

Table 4.3
Viral haemorrhagic fevers causing outbreaks[1]

VHF	Distribution	Natural host/ vector
Lassa Fever	Central/West Africa	rodents (urine)
Junin/Machupo	South America	rodents (urine)
Ebola/Marburg	Central/South Africa	unknown
Crimean-Congo HF *	Africa/Asia	ticks
Rift Valley Fever	Africa	mosquitoes
Dengue HF *	Africa/Americas/Pacific/Europe/Australia	mosquitoes
Yellow Fever	Africa/South America	mosquitoes
HF with Renal Syndrome	Asia/Europe	rodents (saliva and urine)

* HF: Haemorrhagic fever

General control measures are described below, and the measures specific to yellow fever and dengue are dealt with in the next section.

PREVENTION

Highly effective vaccines have been developed, but are available only for yellow fever and Rift Valley fever (only indicated for people at high risk)[3]. In refugee camps, appropriate vector control to prevent mosquito- or tick-borne VHF may be organized in zones at risk, and can be very successful (especially for yellow fever)[4].

As health care workers are at high risk of being infected by patients, the respect of universal precautions is essential in any health care setting, whether an outbreak has been declared or not.

SURVEILLANCE

The early detection of VHF is often missed by a routine surveillance system[1]. It is useful to collect information from health authorities and staff on the eventual occurrence of VHF in the area. If there is a risk of VHF, for instance when refugees arrive in or are coming from an affected area, a general case definition can be included in the health surveillance system to allow quick detection of any VHF outbreak. The patient travel history, possible exposure to other suspected cases, symptoms, and clinical signs provide the most important information.

Case definition for viral haemorrhagic fever[2]:

A suspected VHF case is:

Any patient living in, or with a history of recent travel to a suspected endemic area, who presents with an unexplained and unresponsive high fever, especially with bleeding tendency.

OUTBREAK CONTROL

Outbreak Investigation

Confirmation of VHF outbreak requires laboratory testing, and appropriate specimens should be collected from suspected cases. However, laboratory testing should be kept to the minimum necessary for virus identification, because of the potential risk associated with handling infectious materials[8]. All specimens must be considered as potentially infectious, and very strict safety procedures must be respected during sample collection and analysis. Laboratory staff are at particular high risk of nosocomial infection. Specimens required for confirmation are usually whole blood, and serum is then used for antibody detection or virus isolation[1,5,8]. An alternative method developed by the CDC is based on skin-snip specimen but is used for surveillance only (details available from the CDC). Specimens should be packed in 3 layers, and should be shipped to a specialized referral laboratory[9]. General procedures are described in guidelines[5,6]. The local health authorities should be informed.

General control measures

Control measures should be undertaken in liaison with the local health authorities, and often require the help of experts such as CDC or WHO specialists.

- Respecting universal precautions in health facilities and ensuring adequate barrier nursing are among the most important measures, as health care workers form the group at highest risk of being infected. Protection of staff requires at least the use of gloves, mask, and goggles. Regarding Ebola fever, extended protection is particularly crucial when dealing with patients in the latter stages of the disease - when vomiting, diarrhoea and haemorrhages are present - and involves the use of gown, apron, and rubber boots[2,8].

- Cases should be isolated (see below *Case management*), and their transportation should be limited. Patient contact with non-essential staff and visitors should be prevented; family members should ideally not be involved in patient care, but if this cannot be avoided, caretakers should follow the same protective guidelines as health staff[2].

- Handling of dead bodies should be minimal[2].

- Education of health staff and the patient's family on the above mentioned issues is essential, and training sessions should rapidly be organized for health staff[2].

- Action must be taken to avoid panic in the population, and involves clear public messages. Travel and contacts with people from affected areas should be avoided[2].

- Immunization is useful for controlling outbreaks of yellow fever (immunization against Rift Valley HF is only indicated for people at risk, such as health staff)[7].

- Control of the specific vector, or possibly the animal host, is useful for reducing transmission[7].

Case management

The strict isolation of patients is mandatory; this can be done in a hospital setting when appropriate, or at home when transport of the patient would bring an increased risk of transmission[2]. Patients should be placed under mosquito nets where there is a risk of mosquito-borne disease[7].

Effective antiviral therapy is not available, except for Lassa fever (ribavirin), and treatment is thus symptomatic. The most important measure is the management of fluid and electrolyte balance from the onset, and usually involves the use of perfusions. However, in the treatment of Ebola fever, oral medications and rehydration should be preferred whenever possible to limit the risk of nosocomial transmission.

Immune plasma, obtained from patients who have recovered, may be beneficial, although its use is controversial because it has not yet been scientifically proven[4].

Patients and family members should be informed on the likelihood of sexual transmission during the convalescence period[2].

🔖 Key references

1. WHO. *Emergency preparedness and response. Rapid health assessment in outbreaks of viral haemorrhagic fever, including yellow fever.* [draft]. Geneva: WHO, 1990. ERO/EPR/90.1.4.

2. CDC, WHO, Zairian Ministry of Health. *Barrier nursing handbook. Strategies for managing patients with VHF.* [draft]. CDC, 1995.

Other references

3. Benenson, A. *Control of communicable diseases manual.* 16th edition. Washington DC: American Public Health Association, 1995.

4. Cook, G. *Manson's tropical diseases.* 19th edition. London: WB Saunders, 1996.

5. CDC. *Guidelines for collecting, processing, storing, and shipping diagnostic specimens in refugee health-care environments.* Atlanta: CDC, US Department of Health and Human Services - Public Health Services, 1992.

6. Lacroix, C. *Guide du laboratoire médical.* Paris: Médecins Sans Frontières, 1994.

7. WHO. *Viral haemorrhagic fevers.* Technical Report Serie No. 721. Geneva: WHO, 1985.

8. WHO. Viral haemorrhagic fever. Management of suspected cases. *Wkly Epidemiol Rec,* 1995, 70(35): 249-52.

9. Madeley, C R. *Collection and transport of virological specimens.* Geneva: WHO, 1977.

Yellow fever

Yellow fever has caused many serious epidemics with high mortality rates, especially in Africa. Thirty-three African countries are currently considered at risk of yellow fever outbreaks[4]. Sporadic cases also occur in South America (Amazon basin), where it mainly affects forestry workers.

Yellow fever transmission occurs primarily among non-human primates, with forest mosquitoes serving as vectors (sylvatic cycle: monkey-mosquito-monkey). Sporadic cases occur among humans who are infected when they enter areas of active transmission and are bitten by infected mosquitoes. When these persons then enter urban centres (or refugee camps) and are bitten by specific domestic mosquitoes, especially *Aedes aegypti*, a second cycle may begin (urban cycle: man-mosquito-man), and cause a yellow fever outbreak.

The severity of the disease varies: case fatality rates are lower than 5% among indigenous groups in endemic regions, but may reach 80% among non-indigenous groups or during epidemics[3,6]. Recent epidemics have mainly affected children under 15 years, as adults are often protected by past post-outbreak immunization[4].

Unlike most VHF, effective measures exist to control an outbreak: timely vaccination against yellow fever, combined with vector control measures, may interrupt transmission.

SURVEILLANCE

The general procedures are described under the introductory section on VHFs.

It is usually difficult to distinguish yellow fever from other febrile illnesses and there are many examples of epidemics which were only recognized several months after their onset[1]. In a normal surveillance system, cases of 'jaundice, fatal or non-fatal' should always be recorded. Yellow fever should be suspected when an increased incidence of fatal hepatitis is reported[1]. Further investigation of suspected cases should follow in order to identify the agent (see below).

PREVENTION

An effective vaccine is available: it can be administered to everyone from the age of 2 to 4 months on, and probably protects for life (although boosters are so far recommended every 10 years)[5].

WHO now recommends including the antigen in the regular extended programmes on immunization (EPI) in all countries at risk (currently adopted into the EPIs of 17 countries)[4].

In refugee settings, the national EPI guidelines of the host country should be followed. Vector control measures against *Aedes aegypti* might be considered when the risk of yellow fever is high.

OUTBREAK CONTROL

Laboratory confirmation is absolutely necessary for differential diagnosis and is done by serology (see VHF for procedures). For instance, outbreaks of yellow fever have been suspected and investigated in several refugee situations in East Africa, and have turned out to be resistant malaria (Kenya, 1992), borrelioses (Southern Sudan 1992), rickettsioses and hepatitis (MSF unpublished data). If a WHO reference centre for yellow fever exists in the region, it can carry out the analysis and confirm whether or not yellow fever is present.

- It is recommended to start a mass vaccination campaign as soon as one single case is confirmed in a refugee population. The campaign should cover everybody above 4 months of age[2].

- Vector control by spraying shelters with insecticide, and applying larvicides to breeding sites of *Aedes aegypti* (and/or water containers) contributes to controlling a yellow fever outbreak.

- The treatment of cases is entirely symptomatic. Strict isolation measures are necessary. It is absolutely essential to provide each patient with a mosquito net in order to avoid transmission to other persons; extra attention must be paid to safe nursing procedures.

---

33 African countries at risk for yellow fever:

Angola*, Benin, Burkina Faso*, Burundi, Cameroon*, Cape Verde, Central African Republic*, Chad*, Congo, Côte d'Ivoire*, Equatorial Guinea, Ethiopia, Gabon, Gambia*, Ghana*, Guinea*, Guinea-Bissau, Kenya, Liberia, Mali*, Mauritania*, Niger*, Nigeria*, Rwanda, Sao Tome, Senegal*, Sierra Leone, Somalia, Sudan, Tanzania, Togo*, Uganda, Zaire.

(* = YF antigen included into EPI program)

Data as of October 1991[3]

🔖 Key references

1. WHO. *Emergency preparedness and response. Rapid health assessment in outbreaks of viral haemorrhagic fever, including yellow fever.* [draft]. Geneva: WHO, 1990. ERO/EPR/90.1.4.

2. WHO. *Prevention and control of yellow fever in Africa.* Geneva: WHO, 1986.

Other references

3. WHO/EPI. *The resurgence of deadly yellow fever. Prevention using EPI.* EPI update No. 21. Geneva: WHO, 1992.

4. Yellow fever in 1992 and 1993. *Wkly Epidemiol Rec,* 1995, 70(10): 65-70.

5. WHO. *The immunological basis for immunization. Yellow fever.* Geneva: WHO, 1993. WHO/EPI/GEN/93.18.

6. Benenson, A. *Control of communicable diseases manual.* 16th edition. Washington DC: American Public Health Association, 1995.

Dengue

Dengue is caused by arboviruses, transmitted by *Aedes* mosquitoes, principally *Aedes aegypti*. There are 4 serotypes of dengue virus, and they are all responsible for the same disease. Infection is frequently asymptomatic, or leads to one of the two clinical forms of dengue: dengue fever and dengue haemorrhagic fever[10].

- Dengue fever (DF) is characterized by a high fever and a rash. In emergency settings where diagnostic possibilities are limited, such cases will easily be taken for and treated as malaria[5]. Convalescence might be prolonged, but mortality is rare[10].

- Dengue haemorrhagic fever and dengue shock syndrome (DHF/DSS) are severe illnesses: after a classical dengue pattern, the patient suddenly deteriorates and develops haemorrhages. Eventually s/he might develop shock syndrome. Case fatality rates are high (10%-60%). The current concept of DHF/DSS pathogenesis is that an individual is infected sequentially with two different serotypes, and the haemorrhagic symptoms are probably due to an enhanced immune reaction[10].

Dengue viruses are now endemic in most countries in the tropics. Outbreaks of DF occur in China, Southeast Asia, tropical Africa, Central and South America. DHF outbreaks are limited to Asia, the Caribbean and some countries of South and Central America. So far DHF/DSS is extremely rare in Africa, however human migration patterns can rapidly disperse vectors and viruses into new areas.

The number of dengue cases world wide is increasing rapidly. Major epidemics of what is today already the most important arthropod-borne viral disease may be expected in the years to come.

Classical dengue occurs primarily in children in endemic areas, where 100% of children have been infected by the age of 8 years. The disease is generally not diagnosed as such. The primary infection is mostly mild, except among children between 6 and 9 months in whom a primo-infection may lead to DHF/DSS. Seasonal variations may exist: for instance, in Thailand the number of cases rises considerably in the rainy season.

In refugee settings the risk of outbreaks of dengue fever is likely to increase due to several factors: inadequate water storage/drainage and poor refuse disposal, which may lead to an increase of mosquito breeding sites[8], a lack of acquired immunity among previously unexposed persons who arrive in an endemic area; previous exposure to a different serotype than that present in their country of origin, which could lead to DHF/DSS. For instance, serological evidence of dengue fever has been reported among refugees in Hargeysa (Somalia)[5], and a DHF outbreak has been identified in long-standing refugee camps on the Thai-Cambodian border[5,7].

SURVEILLANCE

In endemic areas, it is important to list dengue fever amongst the possible differential diagnosis of non-specific fever. The clinical case definition of DHF is specific enough to diagnose it in a known endemic area[8,9].

Case definitions for suspected cases of dengue[8]:

- **Dengue fever**: an acute febrile illness characterized by headache, retro-ocular pain, muscle and joint pain, and rash.

- **Dengue haemorrhagic fever**: an acute onset of fever with non-specific symptoms, followed by haemorrhagic manifestations.

When an outbreak is suspected, diagnostic confirmation by serology (haemagglutination inhibition antibody test or ELISA test) should be requested; testing is only available at WHO reference centres. However, control measures should be implemented without waiting for the results[6].

PREVENTION

In refugee settings, the control and treatment of water containers with larvicide (every 2-3 months) to stop the breeding of *Aedes* mosquitoes is often feasible and is an effective approach. Proper solid waste disposal is also necessary[1,2]. Spraying the site with insecticide can be considered but has to be undertaken as soon as the first cases are detected in order to be effective[1]. Since *Aedes* mosquitoes bite during the day, mosquito nets will usually not protect against dengue (unless used in day-time).

Vaccines are still being tested[3]. The production of vaccines against one serotype is possible, but vaccinated individuals may develop DHF/DSS if they become infected with another serotype. A tetravalent vaccine (against 4 serotypes) is currently being tested in Thailand.

TREATMENT

The treatment is symptomatic. For dengue fever, it consists mainly in treatment of fever and pain. In DHF/DSS, the shock often responds to the rapid replacement of fluid losses with Ringer lactate or plasma (and oxygen when available). The patient should be kept under a mosquito net (also in day-time) to prevent transmission[1].

➤ *Key references*

1. WHO. *Dengue haemorrhagic fever: diagnosis, treatment and control.* Geneva: WHO, 1986.

2. PAHO. *Dengue and dengue haemorrhagic fever in the Americas: Guidelines for prevention and control.* Scientific publication No. 548. Washington DC: Pan American Health Organization, 1994.

Other references

3. Ebrahim, G J. Dengue and dengue haemorrhagic fever. *J Trop Pediatr,* 1993, 39(5): 262-3.

4. Cook, G. *Manson's tropical diseases.* 19th edition. London: Saunders, 1996.

5. Botros, B A M, Watts, D M, Soliman A K, Salib, A W et al. Serological evidence of dengue fever among refugees, Hargeysa, Somalia. *J Med Virol,* 1989, 29: 79-81.

6. Knudsen, Le Duc. *Meeting of interested parties on management and financing of the control of tropical diseases other than malaria.* Geneva: WHO, 1993.

7. Elias, C J, Alexander B H, Sokly T. Infectious disease control in a long-term refugee camp: The role of epidemiological surveillance and investigation. *Am. J of Public Health,* 1990, 80(7): 824-8.

8. CDC. Case definition for public health surveillance. *MMWR,* 1990, 39(RR-13): 1-42.

9. Coyette, Y. *Guide clinique et thérapeutique sur la dengue hémorragique.* Phnom Penh: Médecins Sans Frontières Cambodia, 1993.

10. Benenson, A. *Control of communicable diseases manual.* 16th edition. Washington DC: American Public Health Association, 1995.

11. Halstead, S B. The XXth century dengue pandemic: Need surveillance and research. *World Health Stat Q,* 1992, 45(2-3): 292-8.

Japanese encephalitis

Japanese encephalitis is caused by a virus transmitted by mosquitoes, the most important vectors being the *Culex* species. The host for the virus is the pig or certain birds, but humans can be incidentally infected, then becoming an 'accidental host'. Transmission is related to the abundance of mosquitoes and hosts[1]. One to two months after the onset of the rainy season is a common time for epidemics to start[2].

Japanese encephalitis is found in east, south-east and south Asia, where it is the leading cause of viral encephalitis[1]. The most recent outbreaks have occurred in China, Vietnam, Thailand, Nepal, and Sri Lanka. In endemic areas, incidence rates reach 1-10 per 10,000 per year, and the disease mostly affects children; studies of sero-prevalence have revealed that nearly all adults are exposed, and every symptomatic case may hide up to 200 non-symptomatic cases[1]. Mortality is high - the case fatality rate is 25%, with the highest fatality rates among the elderly (up to 60%)[2]. Some 30% of cases are left with neurological sequelae[1,4].

In endemic zones, the risk of disease in refugee settlements may be higher, particularly in rural areas (e.g. near rice fields) during the breeding time for mosquitoes, and among a non-immune population[1]. A lack of acquired immunity in refugee populations may be frequent since the endemic areas are limited to some defined geographic zones.

However, outbreaks of Japanese encephalitis have rarely been reported in refugee populations, probably because of under-reporting; among Bhutanese refugees in Nepal (1992), an outbreak of Japanese encephalitis was detected on a clinical basis, but no laboratory confirmation was possible[3].

SURVEILLANCE

Japanese encephalitis cannot be differentiated on clinical grounds from encephalitis caused by other viruses. The disease may be suspected when 5 to 10 cases of meningo-encephalitis cases appear in the same neighbourhood, particularly in areas of known transmission. Cases should be confirmed by serology (for procedure, see *Viral Haemorrhagic Fevers*).

PREVENTION

Destroying mosquito breeding sites (e.g. by insecticide spraying) is very effective. Other vector control measures include the use of mosquito nets and the spraying of shelters[2].

Different vaccines are currently in use. The newest vaccines (derived from mouse brains) are highly purified; they are produced in several Southeast Asian countries. The immunization schedule comprises 3 doses (day 1, 7 and 30). Mass immunization in refugee camps would be feasible in principle, provided that the financial and material means are available. However, the decision to immunize should balance the risks of disease exposure, the availability of vector control measures, the side effects of vaccination, and the cost of such a programme (the vaccine is expensive, and 3 doses are required)[4]. Non-immunized health staff working in endemic areas should preferably be vaccinated.

CASE MANAGEMENT

Patients must be hospitalized and isolation is not required. Only symptomatic treatment is available.

References

1. Encéphalite japonaise - Vaccin inactivé contre le virus de l'encéphalite japonaise. *Wkly Epidemiolog Rec*, 1994, 69(16): 113-18.

2. Benenson, A. *Control of communicable diseases manual*. 16th edition. Washington DC: American Public Health Association, 1995.

3. Marfin A A, Moore, J, Collins, C, et al. Infectious disease surveillance during emergency relief to Bhutanese refugees in Nepal. *JAMA*, 1994, 272(5): 377-81.

4. CDC. Inactivated Japanese encephalitis virus vaccine. Recommendations of the advisory committee on immunization practices (ACIP). *MMWR*, 1993, 42(RR-1): 1-15.

Typhus fever

Typhus fever is caused by *Rickettsiae* and transmitted through vectors such as lice, fleas or mites. There are several types of typhus fevers, each of them differ by the Rickettsia species, the vector, clinical presentation, epidemiology and control measures (see Table 4.4).

In refugee settings, human-vector contacts are likely to increase (e.g. higher risk of louse-infestation), and outbreaks of epidemic louse-borne typhus, murine typhus, and scrub typhus have been reported[1,3,6,8]. These 3 illnesses are dealt with below.

Table 4.4
Typhus fever (TF) commonly reported in refugee settings: a summary

	Louse-borne TF	**Murine TF**	**Scrub TF**
Agent	*R. prowazeki*	*R. mooseri*	*R. tsutsugamishi*
Vector	body louse	rat flea	mites
Occurrence	epidemic	endemic	sporadic
Areas	highlands, deserts; Burundi Rwanda, Ethiopia	worldwide, where rats are present	Asia (E and S-E)
Severity	high mortality	low mortality	high mortality, sequelae
Action	as soon as lice are detected:	in the post-emergency phase:	
– vector	mass delousing campaign	anti-flea/anti-rat actions	clear vegetation, spraying
– treatment	doxycycline single dose	doxycycline single dose	doxycycline single dose

Epidemic louse-borne typhus fever (LBTF)

LBTF occurs throughout the world. Although it is more common in colder areas, it may also occur in the tropics at high altitudes and in deserts, among louse-infested people. Transmission is through the same body louse that transmits epidemic relapsing fever (LBRF), and the two diseases may co-exist. The most recent cases have been reported in Burundi, Rwanda and Ethiopia and migration through this area may introduce LBTF into areas previously free of the disease[1,2]. LBTF outbreaks may occur whenever a population becomes louse-infected, particularly in endemic areas. Refugee populations are thus at higher risk due to overcrowding and poor hygiene, especially during the rainy season when more clothing and blankets are used[8].

LBTF mortality increases with age: case fatality rates vary from 10% to 40% without treatment[1], and can rise above 50% in the elderly[1,2].

PREVENTION

If lice are present in the refugee population, a delousing campaign and other hygiene measures, described in the section *Relapsing fever*, must take place before an outbreak occurs (either typhus or relapsing fever). In areas at high risk, new arrivals should be screened for the presence of lice on arrival in the settlement, or in out-patient departments whenever this is possible. Safe and effective vaccines are not yet suitable for use at general population level[2].

SURVEILLANCE

Surveillance should primarily monitor lice infestation within the camp. Typhus cases may be suspected on a clinical basis in endemic areas where lice are shown to be present; these cases should be differentiated from louse-borne relapsing fever. However, the clinical picture is not very specific. There is no standard case definition, but the following is an example of a case definition for typhus fever (all types), used in a refugee in-patient service, which can be adapted for any refugee setting:

Example of case definition for typhus fever[3]:

Any case of fever for 4 days or longer, no obvious source of infection, negative malaria smears, and a clinical response to tetracycline within 2 to 3 days of starting treatment.

OUTBREAK CONTROL

Outbreak investigation

Confirmation is required for the first cases, and this must be done by serology. Classical immuno-fluorescence tests cannot differentiate LBTF from other rickettsioses, and only an epidemiological study may be able to identify the responsible vector. Once a typhus outbreak has been confirmed, diagnosis of subsequent cases can be made clinically by senior medical staff, given the complexity and high cost of serological tests.

Vector control

A typhus epidemic should be controlled by a prompt mass delousing campaign. This implies the large-scale use of insecticides which are dusted inside the clothes, treating skin and clothing simultaneously (see *Relapsing fever*, page 338)[8]. Washing clothes may be an effective measure in principle but is usually not easy under camp conditions and does not have a long-lasting effect.

Prophylaxis

Mass prophylaxis with antibiotics is controversial. Although some consider it to be effective in interrupting an outbreak, antibiotic prophylaxis does not prevent the disease but only delays its onset, and provides only short-term protection[2,5,11]. Many authors advise replacing it by prophylactic insecticide application[1,8,9,11]. In refugee settings, resources are better employed in a delousing campaign and improving the level of hygiene.

Case management

The treatment of first choice is a single oral dose of doxycycline. Alternatives are tetracycline or chloramphenicol administered for 3 to 7 days[1,7]. Mild cases can be treated as out-patients while severe cases should be hospitalized after thorough delousing.

Murine typhus fever (MTF)

Murine typhus, also known as flea typhus or endemic typhus, occurs mostly in urban settings, in situations where humans, rats and fleas coexist. It may occur in refugee settings as well, but usually only plays a minor role in overall morbidity[1,3]. However, MTF was a frequent cause of fever of unknown origin in the post-emergency phase among refugees in Thailand and Cambodia (1986-89)[4].

Specific action against MTF is not a priority in the emergency phase because of its low mortality (CFR < 1%). The disease can be controlled by first eliminating fleas, then rats. Treatment is similar to that for LBTF[1].

Scrub typhus

Scrub typhus, also known as mite-borne typhus or rural typhus, occurs mainly in Asia, where it is endemic in small geographical areas ('typhus islands')[1]. Humans become infected by mite bites. It is a severe disease due to its complications, sequelae and high mortality; the case fatality rate ranges from 1% to 60% in untreated cases[1]. Most pregnant women contracting the disease abort and die.

Epidemics may occur in refugee settlements only if they are located in or near a 'typhus island'[1]. The disease was reportedly the second cause of fever in refugee camps on the Thai-Cambodian border in 1988[6].

Control measures are based upon the elimination of mites and the treatment of individuals[9]. Camps should not be installed in known endemic areas. If this is unavoidable, the area should be prepared by clearing vegetation and ground spraying[9]. Clothing and blankets must be impregnated with insecticides. Doxycycline in a single dose is an effective treatment[1].

Key reference

1. Benenson, A. *Control of communicable diseases manual.* 16th edition. Washington DC: American Public Health Association, 1995.

    Other references

2. Perine, P L, Chandler, B P, Krause, D K et al. A clinico-epidemiological study of epidemic typhus in Africa. *Clin. Inf. Dis.*, 1992, 14(5): 1149-58.

3. Brown, A, et al. Murine typhus among Khmers living at an evacuation site on the Thai-Kampuchean border. *Am J Trop Med Hyg*, 1988, 38(1): 168-71.

4. Duffy, P, et al. Murine typhus identified as a major cause of febrile illness in a camp for displaced Khmers in Thailand. *Am J Trop Med Hyg*, 1990, 43(5): 520-6.

5. Cook, G. *Manson's tropical diseases.* 19th edition. London: Saunders, 1996.

6. WHO. *Measles outbreak response. A background document prepared for the Global Advisory Group Meeting.* Washington DC: WHO, 1993. EPI/WHO.

7. Médecins Sans Frontières. *Clinical guidelines, diagnostic and treatment manual.* Paris: Hatier, 1993.

8. Epidemic typhus risk in Rwandan refugee camps. *Wkly Epidemiol Rec*, 1994, 69(34): 259.

9. Lucas, A O, Gilles, H M. *A short textbook of preventive medicine for the tropics.* Bungay (Suffolk): ELBS, 1986.

10. WHO Working Group on Rickettsial Diseases. Rickettsioses: A continuing disease problem. *WHO Bull*, 1982, 60: 157-64.

Relapsing fever

Relapsing fever is a borreliosis (i.e. due to *Borrelia* species) transmitted by two types of vector: lice and ticks. The disease is classically epidemic where it is spread by lice, and endemic where it is spread by ticks[1].

• Louse-borne relapsing fever (LBRF) is caused exclusively by *Borrelia recurrentis*, and transmitted by body lice. Outbreaks occur in limited areas, mainly in Africa, India and South America, with the majority of cases reported in Ethiopia[1,5]. It affects louse-infested populations, and is more frequent in mountainous and cold areas where clothes are worn for long periods without being washed. The related mortality is high (see table below)[10]. Refugee settlements are at high risk of lice infestation because of overcrowding and poor hygiene[1]. Epidemics of relapsing fever have been observed among refugee and displaced populations in Ethiopia[4,5,7], Sudan and Somalia[8], and may coexist with epidemic typhus[4].

• Tick-borne relapsing fever (TBRF) is caused by *Borrelia duttoni*, and is widespread throughout Africa; foci exist in North Africa, Iran, India, Central Asia and South America[1]. TBRF is usually endemic, but occasional outbreaks may occur in limited areas. The related mortality is low[10]. TBRF is not frequently reported in refugee settings; however, it was suspected in displaced persons in Rwanda, in 1993 (MSF unpublished data).

Because of the high case fatality rate, epidemics of LBRF require immediate action. TBRF control measures, on the other hand, are less urgent.

Table 4.5
Relapsing fever in summary

	Louse-borne RF	**Tick-borne RF**
Agent	*Borrelia recurrentis*	*Borrelia duttoni*
Vector	body louse	tick
Occurrence	epidemic	endemic
Areas	Ethiopia, Sudan, India, S. America	mainly Africa
Mortality	CFR high (10-70% w/o treatment)	CFR low
Action required:	if lice already present, before any outbreak:	in post-emergency:
– vector control	– mass delousing campaign	– cut grass, spray houses
– case management	– tetracycline in a single dose	– tetracycline

PREVENTION

The prevention of lice infestation is essential among a refugee population settled in an area at risk of LBRF. Sufficient water and soap should be made available; personal hygiene and the cleaning of shelters must be encouraged. The detection of lice in the community should lead immediately to a delousing campaign, before any louse-borne disease breaks out (such as relapsing fever, epidemic typhus or trench fever). In areas at higher risk (e.g.

Ethiopia), it is advised to check new arrivals systematically for lice during health screening, and carry out delousing for those for whom it is required. As far as the presence of ticks is concerned, no vector control measures have to be implemented as long as TBRF is not an important health problem.

OUTBREAK CONTROL

Outbreak investigation and surveillance

When there is no general outbreak of the disease, borreliosis can easily remain unnoticed because of its non-specific clinical picture, particularly when there is no laboratory facility. However, it can be an important cause of fever of unknown origin[8,9]. Relapsing fever should be suspected when lice are present in endemic areas, and cases suspected on clinical grounds should be differentiated from typhus fever. Confirmation of suspected cases is done by simple microscopy: *Borrelia* may be found in stained thick or thin blood films taken during a febrile attack. This test has a 70% sensitivity and a 100% specificity[10]. *Borrelia* is easy to recognize under the microscope, but *B. recurrentis* cannot be distinguished from *B. duttoni.*

Suspicion of a borreliosis outbreak in a refugee camp should lead to an epidemiological investigation. The case definition must then be established locally, since relapsing fever presents differently from one outbreak to another[8].

Control measures

- Louse-borne relapsing fever

    An epidemic of LBRF cannot be halted without systematic vector control[5,2]. The aim is to reduce lice density, and provide protection against any further infestations[4]. Mass delousing of the refugee population is carried out with the large-scale use of insecticides[1,2]: skin and clothes are treated with dusting insecticide powder[4,11]. Washing clothes is difficult in refugee situations and does not have a long-lasting effect.

    A mass delousing campaign should include[4]:

    – house-to-house screening to assess the level of lice infestation,

    – mass treatment of the population by treatment of clothes with insecticide powder, possibly also treatment of hair by appropriate insecticide or simple shaving,

    – a home spraying campaign,

    – improvement in general hygiene by increasing the water supply, distributing soap and setting up showers and washing-places.

    Delousing campaigns require good logistical organization and are difficult to manage; in Somalia, LBRF remained a problem in camps despite 4 delousing campaigns[8]. Cultural obstacles may prevent the implementation of such a campaign. In these situations, an alternative strategy is active case finding linked with the prompt treatment of cases, and home spraying.

    Mass prophylactic treatment is not recommended[1,3]. However, tetracyclines (e.g. a single dose of doxycycline) may be given after exposure through lice bites; for instance, it has been given during the delousing process to protect against possible infection[3,4,5].

- Tick-borne relapsing fever

Specific control measures are generally not urgent because the related mortality is low. Tick control is the first priority, although this is difficult to achieve, particularly in infested houses. Measures include keeping the grass short in and around the camp, spraying inside shelters, and treating livestock with insecticides[1,2].

Case management

The preferred treatment is a single oral dose of tetracycline or doxycycline (500 mg)[1,7,9]. Procaine penicillin in a single injection may also be given, but it acts more slowly and relapses are more frequent[9]. Therapy sometimes induces a strong adverse reaction after the first dose of antibiotic (Herxheimer reaction) and should therefore be supervised.

Patients with LBRF who are to be hospitalized should be deloused or freed of ticks before admission[1].

🦰 Key references

1. Lucas, A O, Gilles, H M. *A short textbook of preventive medicine in the tropics.* Bungay (Suffolk): ELBS, 1986.
2. OMS. *Méthodes de lutte chimiques contre les arthropodes vecteurs et nuisibles importants en santé publique.* Geneva: WHO, 1984.

Other references

3. Benenson, A. *Control of communicable diseases manual.* 16th edition. Washington DC: American Public Health Association, 1995.
4. Goessens, E. Lice control scheme during an epidemic of relapsing fever in Ethiopia. *Medical News*, 1993, 2(5): 22-6.
5. Sundnes, K O, Haïmanot, A T. Epidemic of louse-borne relapsing fever in Ethiopia. *The Lancet*, 1993, 342(8881): 1192.
6. WHO. Epidemic typhus risk in Rwandan refugee camps. *Wkly Epidemiol Rec*, 1994, 69(34): 259.
7. Bell, L, Griekspoor, A. *Relapsing fever epidemic - displaced civilian shelters - Sept 91, Mekele and Adrigat, Tigray, Ethiopia.* [Internal report]. Brussels, Amsterdam: Médecins Sans Frontières, 1991.
8. Brown, V, Larouze, B, Desvé, G, Rousset, J J, Thibon, M, Fourrier, A, et al. Clinical presentation of louse-borne relapsing fever among Ethiopian refugees in northern Somalia. *Ann Trop Med Parasit*, 1988, 82(5): 499-502.
9. Gebrehiwot, T, Fiseha, A. Tetracyclin vs penicillin in the treatment of louse-borne relapsing fever. *Ethiop Med J*, 1992, 30: 175-8.
10. Mandell, G, Douglas, G, Bennett, J. *Principles and practice of infectious diseases.* London: Churchill Livingstone, 1990: 2141-3.

Typhoid fever

Typhoid fever, caused by the bacteria *Salmonella typhi*, is endemic throughout the world wherever sanitary conditions are poor, but dramatic outbreaks are unusual. Transmission takes place through water and food which have been contaminated by stools, and the degree of infection is directly related to the dose of bacteria ingested. Many infections are mild, atypical or asymptomatic, especially in endemic areas, and healthy carriers contribute significantly to the persistence of *Salmonella typhi* in the community[1,6]. The usual case fatality rate of 10% can be reduced to less than 1% with adequate antibiotic treatment. However, many strains have become resistant to the recommended antibiotics, and multi-resistant strains have been reported in several countries in Asia, the Middle East and Latin America)[1].

In refugee settlements where water supply and sanitation measures are inadequate, transmission of typhoid fever may occur if there are active cases or carriers in the population[1]. Outbreaks of typhoid fever can last over a considerable period of time, occurring as a series of scattered cases, for example, in Kurdish refugee camps in southern Iran in 1991[2].

SURVEILLANCE

Typhoid fever is one of the commonest cause of fever lasting more than a few days in the tropics. However, many cases do not display the classical clinical signs. Since identification of every cause of fever is practically impossible in refugee settings, the disease will always remain under-reported.

Once typhoid fever is known (and confirmed) to be a major health problem, a case definition should be established, but must be adapted to the skills of health staff.

Example of case definition for typhoid fever[1,6]:

Any insidious onset of sustained fever, headache, malaise, anorexia, relative bradychardia, constipation or diarrhoea, and non-productive cough.

OUTBREAK CONTROL

Outbreak investigation

There is no precise epidemic threshold, but the traditional rule of the consecutive doubling of the number of cases over 2 weeks can be used. When an outbreak is suspected, the first cases should be confirmed by laboratory. Serological tests may be used, although these are of limited value for the diagnosis of individual patients[1]. The Widal test has a low sensitivity (60%), but is still acceptable in emergency settings as a diagnostic tool at community level[4]. Newer methods of serodiagnosis have a better sensitivity and specificity[1,6]. The most valuable method is the isolation of the bacteria in the blood or bone marrow (though culture) early in the disease, but is usually not possible in emergency settings. Culture of faeces or urine (after the first week) provides presumptive evidence only in the presence of a characteristic clinical picture. These two methods however have the advantage of allowing sensitivity testing, which is particularly useful in view of the risk of antibiotic resistance[6].

Preventive measures

In refugee settings, preventive measures are similar to those in any other setting.

- Supply of safe drinking water and proper disposal of excreta should be given the highest priority, water points must be treated and well protected[1].
- Personal hygiene should be improved through health education, especially with regards to hand washing[1].
- Mass immunization is not recommended as an epidemic measure[1]: the compliance to the multi-dose vaccine is likely to be poor; the vaccine provides only individual protection and does not restrict transmission[5]; it gives a false sense of security when all efforts should be devoted to the above mentioned measures[1]. However, vaccination might be recommended for health staff.

Case management

In-patient care is preferable during the acute stage of the illness. Patients should receive antibiotic treatment in accordance with current resistance patterns[1]. In some areas, strains have already become resistant to all common antibiotics, and quinolones should be reserved as a last resort. Information on current resistance and treatment schemes should be obtained from the health authorities of the host country.

✎ Key reference

1. Benenson, A. *Control of communicable diseases manual.* 16th edition. Washington DC: American Public Health Association, 1995.

Other references

2. Reisinger, E C, Grasmug, E, Krejs, G J, et al. Antibody response after vaccination against typhoid fever in Kurdish refugee camp. *The Lancet*, 1994, 343(8902): 918-19.
3. Babille, M, De Colombani, P, et al. Post-emergency epidemiological surveillance in Iraqi-Kurdish refugee camps in Iran. *Disasters*, 1994, 18(1): 58-74.
4. Rasaily, R, Dutta, P, Saha, MR et al. Value of a single Widal test in the diagnosis of typhoid fever. *Indian J Med Res*, 1993, 97: 104-7.
5. Bollag, U. Practical evaluation of a pilot immunization campaign against typhoid fever in a Cambodian refugee camp. *Int J Epid*, 1980, 9(2).
6. Cook, G. *Manson's tropical diseases.* 19th edition. London: Saunders, 1996.

Influenza

The importance of influenza resides in the rapidity with which outbreaks evolve, the widespread morbidity, and the seriousness of complications (mainly respiratory infections, e.g. bacterial pneumonia)[3]. Influenza can produce severe outbreaks in the tropics, more frequently in the rainy season. During outbreaks, severe illness and death occur mainly among the weak and the elderly[3].

The extent to which influenza affects refugee populations is probably seriously underestimated because of the lack of diagnostic means[4]. In 1993, influenza was suspected to be the cause of an outbreak among returnees and residents in southern Sudan, with a case fatality rate of 16%[5].

SURVEILLANCE AND OUTBREAK INVESTIGATION

The routine surveillance of influenza is not feasible in practice, because sporadic cases can be identified only by sophisticated laboratory procedures. Indeed, influenza in children cannot be easily differentiated from other respiratory diseases, and it may also be mistaken for chloroquine-resistant malaria in endemic areas[3].

An influenza outbreak may be suspected when there is an outbreak of fever of unknown origin leading to severe respiratory infection and death among the old and weak. Influenza can only be confirmed as the cause of an epidemic by epidemiological studies and virus identification. This can be performed through isolation of the virus in secretions (on nasopharyngeal swabs with a specific transport medium) or through demonstration of a specific serological response[3,6].

OUTBREAK CONTROL

Immunization is not recommended, as this would require a vaccine adapted to the current influenza variant, and would not be cost-effective.

The only action indicated in case of an outbreak is to give special attention to vulnerable groups such as the malnourished and the elderly, and to treat secondary infections as early as possible (see section *Control of acute respiratory infections*, in *7. Control of Communicable Diseases and Epidemics* in Part II).

✎ *References*

1. Bres, P. *Public health action in emergencies caused by epidemics.* Geneva: WHO, 1986.
2. Simmonds, S, Vaughan, P, William Gunn, S. *Refugee community health care.* Oxford: Oxford University Press, 1983.
3. Benenson, A. *Control of communicable diseases manual.* 16th edition. Washington DC: American Public Health Association, 1995.
4. Azinge, N O. A clinical reminder that local epidemics of influenza are common in Africa. *Tropical Doctor*, 1985, 15(4): 199-200.
5. Krug, E, Paquet, C, Fouveau, C, Moren, A. Excessive mortality in the Yambio region, southern Sudan. *Medical News*, 1994, 3(1): 20-3.
6. Duverlie, G, Houbart, L, Visse, B, et al. A nylon membrane enzyme immunoassay for rapid diagnosis of influenza A infection. *J Vir. Methods*, 1992, 40(1): 77-84.

Leishmaniasis

The *Leishmania* parasite causes a number of different diseases, varying from lethal visceral disease to mild, self-healing skin lesions. Clinical manifestations vary according to the different strains and the immunological status of the host. The parasite is transmitted by specific sandfly species. Several classifications of leishmaniasis are in use, based on different strains, mode of transmission, geography ('Old' and 'New World'), or clinical syndromes[1].

From a clinical perspective it is most useful to differentiate between visceral and cutaneous leishmaniasis[4,5]:

- Visceral leishmaniasis or 'kala azar' is characterized by irregular fever, weight loss, splenomegaly, sometimes hepatomegaly and/or lymphadenopathies and anaemia. If untreated, mortality is virtually 100%. The incubation period is very long (from 2 weeks to 2 years, usually around 3 months).

- Cutaneous leishmaniasis has various manifestations: simple cutaneous leishmaniasis usually produces a single, self-healing ulcer; however, multiple lesions are also possible and can cause disfiguring or disabling scars. In the case of the latter, treatment is recommended. In South America, muco-cutaneous leishmaniasis ('espundia') also occurs, which can produce extensive destruction of the oral, nasal and pharyngeal cavities.

Although leishmaniasis occurs in 82 countries around the world, the majority of cases is limited to a few countries[1]. Over 90% of visceral leishmaniasis cases in the world are reported from Bangladesh, Brazil, India and the Sudan; and more than 90% of cutaneous leishmaniasis cases are to be found in Afghanistan, Brazil, Iran, Saudi Arabia and Syria. Within these countries, the disease is usually limited to known, endemic areas[1,3].

Leishmaniasis and refugees

Migration movements from endemic areas appear to be an important factor in some outbreaks[6]. Infected refugees may present symptoms that are unusual for the local health staff. This happened in Sudan from 1988 on, where people fleeing the south of the country, arrived in Khartoum, 900 kilometres from their homes, and were discovered to have kala azar[2,6]. Also in Afghanistan, cases of cutaneous leishmaniasis were found among refugees in Jalalabad who originated from Kabul. Active cases originating from an endemic area are unlikely to transmit the disease in a refugee settlement unless the specific vectors are present.

The opposite situation, where refugees enter an endemic area, may result in an outbreak among non-immune people, with potentially high mortality in the case of visceral leishmaniasis.

DIAGNOSIS AND SURVEILLANCE

- Clinical signs and symptoms are not very specific, especially in the case of visceral leishmaniasis which can be mistaken for tuberculosis, typhoid fever, or chronic malaria[6]. Diagnosis is facilitated if health staff are aware of the occurence of leishmaniasis in the host area, or in the area the refugees came from[3]. It is necessary to confirm suspected cases by a laboratory. The parasite can be isolated through examinations or culture of lymph node, bone-marrow or spleen aspirates, but spleen or bone-marrow puncture may be difficult or even dangerous. Serological tests are simpler and provide quicker results, but they have a lower diagnostic value[3,6].

- Surveillance is best conducted in the treatment unit. The refugees' travel history will have to be recorded carefully in order to find the most likely place of infection and to trace possible local transmission. If the latter is suspected, expert advice should be sought to discuss possible control measures[5].

TREATMENT

Visceral leishmaniasis usually responds well to pentavalent antimonial treatment (e.g. sodium stibogluconate)[4]. Hospitalization is recommended for visceral leishmaniasis - at least in the initial treatment phase - and a special treatment unit may need to be set up. The treatment lasts 15-30 days and is not without side-effects[4,6]. The same drug can be used for cutaneous leishmaniasis if treatment is deemed necessary, e.g. in case of multiple lesions or infection acquired in geographic region where mucosal disease has been reported[5]. Sometimes, infiltration inside the lesion itself may be useful.

📑 References

1. Desjeux, P. Human leishmaniasis: Epidemiology and public health aspects. *World Health Stat Q*, 1992, 45(2-3): 267-75.

2. Zijlstra, E E, Ali, M S, El-Hassan, A M, et al. Kala Azar in displaced people from southern Sudan: Epidemiological, clinical and therapeutic findings. *Trans R Soc Trop Med Hyg*, 1991, 85: 365-9.

3. Desjeux P. *Information on the epidemiology and control of leishmaniasis by country or territory.* Geneva: WHO, 1991. WHO/LEISH/91.30.

4. Cook, G. *Manson's tropical diseases.* 19th edition. London: Saunders, 1996.

5. Benenson, A. *Control of communicable diseases in man.* 16th edition. Washington DC: American Public Health Association, 1995.

6. De Beer, P, El Harith, A, Loyok Deng, L, et al. A killing disease epidemic among displaced Sudanese populations identified as visceral leishmaniasis. *Am J Trop Hyg*, 1991, 44(3): 283-9.

Plague

Plague, an infectious disease caused by *Yersinia pestis*, is a zoonosis affecting primarily wild rodents and their fleas, occasionally causing disease in human beings[1]. Plague is mainly transmitted through flea bites - between wild rodents, from wild rodents to domestic rats, or from rodent to man. Transmission through direct contact with rodents or through ingestion of meat is less common. Airborne transmission (droplets) from man to man may occur in cases of pneumonic plague[1,5].

Human plague thus generally occurs as a result of human intrusion into the animal infection cycle, or from contact between wild rodents and domestic rats (and their fleas); plague is thus a threat in areas of persistent wild rodent infection or natural zoonotic foci of plague[1]. These foci persist in many parts of the world, in Asia, Africa and the Americas, and represent an unpredictable risk for outbreaks of human plague[2,5].

There are 3 main forms of clinical plague[1,2,3]:

1. Bubonic plague, characterized by high fever with 'buboes', is the most frequent form (75%). Buboes - nodes that become swollen, tender and may suppurate - are located in 70%-90% of cases in the inguinal area. The case fatality rate is over 50% in untreated cases.

2. Pneumonic plague may occur as complications arising from bubonic or septicemic plague, or as primary pneumonic plague through person-to-person transmission. This form is highly contagious because of airborne transmission and can result in limited outbreaks or devasting epidemics. The case fatality rate is 100% if left untreated.

3. Septicemic plague may result from a progression of other clinical forms (even with inapparent lymphadenopaty). This form is rapidly fatal in untreated cases.

Plague may become a problem for refugees or returnees in endemic areas due to overcrowding, poor hygienic conditions (if human fleas are playing a role), or when they settle in or enter into contact with areas of wild rodent infection. Cases of plague have been suspected in refugee populations in Malawi and Mozambique[4,5].

Methods of control

OUTBREAK INVESTIGATION

Health staff should be aware of areas where the disease is endemic, and gather surveillance data from the Ministry of Health[2]. Early diagnosis is important, but plague is unfortunately often misdiagnosed.

When cases of plague are clinically suspected, it is essential to have confirmation by identification of the causal agent. Visualizing the organism in microscopic examination of infected fluid (from buboes, blood, cerebrospinal fluid or sputum) is a suggestive - but not conclusive - evidence of plague infection. Diagnosis needs to be confirmed, preferably by culture, or by serology (rise or fall in antibody titre)[1]. The culture may be difficult to obtain, requiring a specimen of fluid taken from a patient before any antibiotic treatment is received, and transported on basic agar medium; precautions have to be taken to avoid contamination.

Once laboratory confirmation has been obtained, clinical diagnosis will be sufficient. A standard case definition has to be determined[5]. Experience in refugee settings has shown that establishing an adequate case definition is difficult; it should be specific enough, for instance it should allow to differentiate buboes from other adenopathies, but must remain easy to use for the health staff.

Sporadic cases in endemic areas do not usually indicate the onset of an outbreak.

PREVENTIVE MEASURES

These measures should aim at reducing the likelihood of people being bitten by infected fleas, having contact with infected tissues or exudate, or being exposed to patients with pneumonic plague[1].

- Anti-flea campaigns[1,5]: if fleas are present in an endemic area, the whole settlement should be treated (houses and out-houses, rodent burrows), and hygienic conditions improved, especially since there is also a risk from other flea-borne diseases (e.g. typhus). National vector programmes should be consulted. In open situations, this may be carried out in expanding circles around known foci. In addition, refugees and their clothing must be dusted with insecticide powder. Although this measure should at least cover patients and close contacts, it is preferable to treat the whole population[1,7].

- Avoid rodent infestation: appropriate food storage and waste disposal is essential in order to limit access to food and shelter by rodents. Rat control should always be preceded by measures to control fleas[1,7].

- Refugees should be adequately educated on the risk of exposure, and informed why these measures have to be taken. This will also help to reduce the risk of panic[9].

- Vaccination (providing protection over 6 months) is not recommended as an outbreak control measure because maximal antibody responses require the administration of multiple doses over several months[8].

- In case of pneumonic plague, those in contact with cases (confirmed or suspected) should receive chemoprophylaxis and be placed under surveillance for seven days, if this is possible[1]. Mass chemoprophylaxis may be envisaged in a refugee setting with high case fatality rates, considering the extreme contagiousness of the disease and the easy access to the population to be covered.

TREATMENT OF CASES

Early treatment of cases is a priority. The first suspected cases should be treated without waiting for laboratory confirmation.

Patients with pneumonic plague must be strictly isolated and precautions against airborne transmission must be taken for health staff and visitors, until 48 hours of appropriate treatment and favourable clinical response. Cases of bubonic plague must not be isolated, but they must be rid of fleas. as well as their clothing. Hospitalization however does improve treatment compliance. Antibiotics (e.g. tetracycline or chloramphenicol) are highly effective when taken early on[1,2,3]. Buboes usually heal spontaneously.

Extra health staff and a special treatment unit will be required. All health staff should receive chemoprophylaxis (doxycycline or tetracycline)[8]. Strict aseptic precautions must be taken in handling dead bodies and exudate.

SPECIFIC MEASURES WITH REGARDS TO POPULATION MOVEMENTS

- Ideally, new arrivals should not be accepted into a refugee settlement affected by plague.

- Refugees or displaced people coming from an area already affected by plague must either be kept in isolation for 7 days (in the case of pneumonic plague) or kept under close surveillance; new arrivals (and their belongings) should be disinfected on entry.

- Repatriation of refugees is not recommended when plague is affecting either the refugee population or the home reception area.

➤ *Key reference*

1. Benenson, A. *Control of communicable diseases manual.* 16th edition. Washington DC: American Public Health Association, 1995.

Other references

2. Cook, G. *Manson's tropical diseases.* 19th edition. London: Saunders, 1996.
3. Médecins Sans Frontières. *Clinical guidelines, diagnostic and treatment manual.* Paris: Hatier, 1993.
4. Bertoletti, G. Bubonic plague outbreak in the refugee camp of Mankhokwe, Malawi. *Medical News*, 1995, 4(2): 21-3.
5. Matthys, F. Plague epidemic in Mutarara district, Mozambique. *Medical News*, 1995, 4(2): 14-20.
6. Butler, G, de Graaf, P, van de Wijk, J. Urban plague in Zaire. *The Lancet*, 1994, 343(8896): 536.
7. Médecins Sans Frontières. *Public health engineering in emergency situations.* Paris: Médecins Sans Frontières, 1994: III/11-III/28.
8. CDC. Human plague - India, 1994. *MMWR*, 1994, 43: 689-91.
9. Mavalankar, D V, Chand, V K, et al. Plague in India. *The Lancet*, 1994, 344(8932): 1298.

Human African trypanosomiasis

Sleeping sickness or human African trypanosomiasis is found exclusively in the inter-tropical region of the African continent (i.e. the area extending from 20° north to 20° south of the equator)[1,2].

It is caused by a parasite, *Trypanosoma*, of which there are two types:
- the *Trypanosoma brucei gambiense* in central and western Africa,
- the *Trypanosoma brucei rhodesiense* in eastern Africa.

It is transmitted by a vector, the *Glossina* or tsetse fly. For the *Trypanosoma gambiense* there is only one single reservoir, i.e. humans, while the *Trypanosoma rhodesiense* shares its cycle with human beings, cattle and wild animals.

In the colonial period and in the period immediately following, the programmes set up to control the major endemic diseases in Africa were able to control most of the foci of infection. But since then, the structural, economic and political problems that plague the African continent have led to a relaxation in control programmes, allowing the resurgence of many transmission foci; in some foci, prevalence is estimated at between 10% and 20% (i.e. in certain parts of Zaire)[4]. According to WHO, out of an exposed population of around 5 million people some 20,000 new cases were recorded during the 80s (which is certainly an under-estimation)[3].

As with malaria, population displacement can contribute towards a rapid reactivation of latent trypanosomiasis foci. Since the disease is always lethal if left untreated, it can become a major public health problem in these situations: the best recent example is the occurrence of a very serious outbreak at the beginning of the 80s in Moyo, in the north-western province of Uganda[6]. Although relatively well-controlled previously, this area became almost entirely depopulated after a change of government in 1979, when most of its inhabitants fled to Sudan and settled in areas where trypanosomiasis is highly endemic. They started to return to Uganda at the beginning of 1986, when some political stability was re-established. A proliferation of tsetse fly and the return of large numbers of people infected in Sudan resulted in an outbreak. Between 1987 and 1992, 6,000 trypanosomiasis cases were treated in Moyo district out of an estimated population of 80,000 inhabitants; prevalence varied from 1% to 30% in each village screened. This focus could be controlled if it were not for a continuous influx of refugees fleeing the civil war in Sudan, where the disease is known to be very active. Trypanosomiasis epidemics easily cross borders in the wake of war[6].

Individual cases, or even outbreaks, of trypanosomiasis should be anticipated in refugees coming from a non-controlled focus, or suspected in an endemic area when individuals present suggestive clinical signs.

In deciding whether to treat trypanosomiasis cases or not, a number of principles should be taken into account.

- The disease evolves slowly with an incubation period varying from 2 to 3 weeks after being infected by a tsetse bite. The symptoms and clinical signs are similar in both *rhodesiense* and *gambiense* trypanosomiasis, except that the illness is usually chronic in *gambiense* with a spontaneous (fatal) evolution over 2 to 3 years or more. The *Rhodesiense* trypanosomiasis has a quicker evolution, usually less than a year. They both inevitably end in death.

- Laboratory confirmation is imperative: every suspected case (clinical or serological) calls for absolute diagnostic certainty - i.e. the isolation of the parasite in lymph nodes, blood or cerebro-spinal fluid - following a complex decisional flow chart that relies on laboratory tests, requiring specific equipment and expertise. Case definition is based on this laboratory confirmation.

- Only confirmed patients should be treated. The treatment still relies on drugs which have been around for a long time, melarsoprol for example. All treatments are costly: the global cost ranges from $50 to $200 per patient (MSF data).

- Active screening is the preferred method for the early detection of cases, as the treatment required in the first stage of the disease is shorter and significantly less dangerous (see *Treatment* below). However, in the first phase of an emergency, or if security conditions do not allow for active screening, it is preferable to treat only passively detected patients.

- During outbreaks, a specialized therapeutic unit is usually necessary because existing in-patient services are very quickly overloaded. For instance, in Moyo, the epidemic led to a doubling, or even a tripling of hospital capacity, involving specialized training for medical personnel.

Disease control programme

A control programme is comprised of several measures.

ACTIVE SCREENING

Based on data provided by hospitals, a map should be drawn up showing the distribution of cases under treatment in different areas (and kept regularly updated); this will enable the identification of priority areas. It is useless, even ethically wrong, to carry out a survey of serological prevalence: every detected case should be treated as quickly as possible, and the efforts and means spent to undertake such a survey would hinder the programme's effectiveness. Using the information contained on this map, mobile teams should conduct an active screening of the population to ensure early detection. Screening relies on the Card Agglutination Trypanosomiasis Test (CATT), which can be carried out on the refugee site by the mobile teams. Every detected patient must be confirmed via isolation of the parasite, and then treated.

TREATMENT

Confirmed patients are treated at hospital level; the drugs used will differ according to the evolutionary stage of the disease[1,2]:

- **Stage 1**: early stage of the disease, invasion of the blood and lymph glands: treatment with suramin or pentamidine.

- **Stage 2**: terminal stage, cerebral trypanosomiasis: treatment with melarsoprol, which provokes lethal side effects in an average of 5 % of cases; DFMO (Difluromethylornithine) is used in case of resistance to melarsoprol.

The protocol may call for pentamidine or suramin, alone or in association with melarsoprol or DFMO.

AWARENESS CAMPAIGNS AND HEALTH EDUCATION

Screening and treatment should be carried out in tandem with a campaign to inform and educate the population at risk; they should take personal measures to protect themselves against tsetse fly bites.

VECTOR CONTROL

Treatment of all cases is not sufficient to control the spread of the disease, especially where *Trypanosoma rhodesiense* is concerned, as the reservoir is not only human. If conditions allow, a programme of vector control by tsetse-fly traps should be implemented, but this is only possible and effective if there is a very high level of community participation[5].

SURVEILLANCE

When an epidemic control programme is launched, a surveillance system should be set up from the outset with two objectives in mind: to draw a map of treatment prevalence based on hospital data, and to monitor the impact of the on-going control programme by following up the disease trends.

Once disease prevalence has been reduced by an effective control programme, a long-term trypanosomiasis surveillance system should be set up and integrated into the existing national health information system of the host country.

✎ *References*

1. Gentilini, M. *Médecine tropicale.* Paris: Flammarion Médecine-Sciences,1993.
2. Cook, G. *Manson's tropical diseases.* 19th edition. London: Saunders, 1996.
3. Arbijn, M, Bruneel, H. Human trypanosomiasis in Zaire: A return to the situation at the start of the century? *Medical News*, 1994, 3(5): 13-15.
4. WHO. *Manual for fighting trypanosomiasis.* Geneva: WHO, 1983.
5. WHO. *African trypanosomiasis: Epidemiology and counter measures.* Technical Report Serie No. 739. Geneva: WHO, 1986.
6. Paquet, C, Castilla, J, et al. Cinq ans de lutte contre la trypanosomiase dans le district de Moyo, Uganda, 1987-1991. *Medical News*, 1993, 2(1): 5-12.

Schistosomiasis

Several species of schistosoma parasites can cause schistosomiasis: *Schistosoma mansoni, S. haematobium* and *S. japonicum* are the major species causing human disease; *S. mekongi* is of importance only in limited areas. *S. mansoni* and *S. japonicum* give rise primarily to hepatic and intestinal manifestations, and *S. haematobium* to urinary manifestations[6].

Schistosomiasis is increasingly reported among refugee populations. Schistosoma have been identified in refugees in Ethiopia, Somalia, Cameroon, Chad, Malawi, Mozambique and Zimbabwe and *S. mekongi* has been reported in Cambodian and Laotian refugees in Thailand, where its possible transmission to the local population has been debated[1,4,5].

However, schistosomiasis is not likely to be a priority health problem in refugee and displaced populations, since the most important pathological effects are complications arising from chronic infection. Only in situations where schistosomiasis is known to be a major health problem in the community, can a control programme be started, provided that the emergency is under control.

PREVENTION

The location of the refugee site is important. If it can be avoided, refugees should not settle in areas where environmental hazards such as schistosomiasis are present[2]. When a non-exposed population arrives in an endemic area, the main preventive measures are to treat surface water with molluscicides and to remove vegetation from surrounding areas. As it is impossible to prevent the population from having direct contact with contaminated water, refugees should be educated and informed about safe bathing, laundering and drinking water facilities[6].

Mass treatment should not be considered in a non-settled population.

SURVEILLANCE

Cases of schistosomiasis will usually not be recognized clinically or reported in routine surveillance activities, with the exception of cases of symptomatic urinary schistosomiasis (haematuria). Diagnosis requires a basic laboratory for stool and urine examination.

DISEASE CONTROL

Ideally, schistosomiasis control programmes should target both host and refugee communities, and be implemented via long-term national projects (e.g. dealing with agriculture and irrigation, water supply, etc.)[3]. However, these programmes are usually outside the scope of refugee relief assistance. It is essential to improve sanitary conditions to decrease transmission. In addition, studies of schistosomiasis prevalence among refugees in Thailand show a high prevalence of other parasitic diseases (60% to 90%), revealing that poor sanitary conditions require more attention than the schistosomiasis problem itself[5].

Individual cases should be treated according to appropriate treatment regimens, which are usually defined at national level.

✎ References

1. WHO. *Implementation of the global strategy for health for all by the year 2000. Second Evaluation.* Geneva: WHO, 1993.

2. Simmonds, S, Vaughan, P, William Gunn, S. *Refugee community health care.* Oxford: Oxford University Press, 1983.

3. WHO. *Schistosomiasis control.* Technical Report Serie No. 728. Geneva: WHO, 1985.

4. Temcharoen, P, Viboolyavatana, J. A Survey on intestinal parasitic infections in Laotian refugees in Ubon province, Northeastern Thailand, with special reference to schistosomiasis. *Southeast Asian J. Trop. Med. Pub. Hlth.*, 1979, 10(4): 552-5.

5. Keittivuti, B, D'Agnes, T, et al. Prevalence of schistosomiasis and other parasitic diseases among Cambodian refugees residing in Bang-Kaeng holding center, Prachinburi province, Thailand. *Am J Trop Med Hyg*, 1982, 31(5): 988-90.

6. Benenson, A. *Control of communicable diseases manual.* 16th edition. Washington DC: American Public Health Association, 1995.

Poliomyelitis

Poliomyelitis is an acute viral infection occurring worldwide that may lead to paralysis, possibly resulting in death or permanent sequellae. Paralytic disease does not occur frequently in infected persons (50-1,000 asymptomatic or minor infections for each case of paralytic disease) but increases in frequency with age at the time of infection[2]. Case fatality rates for paralytic cases vary from 2% to 10% in epidemics[2]. It is a particularly serious health problem in developing countries, where epidemics occur mainly in infants and young children. Transmission is primarily via the faecal-oral route (by inhalation or ingestion) where sanitation is poor; but in outbreaks, transmission through droplets may become more significant. Humans are the only reservoir[2].

WHO has included polio vaccine in the Expanded Programme on Immunization (EPI) with the objective of eradicating the disease by the year 2000.

Population displacements are certainly a factor favouring the circulation of the poliovirus and have been partly responsible for recent outbreaks (Sudan 1993); overcrowding of non-immune groups and the collapse of sanitation measures are other factors responsible for outbreaks[3,4]. Polio outbreaks have been reported in refugee settings, particularly in camps with inadequate sanitation and poor water supplies (e.g. in Thailand in 1980 and in informal settlements in Namibia in 1993-94[5,6]).

PREVENTION

In refugee programmes, EPI activities are implemented when the emergency phase is over and other prerequisites are present (see *Child Health Care in the Post-emergency Phase* in Part III). WHO recommends including the oral poliovirus vaccine (OPV) in the EPI, but injectable vaccines are still used in some countries.

SURVEILLANCE

In highly endemic countries, paralytic poliomyelitis can usually be recognized on clinical grounds. In countries where polio is absent or not frequent, it should be differentiated from other paralytic infections by isolation of the virus from stools[2,3].

Case definition for poliomyelitis[6]:

Any child under 5 years of age with acute flaccid paralysis, for which no other cause can be identified.

In the emergency phase, polio cases are usually not included in the routine surveillance, unless it is known that cases are present. However, as soon as EPI activities are undertaken (post-emergency phase), poliomyelitis should then be included. The occurrence of a paralytic case signifies that the virus is in circulation, and laboratory confirmation is required. This confirmation is performed by isolating the virus on faecal specimens, in an official reference laboratory (information should be gathered from the national EPI). Specimens should be kept below 8°C at all times, and strict precautions must be taken to avoid the spread of poliovirus, i.e. cold chain material used for specimens can no longer be used for vaccines[10]. Special procedures must be followed and these are described in WHO documents[1,10].

OUTBREAK CONTROL

In a camp situation, any acute flaccid paralysis may be considered as the start of a poliomyelitis outbreak. It should prompt immediate outbreak investigation, and early detection of paralytic cases[3].

Control measures must be taken immediately: a mass vaccination with OPV should be instituted as early as possible, and is an effective and rapid way of controlling an outbreak[3]. It should ideally be launched within 2 days of outbreak detection, and completed within 7 days[8]. It generally targets all children under 5 years, but older children may be included if cases occur in higher age groups and resources are sufficient[1,8]. A second round should be carried out after 30 days, regardless of the number of OPV doses received before the outbreak. Administration of other (parenteral) vaccinations should not be continued. All non-emergency surgery and dental extraction should be suspended in the under-five group, until all children have received at least 1 dose of OPV[3].

Improvements must be made in the sanitary conditions and water supply in order to reduce transmission.

CASE MANAGEMENT

If possible, patients should be isolated and all disinfection measures, especially for faeces, should be strictly followed. During the stage of acute illness, only rest and supportive treatment are recommended. After the acute phase, once clinical signs have stabilized, physiotherapy must be introduced when necessary[8].

Key references

1. WHO. *Responding to a suspected polio outbreak: Case investigation, surveillance and control.* Geneva: WHO, 1991. WHO/EPI/POL/91.3.

   Other references
2. WHO. *The immunological basis for immunization. Poliomyelitis.* Geneva: WHO, 1993. WHO/EPI/GEN/93.16.
3. Benenson, A. *Control of communicable diseases manual.* 16th edition. Washington DC: American Public Health Association, 1995.
4. Hull, H, Birmingham, M. *The resurgence of poliomyelitis in Sudan. Final report, 2 December 1993.* [Internal report]. Geneva: WHO/EPI , [n.p.].
5. Horan, J M, Preblud, S R. Poliomyelitis in the Khao I-Dang holding centre, February-March 1980. In: Allegra, D T, Nieburg, P, Brabe, M. *Emergency refugee health care - A chronicle of experience in the Khmer assistance operation 1997-1980.* Atlanta: CDC, 1983: 71-3.
6. Van Niekerk, Vries, J B, et al. Outbreak of paralytic poliomyelitis in Namibia. *The Lancet,* 1994, 344: 661-4.
7. Van Gompel, A. *Health advice for travellers.* Brussels: Medasso, 1996-7.
8. WHO. *Report of the technical consultative group meeting with special focus on poliomyelitis.* Geneva: WHO, 1992. WHO/EPI/POLIO/92.1.
9. WHO. *Guidelines for the prevention of deformities in polio.* Geneva: WHO, 1991. WHO/EPI/RHB/91.1.
10. WHO. *Update on poliomyelitis laboratory network development: collection, storage and shipment of specimens.* Geneva: WHO, 1992. WHO/EPI/RPT 2/92.12.

Whooping cough

Whooping cough or pertussis is a common, highly infectious respiratory disease that predominantly affects children. In unimmunized populations, especially those with underlying malnutrition and multiple gastro-intestinal and respiratory infections, whooping cough is among the most lethal diseases affecting infants and young children. The case fatality rate for hospitalized cases can rise to 14%. In an already malnourished population, the commonly associated weight loss and dehydration due to vomiting may lead to an even higher case fatality rate[1].

The disease is usually underdiagnosed and its prevalence thus underestimated in refugee settings[2]. Pertussis is however a potential problem if introduced into crowded refugee camps with many non-immunized children[4]. It has been observed that outbreaks of whooping cough usually occur once the camp has already been established for some months.

SURVEILLANCE

In the post-emergency phase, a case definition for whooping cough should be established and included in the surveillance system. The CDC case definition is appropriate for use in refugee settings:

Case definition for whooping cough[5]:

Any cough illness lasting at least two weeks with one of the following:
- paroxysms of coughing,
- or inspiratory whoop,
- or post-tussive vomiting.

Health staff should however be aware that in infants under six months, the typical whoop or cough paroxysms are often not present.

DISEASE CONTROL

Prevention

Whooping cough is controlled almost exclusively through immunization. The emphasis should therefore on increasing DTP (diphteria, tetanus toxoid and pertussis vaccines combined) coverage through the Expanded Programme on Immunization (EPI) activities in the post-emergency phase (see *Child Health Care in the Post-emergency Phase* in *Part III*). Three doses at monthly intervals are required to develop a sufficient level of protection. A single dose of pertussis vaccine provides little protection[1].

Case management

There is no effective treatment. Antibiotics have little effect once the paroxysmal phase is established[1]. Feeding and rehydration are the most important measures to be taken. As whooping cough may cause or exacerbate malnutrition, due to the vomiting provoked by coughing, anti-tussive drugs can be a useful adjunct to therapeutic feeding.

It is also useful to educate the population on the transmission and prevention of whooping cough.

OUTBREAK CONTROL

An immunization campaign launched in response to an outbreak cannot be effective, since immunity develops slowly and is never complete (vaccine efficacy of 80% after 3 doses)[1,4]. However, immunization should be completed for those whose schedule is incomplete[4].

Case definition for whooping cough in outbreaks[5]:

Any cough illness lasting at least 2 weeks

Early case detection and management are indicated. Suspected cases should preferably be removed from the presence of young children and infants, especially the unimmunized ones[4]. Since feeding and rehydration are the most important measures, cases may receive special care in a separate feeding unit.

References

1. Muller, A S, Leeuwenburg, J, Pratt, D S. Pertussis: Epidemiology and control. *Bull WHO*, 1986, 64(2): 321-31.

2. Simmonds, S, Vaughan, P, William Gunn, S. *Refugee community health care.* Oxford: Oxford University Press, 1983.

3. WHO/EPI. *Improving routine systems for surveillance of infectious diseases including EPI target diseases: guidelines for national programme managers.* Geneva: WHO, 1995. WHO/EPI/TRAM/93.1: 41-2.

4. Benenson, A. *Control of communicable diseases manual.* 16th edition. Washington DC: American Public Health Association, 1995.

5. CDC. Case Definitions for Public Health Surveillance. *MMWR*, 1990, 39(RR-13): 26-7.

Tetanus

Tetanus occurs world wide and is an important cause of death in rural and tropical areas. Two forms are encountered: neonatal tetanus (NT) and wound-related tetanus. Neonatal tetanus is responsible for over 50% of all tetanus deaths, and causes up to 72% of all neonatal deaths[2]: every year, an estimated 500,000 new-borns die from neonatal tetanus[8]. Case fatality rates are extremely high: 35% to 70% for wound-related tetanus, and up to 85% for neonatal tetanus[1,2]. However, the disease has proven to be almost entirely preventable by immunization with Tetanus Toxoid or TT vaccine, administrated in 3 doses. This vaccine is included in any Expanded Programme of Immunization (EPI).

In refugee settlements, both forms of tetanus can be a serious health problem as several risk factors are often present: disruption of immunization services, traditional practices (e.g. home deliveries and circumcisions) carried out under poor hygiene conditions, and a higher incidence of war-wounded if there is a conflict situation.

PREVENTION

Neonatal tetanus

A combination of 2 strategies is the most effective to prevent neonatal tetanus in refugee settings:
– training traditional birth attendants (TBAs) in clean delivery techniques,
– immunizing women of childbearing age.

Immunization activities aimed at covering all women of childbearing age should be included in ante-natal care in any comprehensive reproductive health programme (see *Reproductive Health Care in the Post-emergency Phase* in Part III)[5]. However, such a programme is only implemented in the post-emergency phase and requires that certain conditions are present.

- In the emergency phase, if neonatal tetanus is frequent, preventive measures should focus on:
  – providing TBAs with basic training in clean delivery techniques, and distributing the necessary equipment to them[3];
  – informing the public about the delivery services available;
  – using alternative strategy to immunize pregnant and lactating women, for instance by including tetanus immunization in supplementary feeding programmes targeting pregnant and lactating women.
- In the post-emergency phase, a comprehensive immunization programme will be implemented in line with EPI recommendations (i.e. the immunization of all women of childbearing age)[5].

Wound-related tetanus

In the case of war wounds, tetanus can be prevented by[7]:
– an early and adequate excision of dead tissue and leaving wounds open;
– administration of penicillin as soon as possible after a wound is received;
– simultaneous administration of anti-tetanus serum (ATS) and tetanus toxoid.

Immunized patients do not need anti-tetanus serum, and should only receive a booster dose of tetanus toxoid. However, most patients in developing countries are not actively immunized and the risk of tetanus among war-wounded is significant. It is therefore safer to consider such patients as non-immunized. This approach towards war-wounded should be maintained both in the emergency and post-emergency phases.

SURVEILLANCE

The diagnosis is mainly clinical. The WHO case definition can be used.

Case definition for neonatal tetanus[5]:

A child with a history of all 3 of the following:
1) normal suck and cry for the first 2 days of life;
2) onset of illness between 3 and 28 days of life;
3) inability to suck, followed by stiffness and/or convulsions.

Morbidity and mortality, as well as vaccination coverage, should be monitored.

CASE MANAGEMENT

The case management of both forms of tetanus requires considerable resources, especially in terms of nursing, which needs to be rigorous and intensive:

- The case management of NEONATAL TETANUS includes disinfection of the umbilical cord, sedation, administration of anti-tetanus serum and antibiotic treatment. Experience in Sudan in 1987-89 suggested ampicillin syrup by nasogastric tube as an alternative to parenteral antibiotics[4,6]. Expressed breast-milk should be administered through the nasogastric tube.

- The case management of WOUND-RELATED TETANUS includes adequate wound excision and disinfection, sedation, administration of intravenous fluids, feeding through nasogastric tube, antibiotic treatment and administration of anti-tetanus serum.

As tetanus is rarely immunizing, all surviving patients should receive tetanus toxoid as well.

🔖 *References*

1. Bres, P. *Public health action in emergencies caused by epidemics.* Geneva: WHO, 1986.

2. Stanfield, J P, Galazka, A. Neonatal tetanus in the world today. *WHO Bull*, 1984, 62(4): 647-69.

3. Benenson, A. *Control of communicable diseases manual.* 16th edition. Washington DC: American Public Health Association, 1995.

4. Van Cutsem, R. *Neonatal tetanus in Anjikoti reception centre, Jan-Dec 1987.* [Internal report]. Brussels: Médecins Sans Frontières, 1988.

5. WHO. *Immunization Policy.* Geneva: WHO, 1986. WHO/EPI/GEN/86.7.

6. Boelaert, M, El Badawi, S, Tibbin, S, Moreno-Reyes, R. An oral treatment schedule for neonatal tetanus in a rural district hospital. *Medical News*, 1994, 3(4): 14-17.

7. Dufour, D, Kromann Jensen, S, Owen-Smith, M, Salmela, J, Stening, G F, Zetterström, B. *Surgery for victims of war.* Geneva: CICR, 1990.

8. WHO/EPI. *Revised plan of action for neonatal tetanus elimination.* Geneva: WHO, 1994.

Scabies

Scabies is a very contagious skin infestation caused by a mite, *Sarcoptes scabiei*. Its presence world wide, irrespective of climate, is closely related to a lack of water and poor hygiene[1,2]. The typical overcrowding and poor hygiene in refugee camps therefore present ideal conditions for scabies infestation[3,4]. Patients frequently present with scabies in out-patient departments (OPD), and a few 'scabies outbreaks' have been reported in refugee populations[4].

It is usually a mild condition; but secondary infections are common, especially in children, and can cause complications (e.g. glomerulonephritis). Although scabies-related mortality is very low, this is a common health problem and should be properly addressed.

PREVENTION

The following measures will contribute to preventing scabies infestation:
– ensuring access to sufficient quantities of water (see *3. Water and Sanitation* in Part II)[5],
– setting up bathing and laundering areas,
– supplying soap in general distributions.

SURVEILLANCE

A high frequency of consultations for scabies and other hygiene-related diseases (e.g. conjunctivitis) may indicate an inadequate supply of water and soap.

CASE MANAGEMENT

Secondary infections have to be treated first. To avoid re-infection, all clothes, blankets and mats should be washed with soap and dried in the sun; the whole family and all close contacts should be treated with a scabicide, preferably at the same time. The treatment of choice for children is the permethrin; in developing countries, the most frequently used scabicide is benzyl benzoate lotion[1,2,3]. It is of the utmost importance that the correct use of these products is clearly explained.

A high caseload of scabies can overload medical consultations. It is therefore advisable in such a situation to have health staff at the OPD triage who identify patients with scabies, and direct them to where they can receive specific treatment (see *Health Care in the Emergency Phase* in Part III).

🖎 *References*

1. I. Cook, G. *Manson's tropical diseases*. 18th edition. London: Saunders, 1987.
2. Médecins Sans Frontières. *Clinical guidelines, diagnostic and treatment manual*. Paris: Hatier, 1993.
3. Benenson, A. *Control of communicable diseases manual*. 16th edition. Washington DC: American Public Health Association, 1995: 385-8.
4. Greco Squarcione, S, Germinario, C, Lo Caputo, S, Binkin, N, Panatta, M. Health response to a large and rapid influx of Albanian refugees in Southern Italy, 1991. *Disasters*, 1991, 17: 61-9.
5. Médecins Sans Frontières. *Public health engineering in emergency situations*. Paris: Médecins Sans Frontières, 1994: I/3-I/8.

Conjunctivitis

Outbreaks of conjunctivitis occur worldwide. The causative agent may be bacterial, viral, or chlamydial. Such agents are transmitted easily by hand or, in the case of viral conjunctivitis, through indirect contact. Mechanic transmission by flies may also occur but their importance as vectors differs from one area to another[3]. In developing countries, outbreaks of bacterial conjunctivitis are associated with overcrowding and poor hygiene. Recent outbreaks have more frequently been caused by viral agents, due to the extensive use of antibiotics[4]. Trachoma, caused by special strains of chlamydia, is a progressive conjunctivitis and a common cause of blindness in endemic areas.

Outbreaks of conjunctivitis are commonly reported in refugee camps as overcrowding, an insufficient water supply, poor sanitation, and exposure to wind and dust provide ideal conditions for it to develop. An outbreak of viral conjunctivitis affected nearly half of the Vietnamese refugee population on Guam in 1977, and the attack rates were highest where the overcrowding and poor sanitation were more severe[2]. Trachoma has been found among refugees and displaced persons in Ethiopia and Sudan, where it was considered a major health problem; in Wad Kowli (Sudan), 90% of the children examined in 1985 between 2 and 12 years of age showed signs of trachoma[6]. However, the initial stages of trachoma are easily confused with common conjunctivitis by untrained health workers.

OUTBREAK CONTROL

The identification of the causal agent is not necessarily recommended since this requires long and expensive investigations, and has no influence on case management. However, an exception should be made for trachoma: if trachoma is suspected in the population, cases must first be assessed clinically, using strict diagnostic criteria as described in WHO guidelines[1]. Once trachoma has been clinically confirmed, a simpler and more sensitive case definition should be introduced.

The most important control measures are listed below.

- The usual sanitation measures, particularly adequate supply of water and soap, are essential. Personal hygiene, such as washing hands and face, should also be encouraged and promoted.

- The organization of health services for the diagnosis and prompt treatment of cases include staff training, case finding, and referral of cases by home-visitors. In some situations, home-visitors may be taught how to apply eye ointment. In refugee camps in Rwanda in 1993, a conjunctivitis outbreak prompted the setting up of health posts to cope with the heavy load of patients.

- Case treatment involves the application of antibiotic eye ointment (usually tetracycline). This is effective for bacterial and chlamydial conjunctivitis, and is indicated for viral conjunctivitis to prevent secondary bacterial infection[5].

- If trachoma is affecting the refugee population, any decision to launch a control programme must be based on the prevalence of trachoma leading to blindness. This will be assessed through a sample survey, following WHO guidelines[1]. Specific control programmes must be restricted to communities where blinding trachoma is highly prevalent[1]. In these populations, active case screening should be pursued if resources are sufficient, and selective treatment should be limited to cases of evolutive trachoma[1].

- The treatment consists in the application of tetracycline ointment over a long period (at least 6 weeks). An intermittent scheme 5 to 10 days of treatment monthly, over a 6-month period, is also recommended by WHO but is not practical in refugee situations[1]. Treatment in the later stages (entropion) is surgical.

Key reference

1. Dawson, C R, Jones, B R, Tarizzo, M L. *Guide for trachoma control.* Geneva: WHO, 1982.

Other references

2. Arnow, P M, Hierholzer, J C, et al. Acute hemorrhagic conjunctivitis: A mixed virus outbreak among Vietnamese refugees on Guam. *Am J Epidemiol*, 1977, 105(1): 68-74.

3. Benenson, A. *Control of communicable diseases manual.* 16th edition. Washington DC: American Public Health Association, 1995.

4. Gentilini, M. *Médecine tropicale.* Paris: Flammarion Médecine-Sciences, 1993.

5. Schwab, L. *Eye care in developing nations.* 2nd edition. Oxford: Oxford University Press, 1990.

6. Hellen Keller International. *Assessment of nutritional blindness and trachoma among young children in five drought-stricken African countries.* HKI, 1985.

Dracunculiasis or Guinea worm

Dracunculiasis is a filariasis infection with current foci in West and East Africa, West India, Pakistan, Iran, Saudi Arabia and Yemen[1,2] It is a debilitating disease, characterized by painful ulcers and abscesses (secondary infection), usually on the feet and legs. This causes considerable suffering and has an adverse impact on food production in affected areas[4].

Contamination is through drinking water infested with certain species of *Cyclops* (water fleas), infected by guinea worm larvae. This parasitosis can be prevented by ensuring safe water supply to the population at risk[4]. The World Health Assembly has adopted a resolution to eliminate dracunculiasis as a public health problem from the world in the 1990s.

Dracunculiasis is not likely to be a priority health problem in refugee or displaced populations since the most important effects are complications from chronic infection. Nevertheless, in refugee populations where dracunculiasis is known to be a major problem, a control programme may be started, providing that the emergency is under control. It is recognized that population displacements can increase the number of cases, if infected people introduce the parasite into the water supply system[4]. In Sudan, an eradication programme, which was started in 1992 under the UN's 'Operation Lifeline Sudan' intervention, provided filter material which reduced the incidence in southern provinces. In spite of this, 95% of cases in Sudan are still notified in that area. An increase in cases probably results from the frequent population movements associated with the civil war, as well as seasonal migrations[3].

SURVEILLANCE

Guinea worm cases can be detected, if their reporting is included in the surveillance system.

Case definition for Guinea worm:

skin ulcers with adult female worm (60 to 100cm) protruding

CONTROL MEASURES

Any guinea worm control programme in refugee settings should be integrated into the long-term national programme of the host country, and should be aimed at both host and refugee communities.

It should be possible to eradicate guinea worm with an effective drinking water control programme covering[2]:

• **Health education**: the population should be informed - for instance through home-visitors - of the need to filter drinking water through fine mesh cloth in order to remove *Cyclops*.

- **Provision of drinking water**: wells should be protected by constructing walls around them to avoid drinking water being contaminated by people already infected.

- **Vector control**: insecticide can be used to kill *Cyclops* in ponds and water tanks.

CASE MANAGEMENT

No more efficient treatment is yet available, except the traditional practice of extracting the adult worm from cutaneous ulcers.

References

1. Cook, G. *Manson's tropical diseases*. 19th edition. London; Saunders, 1996.

2. Benenson, A. *Control of communicable diseases manual*. 16th edition. Washington DC: American Public Health Association, 1995.

3. Dracunculiasis global surveillance summary, 1993. *Wkly Epidemiol Rec*, 1994, 69(17), 121-8.

4. Watts, S J. Human behaviour and the transmission of dracunculiasis: A case study from the florin area of Nigeria. *Int J Epidemiol*, 1986, 15(2): 252-6.

5. Examples of surveillance forms

Population

Place: ....   **Reported by:** ....

From: ..../......./.......   **To:** ..../......./.......
        day/month/year   day/month/year

Population	End of previous week (A)	New arrivals	Departures	End of this week (B)	Average population (A + B) /2
< 5 years old					
All age					

Population is needed to calculate mortality rate and to quantify the needs.

SOURCES: ....

Mortality
• Mortality rate

	Number of deaths			Rate/10,000/day		
	Male	Female	Total	Male	Female	Total
< 5 years old						
All age						

• Causes of mortality

Diseases	< 5 years			> = 5 years			Total			Percentage
	Male	Female	Total	Male	Female	Total	Male	Female	Total	
Non-bloody diarrhoea										
Bloody diarrhoea										
Severe respiratory infections										
Fever unknown/susp.malaria										
Measles										
Susp. meningitis										
War injury										
Malnutrition										
Others										
Total										

Sources: Cemetery ❑   Health facilities ❑   Home visitors ❑   Authorities ❑

Comments: ....

Morbidity summary form

Place: ....   **Reported by:** ....

From: ..../......./.......   **To:** ..../......./.......
        day/month/year   day/month/year

• Table of morbidity

Summary of all the health facilities, OPD, health posts, IPD and feeding centres. Take care to avoid double registration.

DISEASES	< 5 years old	> = 5 years old	TOTAL	INCIDENCE or PERCENTAGE
Non-bloody diarrhoea				
Bloody diarrhoea				
Acute resp.infection				
Fever unknown /susp. malaria				
Measles				
Susp. meningitis				
War injury				
Susp. hepatitis /jaundice				
Others				
Total number of cases				

In the table, only one diagnosis per patient.
Incidence can only be calculated if the population figure is available.

• Is there any epidemic?

Yes ❏   **No** ❏

If yes, fill in the epidemic form.

Note: *Data can be computed by sex in the post-emergency phase.*

Measles vaccination form

Place: ....   **Reported by:** ....

From: ..../......./.......   **To:** ..../......./.......
       day/month/year   day/month/year

• Mass measles vaccination campaign

Yes ❑   **No** ❑

• Routine measles vaccination in health facilities

Yes ❑   **No** ❑

• Measles vaccination coverage

Target population

< 5 years old: ......   **> = 5 years old:** ......

Total target population: ......

No. vaccinated	Mass campaign A		Routine vaccination B		Cumulative measles vaccination coverage*
	No. this week	Cumulative No.	No. this week	Cumulative No.	
< 5 years old					
> = 5 years old					
TOTAL					

* Calculation of the cumulative coverage: A + B/target population

Comments: ....
....
....
....
....

N.B.: This form can also be used for an other mass vaccination campaign; just change the name.

In-patient department

Place: ....   **Reported by:** ....

From: ..../......./.......   **To:** ..../......./.......
day/month/year   day/month/year

• IPD activity and mortality

	Surgical ward	Medical ward	Pediatric ward	Gyn./Obs. ward	Other	Total	
						NR	%
No. of beds							
Admissions							
Discharged							
Deaths							
Total exits*							

* Total exits include discharged + deaths + defaulters + transfers.
  The percentage of mortality is calculated on the total exits.

• IPD: case fatality rate

Pathologies	No. of cases	No. of deaths	Case fatality
	A	B	B/A x 100
Non-bloody diarrhoea			
Bloody diarrhoea			
Severe acute respiratory infec.			
Fever unknown/susp. malaria			
Measles			
Susp. meningitis			
War injury			
Others			
Total			

Comments: ....
....

Surgical activities in war situation

Place: ....   **Reported by:** ....

From: ..../......./.......   **To:** ..../......./.......
day/month/year   day/month/year

• Number of patients operated on

	Number	Per cent
War related		
Other causes		
TOTAL		100%

• Causes of war injuries

	Mines			Total
Civilian patient				
Military patient				
TOTAL				100%

• Site of surgical interventions

	Number	Percent
Abdominal		
Orthopedic		
Thoracic		
Head		
Other		
TOTAL		100%

• Anæsthesia

	Number	Per cent
General + intubation		
Gen. without intubation		
Spinal		
Local		
Other		
TOTAL		100%

Comments: (post-operative infection, etc.) ....
....
....

Human resources versus activity load

Place: ....   **Reported by:** ....

From: ..../......./.......   **To:** ..../......./.......
day/month/year   day/month/year

• Outpatient consultations

Total number of consultations during the week A	Number of days of consultation per week B	Total number of care providers C	No. of consultations per care provider/day A/B/C	Objective
				50 - 70 consultations/ care provider/day

• Surgical interventions

Average number of surgical interventions per day A	Average number of surgeons per day B	No. of surgical interventions per surgeon per day A/B	Objective

• Home visiting

Population A	Number of home-visitors B	Number of persons per home-visitor A/B	Objective
			500 - 1,000 persons per home-visitor

Comments: ....
....
....
....
....

Nutrition forms

Place: ....   **Reported by:** ....

From: ..../......./.......   **To:** ..../......./.......
        day/month /year   day/month /year

• General food distribution

Any food distribution during the week: **Yes** ❑   **No** ❑

Amount in Kcal /person /day that the organization in charge of the distribution is said to have distributed: ....

If a food basket monitoring has been carried out, fill the table below.

Food	Quantity/pers.	Number of days between previous and actual distribution	Quantity/pers./day	Kcal/pers./day
Total				

Comments: ....
....
....
....

• Feeding centre structures and characteristics

Structures	No. of centers	No. of child. end of week	No. of meals/day	Kcal/p/d
TFC				
SFC wet				
SFC dry				
Blanket				

Comments: ....
....
....
....

• Monthly feeding centers admissions and exits

Place: ....   **Reported by:** ....

From: ..../......./.......   **To:** ..../......./.......
     day/month/year   day/month/year

1. Therapeutic feeding

	< 70% W/H or < 110mm MUAC	Oedema	> 70% W/H	> 110cm or > 5 years	TOTAL
TOTAL END OF PREVIOUS WEEK					
New admissions					
Readmissions					
TOTAL ADMISSIONS					
Cured					
Dead					
Defaulters					
Transferred					
TOTAL EXITS					
TOTAL END OF THIS WEEK					

2. Supplementary feeding

	< 80% W/H or < 110mm MUAC	Oedema	> 80% W/H	> 110cm or > 5 years	TOTAL
TOTAL END OF PREVIOUS WEEK					
New admissions					
Readmissions					
TOTAL ADMISSIONS					
Cured					
Dead					
Defaulters					
Transferred					
TOTAL EXITS					
TOTAL END OF THIS WEEK					

Comments: ....
....

• Monthly outcome indicators of feeding programmes

Place: ....   **Reported by:** ....

From: ..../......./.......   **To:** ..../......./.......
      day/month/year   day/month/year

EXITS	THERAPEUTIC		SUPPLEMENTARY	
	Number	**%**	**Number**	**%**
Cured				
Defaulters				
Dead				
Transferred				
Total exits		**100%**		**100%**
* Average length of stay (in days)				
* Weight gain in g/kg/day				

* These indicators are calculated on the cured exits only

Comments: ....
....
....
....
....
....

Water, sanitation and environment

Place: ....   **Reported by:** ....

From: ..../......./.......   **To:** ..../......./.......
        day/month/year   day/month/year

• Water

	No. of litres/day	Population	No. of litres/pers/day	Objective
Water supply				15 litres/p/day

	No. of water points	Population	No. of pers./water point	Objective
Water supply				200 pers./water point

• Sanitation

	No. of latrines	Population	No. of persons /latrine	Objective
Latrines				20 persons/latrine

• Crowding (space/person)

	Surface area in m^2	Population	M^2 per person	Objective
Crowding				30m^2/person

Comments: ....
....
....
....
....
....

Epidemic

Place: ....   **Reported by:** ....

From: ..../......./.......   **To:** ..../......./.......
      day/month/year   day/month/year

Case definition of the disease :   ....
                                             ....
                                             ....

Date	Day	New cases			Deaths		
		< 5 years	> = 5 years	Total	< 5 years	> = 5 years	Total
	1						
	2						
	3						
	4						
	5						
	6						
	7						
Total							

Weekly incidence rate: ....
Number of cases/population x 1,000

Weekly case fatality rate: ....
Number of deaths/No. of cases x 100

Attack rate or cumulative incidence rate: ....
No. of cases since onset epidemic/population x 100

Comments: ....
....
....
....
....

Daily morbidity form

Name of the structure: ....

Date: ..../......./.......   **Reported by:** ....
day/month/year

Diagnosis is only one diagnosis per patient.
The patients who are referred should be written on the column referred and no diagnosis should be written for them.

Diagnostic	< 5 years old	> = 5 years old	Total
Non-bloody diarrhoea			
Bloody diarrhoea			
Acute respiratory infection			
Fever unknown/susp. malaria			
Measles			
Suspicion of meningitis			
War injuries			
Suspicion hepatitis /jaundice			
Other			
Total number of cases			
Number of referred			

Number of care providers: ....

Daily dressing and injections form

Name of the structure: ....

Date: ..../......./.......   **Reported by:** ....
       day/month/year

	< 5 years old	> = 5 years old	Total
Dressing			
Injections			
TOTAL			

Comments: ....
....
....
....
....
....
....
....
....

Weekly evaluation
and
objectives for the next week

1. Specific and main activities developed during the week:

....
....
....
....
....
....
....
....
....
....
....

2. Evaluation of the reached objectives, problems faced, strong and weak points:

....
....
....
....
....
....
....
....
....
....
....

3. Objectives and activities planned for the coming weeks:

....
....
....
....
....
....
....
....
....
....
....

6. Examples of graphs used in surveillance

Proportional mortality among Mozambican refugees in Malawi, 1987-89

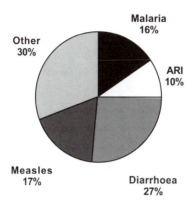

Malaria 16%
Other 30%
ARI 10%
Measles 17%
Diarrhoea 27%

< 5 years

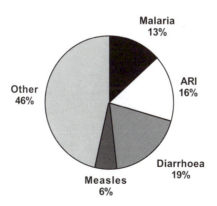

Malaria 13%
ARI 16%
Other 46%
Diarrhoea 19%
Measles 6%

>= 5 years

Source: MSF / Malawian Ministry of Health

Comparison of the evolution
of the Crude Death Rates in two refugee crises

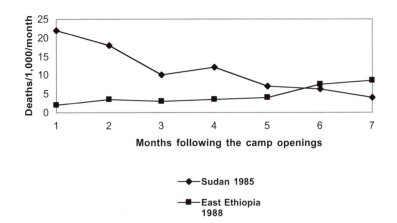

Adpated from: Moren A., Rigal J., *Cahiers Santé*, 1992; 2: 13-2 !

INDEX